Guide to Antibiotics in Urology

Truls E. Bjerklund Johansen • Tommaso Cai
Editors

Guide to Antibiotics in Urology

Springer

Editors
Truls E. Bjerklund Johansen
Department of Urology
Oslo University Hospital
Oslo, Norway

Tommaso Cai
Department of Urology
Santa Chiara Regional Hospital
Trento, Italy

ISBN 978-3-319-92365-9 ISBN 978-3-319-92366-6 (eBook)
https://doi.org/10.1007/978-3-319-92366-6

This Springer imprint is published by the registered company Springer Nature Switzerland AG
The registered company address is: Gewerbestrasse 11, 6330 Cham, Switzerland

The editors dedicate this book to all patients suffering from urinary tract infections unleashed by risk factors due to standard of living, inheritance of host defense defects, or side effects of treatment of other diseases. It is our hope that they will receive antibiotic treatment that does not harm the delicate normal balance between host and microorganisms in their bodies and that effective antibiotic treatment will be available for the foreseeable future.

Preface

According to her death certificate, my great grandmother died of "nephritis chronica" in Norway in 1914. She was in her 40s. Seven childbirths and poor living conditions contributed to her infection risk. At that time, Norway had the highest death rate of tuberculosis in the world, and her nephritis might very well have been caused by tuberculosis. No urine cultures were taken, and there was no antibiotic treatment available for her.

Two generations later, my mother died of urosepsis in 2021 caused by multiresistant Pseudomonas aeruginosa. She was 97 years old and had risk factors related to bladder and intestinal dysfunction. The dysfunctions were caused by adjuvant irradiation of pelvic lymph nodes related to surgery for uterine cancer many years earlier. She received numerous courses of antibiotic treatment for recurrent UTI and had several episodes of urosepsis. Finally, there were no effective antibiotics available for her in our country. Fosfomycin, which would have been the preferred antibiotic, was not available due to national regulations introduced for the sake of antimicrobial stewardship.

In between the two deaths of my female ancestors, there has been an extraordinary development of modern medicine. At the time of my great grandmother's death, there were no medical specialties related to urinary tract infections such as microbiology, infectious diseases, or urology. There were very few doctors, no antibiotics and no intensive care units. As a child, I had to cross the old graveyard outside the old tuberculosis sanatorium to reach school. Every day, I was reminded of tuberculosis as a terrible cause of death. As the standard of living improved, the disease disappeared while we doctors were still treating patients with fresh air.

In the period between the two deaths, numerous antibiotics were developed and used with success to relieve patients of disabling symptoms and save lives. However, limited understanding of the delicate balance between humans and microorganisms, increased number of physicians, as well as marketing pressure from the pharmaceutic industry have brought us to a situation where this lucky period in our history might soon come to an end.

We use to think of ourselves as cohabitants in our own bodies with billions of microorganisms with whom we live in harmony most of the time. Infectious diseases occur when microorganisms enter body parts and cross tissue barriers like the urothelium. This invasion is made possible by virulence factors of the microorganism and is normally prevented by host-protective mechanisms. These mechanisms are influenced by risk factors. Some of them might be eliminated while others remain challenges to antibiotic treatment.

The aims of this book are to provide the reader with understanding of the basic principles of diagnosis, prevention and treatment of urogenital tract infections, and to offer practical guidance on the use of antibiotics.

Stavern, Norway
July 2023

Truls E. Bjerklund Johansen

Acknowledgments

The editors acknowledge the European Section of Infections in Urology (ESIU) and the guidelines panels on urogenital infections in the European Association of Urology (EAU) for permission to reuse material which has been developed by authors of chapters in this book while serving as present and former members of ESIU and the EAU guidelines panels.

Contents

Part I Epidemiological and Microbiological Aspects of Urinary Tract Infections

1 Antimicrobial Resistance in Uropathogens 3
Gianpaolo Perletti and Vittorio Magri

2 Bacterial Resistance: What Is the Epidemiological Scenario? 17
David M. Livermore

3 A Practical Guideline on Sampling and Analysis of Urine and Blood Specimens in Urinary Tract Infections 35
Tommaso Cai and Truls E. Bjerklund Johansen

4 The Antibiogram: From MIC to Breakpoints 43
Carlo Tascini and Sozio Emanuela

5 Classification of Urinary Tract Infections: A Contemporary Guide for Clinical Practice and Research 53
Truls E. Bjerklund Johansen, Zafer Tandogdu, Tommaso Cai, and Kurt G. Naber

6 Novel Antibiotics in Urology 69
Kurt G. Naber, Truls E. Bjerklund Johansen, and Florian M. E. Wagenlehner

Part II Treatment of Low Severity Urinary Tract Infections Without Risk Factors

7 Acute Uncomplicated and Complicated Cystitis: From Empiric Treatment to Antibiogram-Based Tailored Treatment 89
Michael McDonald, Darien Kameh, Mark E. Johnson, Truls E. Bjerklund Johansen, and Vladimir Mouraviev

8 Recurrent Urinary Tract Infection in Young Woman 103
Liliana Mereu and Saverio Tateo

9 Pyelonephritis: In- and Outpatients 115
Gernot Bonkat and Georg Müller

Part III Treatment of Urinary Tract Infections with Risk Factors and Urosepsis

10 Management of Catheter-Associated Urinary Tract Infections 125
András Magyar, Péter Tenke, and Béla Köves

11 Urinary Tract Infections in Kidney Transplant Patients 141
José Medina-Polo, Laila Schneidewind, Fabian P. Stangl, and Truls E. Bjerklund Johansen

12 Management of the Urosepsis Syndrome 153
Florian M. E. Wagenlehner

13 The Treatment of Urinary Tract Infections Caused by ESBL-Producing Gram-Negative Bacteria, Vancomycin-Resistant Enterococci (VRE), and Other Multidrug-Resistant Bacteria 159
Fabian P. Stangl, Jennifer Kranz, Florian M. E. Wagenlehner, Jonas Marschall, Sören Schubert, José Medina-Polo, Laila Schneidewind, and Truls E. Bjerklund Johansen

14 Antibiotic Treatment of Urogenital Tuberculosis 177
Ekaterina Kulchavenya and Truls E. Bjerklund Johansen

15 Bacteriophage Therapy for Urinary Tract Infections 189
Matthew Dunne, Tamara S. Perepanova, and Truls E. Bjerklund Johansen

Part IV Urethritis and Male Accessory Gland Infections

16 Treatment of Urethritis 209
Riccardo Bartoletti, Alessandro Perotti, Matteo Pacini, and Alessandro Zucchi

17 Acute Bacterial Prostatitis 219
Paolo Verze, Massimiliano Creta, Gianluigi Califano, and Alessandro Palmieri

18 Treatment of Epididymitis and Orchitis 229
José Medina-Polo

Part V Antibiotic Prophylaxis and Treatment of Infectious Complications After Urological Procedures

19 Principles of Antibiotic Prophylaxis in Urology: Why, When and How 241
Lars Fredrik Qvigstad, Tommaso Cai, José Medina-Polo, Zafer Tandogdu, and Truls E. Bjerklund Johansen

20 Prevention and Treatment of Urinary Tract Infections After Radical Cystectomy, Diversion, and Reservoirs 261
Mauro Gacci, Sergio Serni, and Jacopo Frizzi

21 Prevention and Treatment of Infectious Complications After Urogenital Prosthesis Surgery 273
Michele Rizzo, Stefano Bucci, Nicola Pavan, Enrica Verzotti, Giacomo Di Cosmo, Paolo Umari, Carlo Trombetta, and Giovanni Liguori

Part VI Practical Guidelines on Antibiotic Treatment of Urinary Tract Infections

22 Practical Guidelines on Antibiotic Treatment of Urinary Tract Infections 281
Truls E. Bjerklund Johansen, Tommaso Cai, Kurt G. Naber, José Medina-Polo, Laila Schneidewind, Gernot Bonkat, Bela Koves, Ana-María Tapia-Herrero, Florian M. E. Wagenlehner, and George G. Zhanel

Part I

Epidemiological and Microbiological Aspects of Urinary Tract Infections

1 Antimicrobial Resistance in Uropathogens

Gianpaolo Perletti and Vittorio Magri

1.1 Background

Urinary tract infections (UTIs) are among the most common infectious diseases in humans. Urinary antiseptics, naturally occurring antibiotics, and synthetic antibacterial agents (AAs) have been used for decades to treat infections like pyelonephritis and cystitis.

Today, about three generations after the introduction of antibiotics into the clinical practice, a return to the "pre-antibiotic era" due to the emergence of multidrug-resistant (MDR) pathogens is becoming "a disturbing possibility" [1]. In fact, we have reached a new crossroad whereby resistance to nearly all antimicrobial classes is increasing to the point that outbursts of infections carried by extremely drug-resistant or even pan-drug-resistant pathogens are happening around the world. In the frame of the Review on Antimicrobial Resistance commissioned by the prime minister of the United Kingdom, it has been foreseen that by year 2050 ten million premature deaths (one every 3 s) will be caused worldwide by pathogen resistance (cancer: about eight million), of which over three million will lose their lives to drug-resistant *E. coli* [2].

Bacterial resistance to antimicrobials is a very intricate subject, whose manifold aspects are determined by a large number of diverse elements. For example, it is known that antibacterial agents show different capacity in inducing resistance in pathogens, and that resistance patterns do not always reflect prescribing patterns [3], though in the urological field it was shown that individuals who have been

G. Perletti (✉)
Section of Medical and Surgical Sciences, Department of Biotechnology and Life Sciences, Università degli Studi dell'Insubria, Varese, Italy
e-mail: gianpaolo.perletti@uninsubria.it

V. Magri
Urology Secondary Care Clinic (UOC Urology), ASST-Fatebenefratelli Sacco, Milan, Italy

T. E. Bjerklund Johansen, T. Cai (eds.), *Guide to Antibiotics in Urology*,
https://doi.org/10.1007/978-3-319-92366-6_1

prescribed antibiotics in primary care had bacteria in the urinary tract resistant to the same antibiotic for up to a year [4]. Moreover, the success of antibacterial therapy relies on specific clinical conditions. For example, the high urinary concentrations of antibacterials toward which a uropathogen shows resistance may be sufficient to treat UTIs but not infections detected in other districts of the body. Such and several other elements, together with the manifold resistance mechanisms that have been so far identified, have increased the complexity of the pathogen resistance scenario and have raised the public awareness about the pandemic threat it represents.

1.2 Principles of Bacterial Resistance to Antimicrobial Agents

When antibacterial agents were first introduced in clinical practice, resistance of exposed pathogens was immediately reported, also because certain resistance determinants were already expressed in the natural milieu where antibiotic-producing organisms were growing.

In fact, throughout their evolution, bacteria have developed natural defense mechanisms against antibiotics produced by co-resident organisms. Such mechanisms are today defined as *intrinsic resistance* determinants. For example, Enterococci express low-affinity penicillin-binding proteins (PBPs) that bind very poorly to beta-lactams. As a result, minimum inhibitory concentrations (MICs) for these agents in *Enterococcus faecalis* and *Enterococcus faecium* are in general 2–8 mg/L and 8–16 mg/L, respectively [5].

However, clinicians and scientists are more frequently and more significantly confronted with the phenomenon of *acquired resistance*, occurring in pathogens which were at first susceptible to a given antibacterial agent. Acquired resistance occurs as the result of the rapid development of mutations at the chromosomal level, or through the horizontal exchange of genetic resistance determinants, occurring more commonly via bacterial conjugation, but also by transformation (i.e., by transfer of naked DNA), or by phage transduction.

Transferrable genetic resistance determinants are most commonly carried by *transposons* and *plasmids*, and incorporation of resistance gene cassettes into target chromosomes may be facilitated by *integrons*, which encode specific recombinases catalyzing the exchange of genetic material by site-specific recombination reactions. For example, co-trimoxazole resistance is transmitted by all these three mobile elements, which are commonly causing overexpression of dihydrofolate reductase and dihydropteroate synthase by the transferable *dhfr1* and *sul1(Tn21* transposon*)/sulI2(IncQ/pBP1* plasmids*)* genes, respectively.

Resistance to a specific antibacterial agent often results in resistance to other, often chemically unrelated agents, due to the co-expression of multiple resistance genes within the same operon.

The transition of chromosomal resistance determinants multidrug-resistant plasmid cassettes is a well-characterized phenomenon. For example, whereas in earlier years transmission of fluoroquinolone resistance was mainly chromosomal, more recently genetic resistance determinants like the efflux pumps OqxAB and QepA and the modified aminoglycoside acetyltransferase AAC(6′)-Ib-cr now reside in plasmids, also containing elements conferring resistance to beta-lactams, tetracyclines, aminoglycosides, sulfonamides, trimethoprim, and rifampin.

Resistance mechanisms may be transmitted across species (as happens, e.g., between *Klebsiella* spp. and *Pseudomonas aeruginosa*), but appear to be species-specific in some cases. For example, whereas beta-lactamase expression occurs mainly in Gram-negative bacteria, resistance to beta-lactams in Gram-positive organisms occurs more frequently through mutational modification of PBPs.

Resistance of pathogens to antibacterial agents occurs in most cases by way of (1) increased efflux of the drug from the cell, (2) decreased cell wall permeability to the drug, (3) activity of enzymes modifying or disrupting the drug, (4) bypass of drug-induced metabolic blockades within bacterial cells, (5) protection, mutation, overexpression, or modification of the drug targets.

Explanatory examples of special interest to urologists and to specialists involved in UTI diagnosis and treatment will be briefly described in the following paragraphs.

1. A variety of mechanisms, showing different degrees of drug specificity, regulate the *efflux of antimicrobials* from bacterial cells. Various drugs, such as fluoroquinolones, beta-lactams, macrolides, and tetracyclines, are substrates of such mechanisms. Efflux pumps belong to five families: the major facilitator superfamily (MFS), the adenosine triphosphate (ATP)-binding cassette (ABC) family, the resistance-nodulation-division (RND) family, the small multidrug resistance (SMR) family, and the multidrug and toxic compound extrusion family [6]. For example, tetracyclines are extruded against protons by means of Tet efflux pumps belonging to the MFS, but are also extruded by other efflux mechanisms, as in *Enterobacteriaceae* and *P. aeruginosa* tetracyclines are extruded by means of RND efflux pumps like AcrAB-TolC and MexAB-OprM, respectively [7]. RND pumps also act as proton antiporters, are typically expressed in *E. coli*, and can extrude a variety of other drugs like fluoroquinolones, beta-lactams, chloramphenicol, and macrolides.
2. Porins are beta-barrel proteins allowing transmembrane exchange of solutes with various degrees of specificity. Alterations in structure or expression of porins are most commonly responsible for *decreased cell wall permeability* to antimicrobials. Typical porins conferring resistance to *P. aeruginosa* or *K. pneumoniae* are, for example, OprD and OmpK25/36, respectively. Notably, porin alteration concurs, together with other mechanisms, to carbapenem-resistant phenotypes [7].
3. A variety of enzymes can induce *modifications to drug molecules* or can disrupt their structure, mainly by hydrolysis. Enzymes belonging to the first category include aminoglycoside acetyltransferases (AAC(6′)-I) expressed by both Gram-negative and Gram-positive bacteria, adenylyltransferases, and phosphotransferases. Bifunctional enzymes (acetyl- and phosphotransferases) are also frequently found in resistant organisms [8]. The genes encoding such resistance determinants are carried in most case by mobile genetic elements, but, as happens in

Enterococcus faecium, they are also expressed chromosomally. *Enterobacteriaceae* express very frequently AAC(6′)-I, together with *P. aeruginosa* and *Acinetobacter*. A plasmid-harbored mutated version of AAC(6′)-I, encoded by *AAC(6′)-Ib-cr*, has evolved to acetylate certain fluoroquinolones at a specific site of their piperazine ring.

Beta-lactamases can hydrolyze the cyclic amide bond of the four-membered lactam ring of beta-lactam agents, thus disrupting their inhibitory activity on the final phase of bacterial cell wall peptidoglycan biosynthesis. The activity of beta-lactamases has been characterized as early as 1940 [9], and from that moment on, discovery of new beta-lactams was invariably followed by the development of hundreds of chromosomal or transferable bacterial genes (*bla*) encoding more and more potent beta-lactamases [10]. Today, extended-spectrum beta-lactamases and carmapenemases are top worldwide medical emergencies. These resistance determinants will be described in greater detail in Sect. 1.3.1.

4. A typical example of resistance achieved through *bypass of the metabolic target of antimicrobial agents* is the resistance to sulfonamides. It is known that bacteria rely on their own enzymatic machinery for folate synthesis, and that sulfonamides act as competitive inhibitors of a major component of this machinery, the enzyme dihydropteroate synthase (DHPS). Thus, resistant pathogens can bypass this metabolic blockade by overexpressing DHPS through mutations in the promoter region of the DNA encoding such enzyme. Overproduction of dihydropteroic acid can overcome the ability of sulfa drugs to block folate production. An alternative "bypass" to such blockade is the acquisition of the ability to incorporate tetrahydrofolic and folinic acids from the environment, typically shown by Enterococci [11].
5. Resistance to antibacterial agents can be achieved by *protection, mutation, or modification of drug targets*. Glycopeptides (vancomycin, teicoplanin) bind the D-Ala–D-Ala portion of the pentapeptides of the peptidoglycan precursor and block the formation of peptide cross-links and bacterial wall synthesis. Vancomycin resistance in Enterococci involves the acquisition of a "cluster" of genes (located in most cases on Tn-3 transposons harbored within conjugative plasmids) encoding an enzymatic machinery that modifies the synthesis of peptidoglycans. The destruction of the normal D-Ala–D-Ala portion to prevent vancomycin binding to the cell wall precursors is one of the manifold mechanisms whereby such machinery can induce resistance to glycopeptides [12]. Bacterial resistance to fluoroquinolones occurs frequently via *protection or mutation of the target* of this class of agents, i.e., DNA gyrase and topoisomerase IV. The *qnr* gene product, expressed in the form of variant alleles (qnr A, B, C, D, S, VC, with comparable mechanism of action), is a pentapeptide repeat protein acting as a DNA homologue, able to bind to the DNA-binding sites of DNA gyrase and topoisomerase IV [13]. Well-characterized gyrase or topoisomerase-IV mutants conferring resistance to fluoroquinolones are, for example, *gyrA*, *gyrB*, *parC*, and *parE* [14].

The next section of this chapter will expand on some of the most worrisome resistance mechanisms among the ones described above, based on the type of pathogen expressing such determinants.

1.3 Emerging Resistance Threats

Antimicrobial resistance has been defined by the World Health Organization as "one among of the biggest threats to human health." Resistant Gram-negative pathogens like *Klebsiella pneumoniae*, *Escherichia coli*, and *Enterobacter* spp., involved in bacteremia, urinary tract infections, pneumonia, and intra-abdominal infections, but also multi-resistant Gram-positive Enterococci and Staphylococci are today the main driving force of such threat. Information and awareness thereof are thus of great significance to urologists and infectious disease specialists.

1.3.1 Gram-Negative Pathogens

1.3.1.1 Extended-Spectrum Beta-Lactamases (ESBLs), Carbapenemases

The most worrisome threats in the field of antibacterial therapy are represented by the worldwide surge of ESBL-producing multidrug-resistant (MDR) and carbapenemase-producing extensively drug-resistant *Enterobacteriaceae*.

ESBLs can be defined in different ways. Basically, ESBLs are a group of plasmid-transmissible enzymes, originated in the 1980s from a single-nucleotide mutation in the *blaSHV* gene, resulting in an altered structure of the catalytic serine site conferring a broader substrate spectrum and enabling these enzymes to hydrolyze antibiotics belonging to the penicillin, monobactam, and extended-spectrum cephalosporin groups.

The currently most common class variants of ESBLs are the CTX-M-type, TEM, sulfhydryl variable (SHV), and oxacillin (OXA) beta-lactamases, showing hundreds of genetic variants. The former is the most prevalent ESBL types globally, and has been found in association with insertion sequences (IS*Ecp1*) and transposable elements like Tn-*402* transposons, and can be included in a broad panel of phage-like and conjugative plasmids (reviewed in: [7]). ESBLs can be inhibited to various extents by beta-lactamase inhibitors like clavulanic acid, tazobactam, or sulbactam.

The therapy of choice for infections caused by ESBL-producing members of the *Enterobacteriaceae*—mainly *E. coli* and *K. pneumoniae*—is a carbapenem. However, the raise of worldwide carbapenem resistance in *Enterobacteriaceae* showing a multidrug-resistant phenotype is dramatically decreasing the therapeutic possibilities against such pathogens, both in adult and pediatric populations [15].

Comparison between the worldwide map of carbapenem resistance published by Nordmann et al. in the year 2014 [16] and a previous map released by the same authors in the year 2009 [17] gives a tangible impression of the dramatic surge of resistance to carbapenem antibiotics. Briefly, whereas in 2009 the spread of the

Klebsiella pneumoniae carbapenemase (KPC) in the USA was defined as *sporadic* in half of the federal states and *less than sporadic* in the rest of the states, in 2014 the whole of the USA has become affected by *endemic* isolation of KPC. The concern caused by such emerging resistance trend is due to the fact that carbapenemases are lactamases able to breakdown almost all beta-lactam antibiotics including in first place carbapenems that are today last-resource weapons in the struggle against Gram-negative complicated and life-threatening infections. Resistance to carbapenemases is in most cases mediated by horizontally transferable genetic elements (e.g., plasmidic or chromosomal integrons, transposons), also containing a multiplicity of resistance determinants, often conferring a multidrug- or extensively drug-resistant phenotype to carrier pathogens. Urinary catheters, mechanical ventilation, and previous exposure to broad-spectrum antibacterial agents and surgical procedures like transplantations are known risk factors for infection with carbapenem-resistant *Enterobacteriaceae* (CREB).

The 2016 report of the by the European Centre for Disease Prevention and Control reported that *K. pneumoniae* (KP) is the most prominent pathogen among carbapenemase-producing pathogens [18]. High mortality rates have been attributed to carbapenemase-resistant KP. A meta-analysis has shown that the mortality rate was as high as 42.1% in patients infected with carbapenemase-resistant KP, versus 21.2% in those infected with carbapenem-susceptible KP [19]. Moreover, the mortality of patients with UTIs was 13.5%, raising to 43.1% in intensive care unit cases. When the severity of infection was classified according to the resistance determinants, the mortality was 47.66% in patients infected with KPC-producing KP and 46.71% in those infected with VIM-producing KP. As far as the geographic distribution is concerned, the mortality reported in studies from North America, South America, Europe, and Asia was 33.2%, 46.7%, 50%, and 44.8%, respectively [19]. Concerning the specific mortality related to UTIs, a careful study by Hauck et al. reported that a *net excess hospital mortality* was not observed in hospitalized patients with UTI, compared to control populations [20].

Several groups of carbapenemases have emerged in the last decade, showing different efficiency in their hydrolytic activity as well as distinct catalytic site structures, which direct their assignment to different classes.

Class A enzymes include among others (SME, IMI, GES-5) the plasmid-encoded *K. pneumoniae* carbapenemase (KPC), which has an active serine in its catalytic site, and which is only weakly inhibited by clavulanate and tazobactam. Class A carbapenemases can hydrolyze virtually all beta-lactam agents, including carbapenems, penicillins, broad-spectrum cephalosporins, and monobactams. However, cefamycins and ceftazidime are only weakly hydrolyzed by these enzymes [17]. KPC genes are frequently located within the IncFIIK2, IncF1A, IncI2 plasmids and Tn4401 transposon and are at the moment the most common transmissible class A genes in *Enterobacteriaceae* worldwide [21]. Notably, strains of KP harboring the bla_{KPC} gene, which is present in plasmids showing various structures and dimensions, are very often co-resistant to co-trimoxazole, fluoroquinolones, and aminoglycosides [22]. Many variants of KPC have been isolated worldwide in various settings, including acute care facilities, intensive care units, and tertiary care hospitals, but are also increasingly found in community-acquired infections. In Europe, their diffusion is endemic in Greece, Italy, and Poland [17]. KPC are classified on the basis of their variant amino acid sequences, KPC-2 and-3 variants having been isolated worldwide. Importantly, KPC-producing uropathogens are often difficult to identify, as routine disc-diffusion tests report them as carbapenem-susceptible or borderline-intermediate. Indeed, it is known that the resistant phenotype in these cases is fully expressed when other resistance determinants, for example, outer membrane permeability defects or efflux pumps, are compresent.

The most representative family of genes encoding for *class C beta-lactamases* is AmpC, a penicillinase/cephalosporinase harbored in chromosomes of *Enterobacter* spp. Class C enzymes do not include carbapenemases, are not inhibited by clavulanic acid, and show poor activity against monobactams.

The *D class* includes over 400 serine oxacillinase-type OXA beta-lactamases, divided into several subgroups and often found within the IncL/M, Tn1999, and IS1999 mobile genetic elements. OXA-48 and its derivative variants are commonly identified in *K. pneumoniae*, *E. coli*, and *E. cloacae*, and are today disseminated throughout Europe, Mediterranean countries, and the world [23]. OXA enzymes can breakdown penicillins at high rate, carbapenems at a low level, and expanded-spectrum cephalosporins to a limited extent. Despite such weak carbapenemase activity, carbapenem resistance may result from the combined action of an OXA-type carbapenemase with other mechanisms such as mutated porins or overexpressed efflux pumps [24].

Unlike class A and D serine enzymes, class B metallo beta-lactamases (MBL) require zinc for their catalytic nucleophilic reaction directed toward the beta-lactam ring. These enzymes, expressed in *Enterobacteriaceae* (including *Klebsiella oxytoca*) and in *P. aeruginosa*, can hydrolyze a broad range of beta-lactams (with the exception of aztreonam, but not in all strains) and are known to be resistant to all beta-lactamase inhibitors so far produced [17]. Transferable MBL genes include the New Delhi MBL (NDM, found in IncA/C, ISAba125, and other mobile genetic elements), the Verona Integron-encoded MBL (VIM, found in IncN, IncI1, and other mobile genetic elements), the IMP beta-lactamase (found in IncL/M, IncA/C, and other mobile genetic elements), and the German Imipenemase (GIM-1) MBL, detected in Germany in *E. cloacae*, *K. oxytoca*, and *E. coli* isolates [22, 25, 26]. The NDM enzymes share little amino acid identity with other MBLs, and hydrolyze carbapenems to various extents, with the NDM-4, NDM-5, and NDM-7 variants showing increased breakdown activity. NDMs are often co-expressed with other carbapenemases (OXA-48, VIM, and KPC), and are almost always associated with various resistance determinants, such as plasmid-borne AmpC cephalosporinases, clavulanic acid-inhibited ESBLs, and determinants conferring resistance to aminoglycosides (e.g., 16S RNA methylases), quinolones (e.g., Qnr), macrolides (esterases), rifampicin, chloramphenicol, and co-trimoxazole [22]. Thus, basically most NDM-expressing pathogens show residual susceptibility only to colistin or fosfomycin, which represents a very limited choice among last-resource agents.

1.3.1.2 Polymyxin Resistance Determinants

The mobilized colistin resistance *mcr-1* gene encodes a phosphatidylethanolamine transferase, which modifies cell membrane lipid A to decrease its affinity to colistin. The *mcr-1* gene has been detected in *E. coli*, *Klebsiella* spp., and *Enterobacter* spp. [27]. The increasing diffusion of this plasmid-borne, cross-species transferable resistance gene, likely facilitated by the usage of colistin as cattle fattening agent in Asia and elsewhere, will soon compromise the efficacy of this last-resort antibiotic for treatment of carbapenem-resistant *Enterobacteriaceae*.

1.3.1.3 Plasmid-Mediated Fluoroquinolone Resistance

Plasmid-mediated fluoroquinolone (FQ) resistance (PMQR) in *Enterobacteriaceae* is dramatically increasing worldwide, and in many countries quinolones are no longer recommended as drugs of choice for treatment of UTIs and other uro-genital infections like prostatitis. International guidelines from the Infectious Diseases Society of America, the European Society for Microbiology and Infectious Diseases and other agencies no longer recommend empirical administration of fluoroquinolones in areas showing resistance rates higher than 10% (raised to 20% in the Asia-Pacific region) [28, 29].

As mentioned in the previous section, FQs interfere with the activity of bacterial gyrase (main target in Gram-negative pathogens) and topoisomerase IV (main target in Gram-positive organisms), which are essential for DNA replication and cell duplication. Mutations (e.g., *gyr*A, *gyr*B, *par*C, *par*E) occurring on the *quinolone resistance determining regions* of genes encoding these type II topoisomerases are the most common chromosomal determinants of FQ resistance [14]. Determinants of PMQR also include (1) the *qnr* genes, whose *pentapeptide-repeat* product protects DNA gyrase from the interaction with FQs, (2) the variant aminoglycoside acetyl-transferase *aac (6′)-Ib-cr*, which acetylates and inactivates the piperazine ring of certain FQs, (3) the *qep*A-encoded efflux pumps, sharing sequence homology with MFS 14-transmembrane transporters, and (4) the *oqxAB*-encoded efflux pumps, very common in *K. pneumoniae* and *E. coli*-borne plasmids, but also on bacterial chromosomes [30–33].

Determinants of PMQR are commonly associated with genes encoding ESBLs, AMP-C beta-lactamases, and other genetic elements conferring resistance to various antibacterial agents. *qnrA1, A3, A6, B2, B4, B6*, and *B10* are associated with the mobilizing element insertion sequence ISCR, whereas *qnrB1* and *B20* are associated with IS26 and Orf1005. The *aac (6′)-Ib-cr* enzyme-encoding gene is often found in association with *qnr*B and *blaCTX* in a cassette within an IS26 transposon. *qep*A and the OqxAB-encoding genes are also often mobilized by IS26 transposons.

In Europe, the areas most affected by increasing resistance trends are the Mediterranean countries, together with Mediterranean North African regions. A comprehensive systematic review by Yanat and coworkers included a map describing the geographic distribution of high-rate PMQR, extending to the entire Mediterranean area, including Spain, Tunisia, Italy, France, Algeria, Egypt Morocco, Greece, Slovenia, Croatia, and Turkey [34].

1.3.1.4 *Pseudomonas aeruginosa*

Multidrug-resistant (MDR) *P. aeruginosa* (PA) is steadily expanding worldwide. Isolates of MDR PA show resistance to third-generation cephalosporins, carbapenems, aminoglycosides, and fluoroquinolones, whose determinants are expressed within transposons, plasmids, and integrons. It has been reported that ESBL typically found in *Enterobacteriaceae* (e.g., PER-1, VEB, GES, and BEL-1) are gradually spreading to PA [35]. Similarly, the KPC carbapenemase, previously found exclusively in *Enterobacteriaceae*, as well as several metallo-beta lactamases (IMP, VIM, SPM) are increasingly found in PA [35, 36]. In this context, Nordmann and coworkers foresee that pan-drug resistance in ICU-acquired PA will be increasingly reported worldwide [35].

1.3.2 Gram-Positive Cocci

Enterococci, the third most frequently isolated pathogens in the hospital setting, are among the most common etiological determinants of urinary tract infections. In these species, expression of penicillinase resistance determinants is infrequent, though Enterococci are intrinsically resistant to cephalosporins via expression of penicillin-binding proteins (PBP) showing low affinity for these antibiotics (MIC range: 2–16 mg/L for Enterococci). Resistance to ampicillin and similar agents is mainly present in *E. faecium*, also due to the presence of low-affinity PBP. Enterococci may also acquire beta-lactamases via horizontal transfer of *bla* genes or similar.

The ability of Enterococci to uptake folic acid from the surrounding milieu makes them naturally resistant to co-trimoxazole. *E. faecalis* is also intrinsically resistant to lincosamides, though this characteristic is probably of lesser importance in the management of UTIs, as agents like clindamycin are mainly excreted through the biliary system.

Enterococci are intrinsically non-susceptible to aminoglycosides due to inability of these to enter coccal cells in the absence of a cell wall synthesis inhibitor. Hence, co-administration of a penicillin confers a synergic and rapidly bactericidal action to this antibiotic combination. Nevertheless, as described in the previous section, Enterococci can become resistant to aminoglycosides mainly by acquisition of modifying enzymes like phosphotransferases and nucleotidyltransferases. Importantly, acetyltransferases (AAC) like AAC(6′)-Ii are ubiquitous among *E. faecium*. As mentioned above, high-level aminoglycoside resistance occurs through acquisition of a bifunctional resistance determinant encoding a phosphotransferase and an acetyltransferase, *aph(2″)-Ia-aac(6′)-Ie* [37].

Conjugation in Enterococci is made easy by pheromone-stimulated production of *aggregation substance*, which facilitates cell–cell contact by interacting with the *enterococcal binding substance*, thus resulting in horizontal exchange of resistance determinants [5].

Three types of transposons facilitate gene exchange in Enterococci: Tn3, composite, and conjugative transposons. An example of the former is the common Tn917, conferring resistance to macrolides, lincosamides, and dalfopristin.

Acquired resistance to glycopeptide antibiotics is given by five determinants (clusters): VanA, VanB, VanD, VanE, and VanG, responsible for the expression of peptidoglycan pentapeptide precursors (PPP) showing decreased binding affinity for vancomycin and other glycopeptides. In particular, VanA-type Enterococci are also resistant to dalbavancin, a last-generation glycopeptide, but retain susceptibility to oritavancin, possibly due to the dual mechanism of action—including transglycosidase inhibition—shown by this second-generation agent [38]. Horizontal transfer of Van genes may occur via Tn-1546 transposons, which are found in conjugative and non-conjugative plasmids [5].

In Gram-positive cocci including Enterococci, resistance to fluoroquinolones is given by mutations occurring in the gyrase and topoisonerase-IV *GyrA* and *ParC* genes, with higher MICs achieved by cumulative mutations in both genes [39].

The synergistic bactericidal activity of the streptogramin combination quinupristin/dalfopristin (QD) is due to the binding of the two agents to different domains of the 50S ribosomal subunit of vancomycin-susceptible or -resistant *E. faecium. E. faecalis* is resistant to these streptogramins in most cases, due to the activity of the Lsa efflux pump, which is probably expressed constitutively by this species. Streptogramin resistance is also mediated by drug-modifying enzymes. Quinupristin resistance in Enterococci is given by acetyltransferases encoded by plasmid-mediated *vatD and vatE* genes, whereas dalfopristin resistance is mediated by lyases encoded by *vgb(A)* and *vgb(B)* genes [38].

Resistance to the oxazolidinone linezolid is acquired via mutations in the target genes encoding the 23S ribosomal RNA. In particular, the G2576T point-mutation has been detected in Enterococci in several countries [40, 41], whereas the transferable *cfr* gene, identified in *E. faecalis,* encodes a rRNA methyltransferase which prevents the binding of linezolid through modification of the linezolid binding region of the 23S rRNA.

1.4 Recommendations and Future Perspectives

- Detailed diagnostic guidelines, treatment algorithms, and expert recommendations are regularly published and upgraded worldwide (e.g., [42, 43]). Strict adherence to such guidelines and recommendations is encouraged by national and international health organizations, by academic institutions, and by scientific/medical societies.
- Strict stewardship strategies, aimed at selecting types, optimal dosages, and combinations of antibacterial agents aimed at minimizing the emergence and spread of chemoresistance should be applied worldwide, and modifiable practice patterns should be implemented in those countries where bad prescription practices, negligent dispensation attitudes, and incorrect patient compliance are highly prevalent.
- To date, available options for treatment of CREB infections are limited to polymyxins and aminoglycosides, but toxicity and adverse effects of these agent classes often hinder the implementation of effective therapeutic protocols.

- Many *in vitro* studies have shown that combination therapy with various classes of antibacterial agents shows enhanced cure rates of infections caused by CREB. These protocols may include aminoglycosides, aztreonam, colistin, rifampicin, tigecycline, or fosfomycin (e.g., [44]). Several studies seem to univocally show that combination therapy with two or more *in vitro*-active agents are associated with lower mortality than treatment with a single *in vitro*-active agent. Presentation of various possible combination regimens is beyond the scope of this chapter.
- Research focusing on suppressive drug combinations, a seemingly paradoxical phenomenon showing that selection of resistant mutants can be inverted by administration of hyper-antagonistic combinations of antibacterial agents, produced interesting preliminary results and should be further investigated, though it is still early to imagine how such findings will be implemented in the clinics [45, 46].

References

1. Nolan LK, Li G, Logue CM. Origin and dissemination of antimicrobial resistance among uropathogenic *Escherichia coli*. Microbiol Spectr. 2015;3:5.
2. https://amr-review.org/sites/default/files/160525_Final%20paper_with%20cover.pdf.
3. Edlin RS, Copp HL. Antibiotic resistance in pediatric urology. Ther Adv Urol. 2014;6:54–61.
4. Costelloe C, Metcalfe C, Lovering A, Mant D, Hay AD. Effect of antibiotic prescribing in primary care on antimicrobial resistance in individual patients: systematic review and meta-analysis. BMJ. 2010;340:c2096.
5. Hollenbeck BL, Rice LB. Intrinsic and acquired resistance mechanisms in enterococcus. Virulence. 2012;3:421–33.
6. Kumar S, Varela MF. Biochemistry of bacterial multidrug efflux pumps. Int J Mol Sci. 2012;13:4484–95.
7. Munita JM, Arias CA. Mechanisms of antibiotic resistance. Microbiol Spectr. 2016;4:2.
8. Culebras E, Martínez JL. Aminoglycoside resistance mediated by the bifunctional enzyme 6′-*N*-aminoglycoside acetyltransferase-2″-*O*-aminoglycoside phosphotransferase. Front Biosci. 1999;4:D1–8.
9. Abraham EP, Chain E. An enzyme from bacteria able to destroy penicillin. Nature. 1940;46:837.
10. Frère JM, Sauvage E, Kerff F. From "An enzyme able to destroy penicillin" to carbapenemases: 70 years of beta-lactamase misbehaviour. Curr Drug Targets. 2016;17:974–82.
11. Flensburg J, Sköld O. Massive overproduction of dihydrofolate reductase in bacteria as a response to the use of trimethoprim. Eur J Biochem. 1987;162:473–6.
12. Arias CA, Murray BE. The rise of the enterococcus: beyond vancomycin resistance. Nat Rev Microbiol. 2012;10:266–78.
13. Aldred KJ, Kerns RJ, Osheroff N. Mechanism of quinolone action and resistance. Biochemistry. 2014;53:1565–74.
14. Yoshida H, Bogaki M, Nakamura M, Nakamura S. Quinolone resistance-determining region in the DNA gyrase gyrA gene of *Escherichia coli*. Antimicrob Agents Chemother. 1990;34:1271–12.
15. Lukac PJ, Bonomo RA, Logan LK. Extended-spectrum β-lactamase-producing Enterobacteriaceae in children: old foe, emerging threat. Clin Infect Dis. 2015;60:1389–97.
16. Nordmann P, Poirel L. The difficult-to-control spread of carbapenemase producers among Enterobacteriaceae worldwide. Clin Microbiol Infect. 2014;20:821–30.

17. Nordmann P, Cuzon G, Naas T. The real threat of *Klebsiella pneumoniae* carbapenemase-producing bacteria. Lancet Infect Dis. 2009;9:228–36.
18. https://ecdc.europa.eu/sites/portal/files/documents/AMR-surveillance-Europe-2016.pdf.
19. Xu L, Sun X, Ma X. Systematic review and meta-analysis of mortality of patients infected with carbapenem-resistant *Klebsiella pneumoniae*. Ann Clin Microbiol Antimicrob. 2017;16:18.
20. Hauck C, Cober E, Richter SS, Perez F, Salata RA, Kalayjian RC, Watkins RR, Scalera NM, Doi Y, Kaye KS, Evans S, Fowler VG Jr, Bonomo RA, van Duin D, Antibacterial Resistance Leadership Group. Spectrum of excess mortality due to carbapenem-resistant *Klebsiella pneumoniae* infections. Clin Microbiol Infect. 2016;22:513–9.
21. Patel G, Bonomo RA. "Stormy waters ahead": global emergence of carbapenemases. Front Microbiol. 2013;4:48.
22. Logan LK, Weinstein RA. The epidemiology of carbapenem-resistant Enterobacteriaceae: the impact and evolution of a global menace. J Infect Dis. 2017;215(suppl_1):S28–36.
23. Poirel L, Potron A, Nordmann P. OXA-48-like carbapenemases: the phantom menace. J Antimicrob Chemother. 2012;67:1597–606.
24. Walther-Rasmussen J, Høiby N. OXA-type carbapenemases. J Antimicrob Chemother. 2006;57:373–83.
25. Wendel AF, Brodner AH, Wydra S, Ressina S, Henrich B, Pfeffer K, Toleman MA, Mackenzie CR. Genetic characterization and emergence of the metallo-β-lactamase GIM-1 in Pseudomonas spp. and Enterobacteriaceae during a long-term outbreak. Antimicrob Agents Chemother. 2013;57:5162–5.
26. Hamprecht A, Poirel L, Göttig S, Seifert H, Kaase M, Nordmann P. Detection of the carbapenemase GIM-1 in *Enterobacter cloacae* in Germany. J Antimicrob Chemother. 2013;68:558–61.
27. Gao R, Hu Y, Li Z, Sun J, Wang Q, Lin J, Ye H, Liu F, Srinivas S, Li D, Zhu B, Liu YH, Tian GB, Feng Y. Dissemination and mechanism for the MCR-1 Colistin resistance. PLoS Pathog. 2016;12:e1005957.
28. Gupta K, Hooton TM, Naber KG, Wullt B, Colgan R, Miller LG, Moran GJ, Nicolle LE, Raz R, Schaeffer AJ, Soper DE, Infectious Diseases Society of America; European Society for Microbiology and Infectious Diseases. International clinical practice guidelines for the treatment of acute uncomplicated cystitis and pyelonephritis in women: a 2010 update by the Infectious Diseases Society of America and the European Society for Microbiology and Infectious Diseases. Clin Infect Dis. 2011;52:e103–20.
29. Hsueh PR, Hoban DJ, Carmeli Y, Chen SY, Desikan S, Alejandria M, Ko WC, Binh TQ. Consensus review of the epidemiology and appropriate antimicrobial therapy of complicated urinary tract infections in Asia-Pacific region. J Infect. 2011;63:114–23.
30. Tran JH, Jacoby GA, Hooper DC. Interaction of the plasmid-encoded quinolone resistance protein Qnr with *Escherichia coli* DNA gyrase. Antimicrob Agents Chemother. 2005;49:118–25.
31. Robicsek A, Strahilevitz J, Jacoby GA, Macielag M, Abbanat D, Park CH, Bush K, Hooper DC. Fluoroquinolone-modifying enzyme: a new adaptation of a common aminoglycoside acetyltransferase. Nat Med. 2006;12:83–8.
32. Yamane K, Wachino J, Suzuki S, Kimura K, Shibata N, Kato H, Shibayama K, Konda T, Arakawa Y. New plasmid-mediated fluoroquinolone efflux pump, QepA, found in an *Escherichia coli* clinical isolate. Antimicrob Agents Chemother. 2007;51:3354–60.
33. Hansen LH, Johannesen E, Burmølle M, Sørensen AH, Sørensen SJ. Plasmid-encoded multidrug efflux pump conferring resistance to olaquindox in *Escherichia coli*. Antimicrob Agents Chemother. 2004;48:3332–7.
34. Yanat B, Rodríguez-Martínez JM, Touati A. Plasmid-mediated quinolone resistance in Enterobacteriaceae: a systematic review with a focus on Mediterranean countries. Eur J Clin Microbiol Infect Dis. 2017;36:421–35.
35. Nordmann P, Naas T, Fortineau N, Poirel L. Superbugs in the coming new decade; multidrug resistance and prospects for treatment of *Staphylococcus aureus*, enterococcus spp. and *Pseudomonas aeruginosa* in 2010. Curr Opin Microbiol. 2007;10:436–40.
36. Villegas MV, Lolans K, Correa A, Kattan JN, Lopez JA, Quinn JP, Colombian Nosocomial Resistance Study Group. First identification of *Pseudomonas aeruginosa* isolates produc-

ing a KPC-type carbapenem-hydrolyzing beta-lactamase. Antimicrob Agents Chemother. 2007;51:1553–5.
37. Mederski-Samoraj BD, Murray BE. High-level resistance to gentamicin in clinical isolates of enterococci. J Infect Dis. 1983;147:751–7.
38. Woodford N. Biological counterstrike: antibiotic resistance mechanisms of gram-positive cocci. Clin Microbiol Infect. 2005;11(Suppl_3):2–21.
39. Korten V, Huang WM, Murray BE. Analysis by PCR and direct DNA sequencing of gyrA mutations associated with fluoroquinolone resistance in *Enterococcus faecalis*. Antimicrob Agents Chemother. 1994;38:2091–4.
40. Auckland C, Teare L, Cooke F, Kaufmann ME, Warner M, Jones G, Bamford K, Ayles H, Johnson AP. Linezolid-resistant enterococci: report of the first isolates in the United Kingdom. J Antimicrob Chemother. 2002;50:743–6.
41. Bersos Z, Maniati M, Kontos F, Petinaki E, Maniatis AN. First report of a linezolid-resistant vancomycin-resistant *Enterococcus faecium* strain in Greece. J Antimicrob Chemother. 2004;53:685–6.
42. Wagenlehner FM, Schmiemann G, Hoyme U, Fünfstück R, Hummers-Pradier E, Kaase M, Kniehl E, Selbach I, Sester U, Vahlensieck W, Watermann D, Naber KG. National S3 guideline on uncomplicated urinary tract infection: recommendations for treatment and management of uncomplicated community-acquired bacterial urinary tract infections in adult patients. Urologe A. 2011;50:153–69.
43. http://uroweb.org/guideline/urological-infections/.
44. Tängdén T, Hickman RA, Forsberg P, Lagerbäck P, Giske CG, Cars O. Evaluation of double- and triple-antibiotic combinations for VIM- and NDM-producing *Klebsiella pneumoniae* by in vitro time-kill experiments. Antimicrob Agents Chemother. 2014;58:1757–62.
45. Singh N, Yeh PJ. Suppressive drug combinations and their potential to combat antibiotic resistance. J Antibiot (Tokyo). 2017;70:1033–42.
46. Chait R, Craney A, Kishony R. Antibiotic interactions that select against resistance. Nature. 2007;446:668–71.

Bacterial Resistance: What Is the Epidemiological Scenario?

2

David M. Livermore

2.1 Introduction: the Nature of Resistance

Antibiotics kill susceptible bacteria while leaving resistant ones to survive and to accumulate. The initial emergence of resistance is random, contingent of chance genetic events. Its subsequent accumulation reflects the extent of selection pressure, meaning the weight of antibiotic use, the strength or weakness of infection control, and the fitness of the strains that have acquired resistance.

At a genetic level, resistance can arise via mutations—DNA copying errors—that engender resistance in a previously-susceptible strain or species, or by transfer of mobile DNA, in the form of transposons or plasmids carrying resistance genes. Plasmids existed in the pre-antibiotic era but have since become major vectors of resistance, recruiting and spreading genes from organisms which, of themselves, have little or no clinical relevance [1]. For example, (1) many of the genes that encode aminoglycoside-modifying enzymes were mobilized to plasmids from aminoglycoside-producing streptomycetes [1, 2]; (2) the genes encoding the (now predominant) CTX-M extended-spectrum β-lactamases (ESBLs), responsible for cephalosporin resistance originated in environmental *Kluyvera* spp. [2], and (3) those encoding OXA-48 carbapenemases were recruited from free-living *Shewanella* spp. [3].

Over time, the accumulation of mutations and or resistance plasmids can lead to historically susceptible species becoming broadly resistant, with the drug "lost," as with *Escherichia coli* in the case of ampicillin or *Staphylococcus aureus* and penicillin [4].

Resistance can also accumulate because inherently resistant species became more important at the expense of more susceptible ones. This is important in the case of opportunistic gram-negative infections in vulnerable hospitalized patients,

D. M. Livermore (✉)
Norwich Medical School, University of East Anglia, Norwich, UK
e-mail: d.livermore@uea.ac.uk

T. E. Bjerklund Johansen, T. Cai (eds.), *Guide to Antibiotics in Urology*,
https://doi.org/10.1007/978-3-319-92366-6_2

where *Enterobacter*, *Klebsiella*, and *Pseudomonas* spp. have gained importance over time, but is less so in the case of UTIs, where *Escherichia coli* has remained the principal pathogen since before the antibiotic era [5].

2.2 Resistance and the Pathogens of UTI

E. coli accounts for around 65–90% of UTIs, regardless of whether these are complicated or uncomplicated, affect the lower or upper urinary tract, and are community- or hospital-acquired [5].

As a species, *E. coli* has little inherent resistance except to antibiotics that cannot penetrate gram-negative bacteria in general or which are very rapidly effluxed (e.g., macrolides, clindamycin, oxazolidinones, glycopeptides, rifampin, and fusidic acid) [6]. Rather, most resistance to UTI-relevant β-lactams, aminoglycosides, and antifolates arises from plasmid acquisition; most resistance to fosfomycin and fluoroquinolones arises via mutation (Table 2.1; Refs. [7–20]).

Among other important gram-negative uropathogens, *Klebsiella* spp., *Enterobacter* spp., and *Pseudomonas aeruginosa* all have greater inherent resistance than *E. coli* owing to (1) the production of more potent chromosomally encoded β-lactamases and (2) slower uptake, reflecting a less favorable (from the clinician's standpoint) balance of uptake and efflux, with efflux particularly important in the case of *P. aeruginosa* (Table 2.2) [6, 7, 21]. *Proteus mirabilis*, another frequent gram-negative uropathogen, is inherently more susceptible than *E. coli* to many β-lactams and fluoroquinolones, but is inherently resistant to colistin, tetracyclines, and nitrofurantoin (Table 2.2) [22–24].

Non-*E. coli* Enterobacteriaceae, including *Klebsiella*, *Enterobacter*, and *Proteus* spp., as well as rarer uropathogens such as *Serratia*, *Morganella*, and *Providencia* spp. commonly acquire the same plasmid-mediated resistances as *E. coli*; plasmid-mediated resistance is rarer in *P. aeruginosa*, with mutational mechanisms—notably, upregulation of efflux and hyperproduction of chromosomal AmpC β-lactamase—much more important (Table 2.2) [24].

Among frequent gram-positive uropathogens, *Enterococcus faecalis* remains almost universally susceptible to ampicillin, but with universal inherent resistance to cephalosporins and mecillinam owing to target insensitivity [23]; *Staphylococcus saprophyticus* is often resistant to unprotected ampicillin but typically remains susceptible to amoxicillin/clavulanate.

Table 2.1 Major mechanisms of resistance among *E. coli* isolates to UTI-relevant antibiotics

Drug class affected	Major plasmid-mediated mechanisms	Major mutational mechanisms
Ampicillin [7]	TEM, SHV, OXA β-lactamases	Upregulation of chromosomal AmpC β-lactamase, by loss of terminator codons
Mecillinam [8]	ESBLs (variable, with type SHV-5 strongly active, CTX-M-15 moderately active, and CTX-M-9/14 minimally active)	Multiple mutations affecting the stringent response and thereby compensating for inhibition of penicillin-bring protein-2 by mecillinam
Cephalosporins (first generation) [7, 9]	TEM, SHV β-lactamases (marginal) ESBLs (mostly CTX-M types)	Upregulation of chromosomal AmpC β-lactamase, by loss of terminator codons
Cephalosporins (3/4 generation) [7, 9]	ESBLs (mostly CTX-M types); plasmid-mediated AmpC β-lactamases	Upregulation of chromosomal AmpC β-lactamase, by loss of terminator codons; compromises third-generation analogs only
Amoxicillin/clavulanate and piperacillin/tazobactam [10, 11]	Hyperproduction of TEM β-lactamases; OXA-1 or plasmid-mediated AmpC β-lactamases; mutant TEM β-lactamases with reduced inhibitor binding	Upregulation of chromosomal AmpC β-lactamase, by loss of terminator codons
Carbapenems [9, 12, 13]	Metallo-carbapenemases (NDM, VIM, IMP)[a], also KPC[a], and OXA-48-like[b] serine β-lactamases	Porin loss together with plasmid-mediated ESBLs or AmpC enzymes or upregulation of chromosomal AmpC β-lactamase, by loss of terminator codons
Trimethoprim [14, 15]	Multiple trimethoprim-resistant dihydrofolate reductases, compensating for inhibition of corresponding chromosomal enzymes	
Sulfonamide [15]	Sul1/2 sulfonamide-resistant dihydropteroate synthases, compensating for inhibition of corresponding chromosomal enzymes	Mutations affecting chromosomal dihydropteroate synthase
Fluoroquinolones [16]	Qnr efflux pumps and mutant AAC(6′)-1b-cr, augmenting resistance, though unable to cause resistance as sole mechanism	Mutations affecting both DNA gyrase and topoisomerase IV
Aminoglycosides [17, 18]	Enzymes modifying aminoglycosides by acetylation, nucleotidylation, or phosphorylation. Amikacin is compromised by fewer such enzymes than gentamicin or tobramycin Methyltransferase enzymes modifying rRNA to block binding of all relevant aminoglycosides	Rare
Fosfomycin [8, 19]	FosA enzymes, adding glutathione to fosfomycin and thereby inactivating the drug	Loss of hexose and triose sugar transporters ordinarily exploited by fosfomycin for uptake across the cytoplasmic membrane
Nitrofurantoin [8, 20]		Mutations to nitroreductase-encoding *nfsA* and *nfsB* genes

[a]Also confer resistance to penicillins, penicillin/β-lactamase-inhibitor combinations, and cephalosporins
[b]Also confer resistance to penicillins, penicillin/β-lactamase-inhibitor combinations, not cephalosporins

Table 2.2 Inherent and acquired resistance in important uropathogens besides *E. coli*

Species or genus	Inherent resistances, present in all/almost all isolates [22, 23]	Acquired resistances
Klebsiella spp., except *K. aerogenes*	Ampicillin, owing to chromosomal SHV-like β-lactamases; nitrofurantoin; fosfomycin at doses used for oral therapy	As *E. coli*, Table 2.1
Enterobacter spp., also *K. aerogenes* and *Citrobacter freundii*	Ampicillin, amoxicillin/clavulanate, and first-generation cephalosporins owing to chromosomal AmpC β-lactamases; nitrofurantoin; fosfomycin at doses used for oral therapy	As *E. coli*, Table 2.1; heightened risk of mutational hyperproduction of chromosomal AmpC β-lactamases leading to cephalosporin resistance
Proteus mirabilis	Nitrofurantoin (high level); tetracyclines; colistin	As *E. coli*, Table 2.1
Serratia, Morganella, and *Providencia* spp.	Ampicillin, amoxicillin/clavulanate, and first-generation cephalosporins owing to chromosomal AmpC β-lactamases; nitrofurantoin (high level); fosfomycin at doses used for oral therapy; colistin	As *E. coli*, Table 2.1; heightened risk of mutational hyperproduction of AmpC β-lactamases leading to cephalosporin resistance *Serratia* only, heightened risk of hyperproduction of chromosomal AAC(6′)-Ic conferring aminoglycoside resistance
Pseudomonas aeruginosa	All *except* piperacillin/tazobactam, ceftazidime, cefepime, imipenem, meropenem, ciprofloxacin, aminoglycosides, and colistin	Mostly via mutation: hyperproduction of chromosomal AmpC compromises piperacillin/tazobactam and ceftazidime; upregulation of various efflux pumps compromise all agents except imipenem and colistin; loss of porin OprD compromises imipenem and meropenem; reduced cytoplasmic membrane transport compromises aminoglycosides; mutations to DNA gyrase and topoisomerase IV compromise fluoroquinolones [6, 24]

2.3 Prevalence of Resistance

The likelihood of resistance in a clinical isolate depends on time, place, and risk factors pertinent to the specific patient. Owing to the great limitations of resistance surveillance for UTIs, described in the next section, it is not helpful to provide long catalogues of reported resistance rates by country or region. Rather, it is better to stress general principles, and to encourage development of better local surveillance to guide empirical therapy and international comparisons. What these systems need to deliver, and how to achieve this, is outlined at the end of this chapter.

There is no doubt that resistance to relevant antibiotics has accumulated substantially in relevant uropathogens. At introduction, ampicillin (1963), trimethoprim and co-trimoxazole (1968), and ciprofloxacin (1984) were active against 90–>99% of *E. coli* [25–27]. Trimethoprim and ciprofloxacin were also widely active against other relevant Enterobacterales, with ciprofloxacin additionally covering *P. aeruginosa*. Subsequently, each of these agents has been massively undermined by resistance, with reported resistance rates (whatever their deficiencies) widely exceeding 20% and, in the case of ampicillin, up to 70%, both for urinary *E. coli* in general and even for community cystitis [28]. In the case of ampicillin, the major factor driving the accumulation of resistance was the spread of plasmids encoding bla_{TEM}, the determinant of TEM-1 β-lactamase, first seen as early as 1965 (Table 2.1) [7, 29]. In the case of trimethoprim, the issue is the spread of plasmids carrying *dfr* genes, encoding alternative dihydrofolate reductase enzymes, which compensate for inhibition of their chromosomally-mediated counterpart, which is targeted by the drug [14]. These alternative dihydrofolate reductases are often encoded by plasmids that also carry *sul1* or *sul2* genes, encoding alternate dihydropteroate synthetase enzymes that confer sulfonamide resistance, thereby compromising both components of co-trimoxazole [14, 15]. For ciprofloxacin, the major issue is the accumulation of multiple mutations affecting the *gyrA* and *parC genes* [16], and the global proliferation of "high risk" lineages that have these lesions, notably *E. coli* Sequence Type ST131 (below) [30]. Plasmid-mediated genes (*qnr* and *aac6′-Ib-cr*) can augment fluoroquinolone resistance but, of themselves, cause only reductions in susceptibility [16].

Cephalosporins, irrespective of "generation," have been undermined, by the spread of ESBLs. Until year 2000 these were principally mutants of the long-established TEM-1 and SHV-1 penicillinases, mostly seen in nosocomial *Klebsiella* spp. and rarely in *E. coli*. Since 2000 there has been massive spread of CTX-M ESBLs, particularly CTX-M-15, including in community *E. coli* [7, 31]. As with fluoroquinolone resistance, there is a strong link to the Sequence Type (ST)131. CTX-9/14 ESBLs are frequent too; in the early 2000s they were more prevalent than CTX-M-15 among *E. coli* in the Far East, whereas CTX-M-2 initially dominated in Argentina; subsequently, CTX-M-15 enzyme has become globally dominant, again substantially reflecting its link (below) to ST131 [32].

Penicillin-β-lactamase inhibitor combinations too have been undermined, though the issue is complicated both by the multiplicity of mechanisms and EUCAST's use of different amoxicillin/clavulanate breakpoints for uncomplicated cystitis (32 + 2 mg/L) and systemic infections (8 + 2 mg/L) [33]. Correlates of resistance include (1) mutations that reduce inhibitor binding to TEM enzymes; (2) co-production of inherently inhibitor-resistant β-lactamases, principally OXA-1; and (3) hyperproduction of TEM-1 enzyme, overwhelming the inhibitor as well as (4) mutations affecting antibiotic uptake [10, 11, 34].

The accumulation of resistance to β-lactams, trimethoprim and its sulfonamide combination, and fluoroquinolones is of vital importance because (1) they are, or have been, the "standard of care" for UTIs, (2) they have oral formulations, suitable for community use, and (3) most critically, they are widely effective in ascending infections, meaning both that they can be used to treat these, and that they can prevent adverse progression from established lower UTIs.

Other UTI antibiotics—nitrofurantoin, fosfomycin, and mecillinam—have much lower rates of resistance, below 10% in most jurisdictions, are suitable for oral administration, and are now widely recommended as first-line therapies for uncomplicated UTIs [35]. However, they have important limitations compared with agents that are now widely compromised by resistance [36]. In particular, (1) they are only active in cystitis and are not suitable for ascending infections; (2) fosfomycin and nitrofurantoin have convincing activity and breakpoints only for *E. coli*; (3) mecillinam is compromised by some ESBLs, and its efficacy against producers is debatable, perhaps contingent on enzyme type and quantity [37, 38]; and (4) nitrofurantoin is constrained by age-related decline in renal function, which may prevent adequate levels being attained in the urine. Drugs that retain wide activity, including against ESBL producers and in ascending infections, include carbapenems, fosfomycin (given intravenously at considerably higher dosage than the oral formulation), amikacin, and newer cephalosporin/β-lactamase inhibitor combinations. These, however, are only available as parenteral formulations, limiting their utility to hospital settings, with the sole exception that once-daily ertapenem and amikacin are suitable for out-patient parenteral therapy (OPAT). Further limitations are that (1) aminoglycoside resistance, including to amikacin, is prevalent in some countries [39], and (2) there is a slow diffusion of carbapenemases among Enterobacterales, undermining carbapenems [12, 13, 40]. Two oral penems/carbapenems, sulopenem [41] and tebipenem [42], which might have provided convenient treatments for ascending infections due to ESBL producers have recently been denied licenses by the FDA, with additional trials demanded in both cases. These trials have now been initiated.

As a rule of thumb, and subject to all the caveats on data quality outlined in the next section, the general pattern is for antibiotic resistance, including in UTIs, to be most prevalent in newly prosperous developing country—India particularly—but also across in the Middle East and much of East and Southeast Asia (Fig. 2.1) [43–45]. These jurisdictions typically have heavy usage, increasing selection pressure, together with lax controls on availability, including, in some cases, over-the-counter sales of UTI-relevant antibiotics [46]. In Europe, resistance rates are widely higher

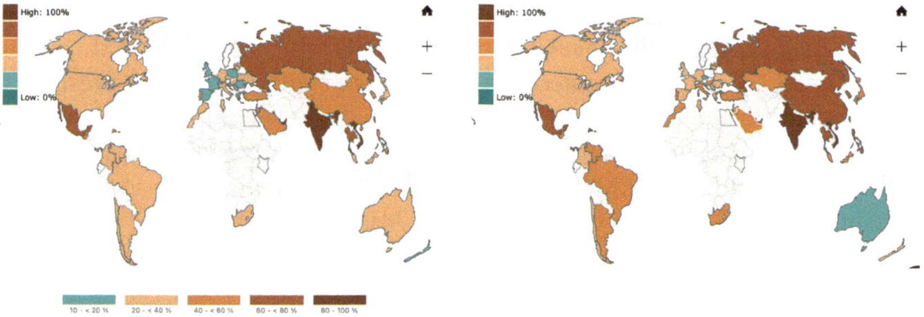

Fig. 2.1 Prevalence of resistance among *E. coli* from hospital-onset UTIs to (left) ceftriaxone and (right) ciprofloxacin; EUCAST criteria, 2015–2019 pooled data, Merck SMART surveillance. **This SMART data image is reproduced with permission of Merck & Co., Inc., Rahway, NJ, USA, and its affiliates. All rights reserved.** (Data from https://globalsmartsite.com; [44] see also Karlowsky et al. [45])

in the South and East and lower in the North (Scandinavia, particularly) and Northwest. US rates are mid-ranking by European standards, while Canadian and Australasian rates are generally low. CTX-M ESBLs came late to the USA but subsequently have spread extensively there, as previously in Europe, Asia, and Latin America [7, 32].

2.4 Three Great Problems with Resistance Surveillance Data for UTIs

It is commonplace for hospitals, countries, or supra-national studies to publish "antibiograms" summarizing rates of resistance among isolates from different infection types. Figure 2.1 provides examples of supra-national surveillance, while an example of a local antibiogram can be found, for example, here [47].

Hospital antibiograms guide empirical therapy, which must be given during the 48–72 h between clinical diagnosis and laboratory data on any isolate's antibiotic susceptibility becoming available. National and international resistance rates provide a benchmark for individual hospitals, which can see if their rates are "high" or "low" compared with peers, both nationally and internationally. Such summaries are most representative, and most useful, for severely-ill patients in hospitals, who reliably have microbiological investigations. Consequently, many surveillances concentrate on bloodstream infections.

For non-bacteremic infections, including community UTIs, three major problems arise. First, laboratory testing may only be undertaken on a biased subset of infections, with the degree of bias varying between countries and sites. Secondly, the hazard of resistance varies among patients with the same type of infection according to their individual history and risk factors. Thirdly, antibiograms pool data for all isolates tested or, at best, only distinguish between hospital and community infections, failing to stratify according to the type of UTI, whereas this may affect the likelihood of resistance.

The result of these issues, explored in detail below, is that bald assertions along the lines of "A quarter of our urinary *E. coli* are resistant to ciprofloxacin" are akin to saying that "20% of our population are bald or balding," but omitting to mention that baldness is a correlate of male aging, and is extraordinarily rare among young women.

2.4.1 Biased Sampling

Hospitalized patients with a suspected UTI typically have a urine sample taken for investigation, at least in developed countries. Culture and susceptibility testing are then performed if microscopy or particle analysis, for example, by flow cytometry, indicates significant numbers of leukocytes and bacteria. Consequently, susceptibility data are potentially comprehensive, and—if the issues (below) of stratification by patient risk and UTI type can be resolved—should provide a good representation of true resistance rates.

The situation is very different for community UTIs. Here, it is typical for treatment to be entirely empirical, based upon clinical symptoms and without laboratory investigation. In many cases, culture and susceptibility testing are requested only after a first empirical antibiotic treatment fails. The result is that, for cystitis, laboratory investigation is biased toward treatment failures and difficult cases. These, by their nature, overestimate resistance. This point was illustrated by the studies of McNulty et al. [48], who found a resistance rate of 13.9% to trimethoprim among consecutive urinary isolates from women presenting with cystitis to general practitioners in Norwich and Gloucester (UK), as compared with 24.5–27.0% among urinary isolates routinely passing through the Norwich and Gloucester clinical laboratories.

These studies were done almost two decades ago, when trimethoprim resistance was less prevalent than now, but there is no reason to suppose that the underlying patterns have since changed: there have been no subsequent recommendations that all cystitis cases should have routine microbiology done. Rather, at least in the UK, it has become easier to obtain a prescription for cystitis treatment online or by telephone consultation, without physical examination or sampling.

Notably, McNulty also showed that cystitis patients with pathogens resistant to empirically-prescribed trimethoprim were more likely to reconsult (39% vs. 6%), more likely to receive further antibiotics (39% vs. 4%), and more likely to have significant bacteriuria 1 month after therapy (41% vs. 20%). In short, resistance mattered, being associated with clinical failure, but its prevalence was overestimated by routine data. The extent of this over-estimation seems certain to vary between countries. Microbiological culture is especially unlikely in countries where antibiotics can be accessed without prescription, increasing this bias. Even in countries with more restricted access, including the UK, the bias will likely have been increased by the growth of internet pharmacies, which prescribe antibiotics following a brief online "consultation" [49], and by the COVID pandemic, which has greatly increased telephone, rather than face-to-face, general practitioner (GP) consultations [50]. Both these modes of prescribing reduce the likelihood of urine microscopy and culture (or even dipstick testing) being performed.

2.4.2 Patient-Related Risks of Resistance

Factors that increase the likelihood of a resistant pathogen include recent prior hospitalization(s), prior antibiotics, and travel to countries with high rates of resistance. A patient with recurrent infections reflecting structural abnormalities is more likely to host a resistant uropathogen than in a young woman experiencing her first episode of cystitis. Yet data for these two patients typically are bundled together in an antibiogram for urinary isolates.

The effect of prior therapy is well illustrated by the work of Donnan et al. (Table 2.3) [51], showing that the probability of resistance to trimethoprim in community UTIs increased with the number of prior prescriptions of trimethoprim and other antibiotics. Other factors associated with a greater likelihood of resistance included age, time, and sex.

International movement exposes travelers to different water- and food-associated *E. coli*. Some cause traveler's diarrhea. Others, with uropathogenic potential, establish in the gut flora. Travel-associated colonization was shown by Tängdén et al. who performed rectal swabs, pre- and post-travel, on 105 Swedish volunteers [52]. Twenty-four became colonized by ESBL-producing *E. coli* during their travels, including 7/8 who went to India and 10/34 traveling to East Asia. Those who went to India largely acquired *E. coli* with CTX-M-15 β-lactamases, whereas those who went to East Asia predominantly acquired strains with CTX-M-9/14 enzymes, matching the ESBL types then prevalent in these regions. Twenty-one of the 24 colonized patients had a 6-month follow-up, and five remained persistently colonized. The relevance is shown by the separate work of Pitout et al. in and around Calgary (Canada), who found that, for post-travel UTIs due to ESBL-*E. coli*, the enzyme type most often corresponded to that prevalent in the region visited (Table 2.4) [53]. Thus, travelers to Europe, South Asia, and the Middle East predominantly had infections due to *E. coli* with CTX-M-15 enzymes; those to East Asia had infections due to strains with CTX-M-9/14 enzymes, and those who went to the USA mostly had infections due to *E. coli* strains with TEM and SHV-type ESBLs.

Table 2.3 Risk of resistance to trimethoprim in UTI

	Odds ratio	*p*
Older (+10 years)	1.15 (1.13–1.17)	<0.001
Year (1996 vs. 1995)	2.68 (2.14–3.35)	<0.001
Sex (male vs. female)	0.70 (0.59–0.82)	<0.001
Deprivation score	0.99 (0.97–1.00)	0.096
More urines sent to lab	1.04 (0.99–1.10)	0.106
More trimethoprim prescriptions + 1	1.22 (1.16–1.28)	<0.001
More prescriptions, other antibiotics + 1	1.18 (1.06–1.32)	0.002
Benzodiazepime, SSRI, oral contraceptive prescriptions		All >0.2
Hormone replacement therapy	0.79 (0.64–0.97)	0.0208

Data from Donnan et al. [51]

Table 2.4 ESBL types in *E. coli* UTIs in relation to regions previously visited by travelers

	ESBL type				
Country visited and no visitors with subsequent UTI	CTX-M-15	CTX-M-14	Other CTX-M	TEM ESBL	SHV ESBL
US (31)	7	3	2	9[a]	10[a]
S. America (16)	7	1	2	3	3
Africa (5)	5	0	0	0	0
East Asia (15)	2	8[a]	4	0	1
Mid-East (9)	8[a]	0	1	0	0
Europe (12)	9[a]	1	0	1	1
South Asia (17)	17[a]	0	0	0	0

Data from Pitout et al. [53]
[a]Corresponds to predominant ESBL type in country visited

2.4.3 Type of UTI

The final deficiency of resistance surveillance for UTIs stems from the fact that laboratories generate antibiograms from their Laboratory Information Management Systems and not from their main clinical databases, where full patient data are held. As a result, resistance data become dissociated not only from important patient-related predictors of resistance (above), but also from whether the infection is localized to the lower urinary tract or is ascending, and whether or not it is "complicated," for example, by anatomical obstruction.

Little is published comparing resistance rates in different UTI strata. Some hint of the problem can, however, be gleaned from comparing resistance rates for bloodstream *E. coli* (from ECDC EARS-NET surveillance) [54] most of which have a urinary origin, with those for *E. coli* from community cystitis (from a recent multinational study) [55], as illustrated in Table 2.5. In 12/15 comparisons the resistance rates are higher, often substantially so, among the bacteremia isolates. The sole major exception (UK, cefpodoxime) is clearly a rogue result, for all personal experience shows that the UK rate for third-generation cephalosporin resistance in *E. coli* from cystitis is nowhere near so high as 27.5%.

Greater resistance among bloodstream isolates is despite the fact that patients with suspected bacteremia should routinely have microbiological investigation, whereas the microbiological investigation of cystitis is prone to be biased to patients with prior treatment failure and a greater likelihood of resistant pathogens (above). Accordingly, it is likely that the true differential in resistance rates is greater than Table 2.5 suggests.

Greater resistance among bloodstream isolates plausibly may be because (1) the strains of *E. coli* most capable of causing ascending infections, with bloodstream overspill, are more often resistant than the generality of strains causing cystitis, and/or (2) bacteremias commonly reflect the failure of prior therapy to cure a more localized primary infection, often precisely because it is caused by a resistant strain. In either case, the role of ST131 *E. coli* (below) is highly pertinent.

Either of these hypotheses, which are not mutually exclusive, implies that rates of resistance among isolates in ascending UTIs are likely to be intermediate between

Table 2.5 Rates of resistance to ampicillin, cefpodoxime, and ciprofloxacin and *E. coli* from cystitis and bacteremias, 2019 data

	Ampicillin		Cefpodoxime		Ciprofloxacin	
	Lower UTI in women	Bacteremia	Lower UTI in women	Bacteremia	Lower UTI in women	Bacteremia
Italy	52.0	68.1	21.8	30.9	32.3	40.6
Spain	51.7	61.2	6.4	14.1	16.8	29.5
United Kingdom	63.8	59.8	27.5	11.9	15.0	17.8
Belgium	48.0	56.5	11.7	10.0	14.4	19.1
Russia	47.8	65.3	20.1	47.8	23.2	50.2

Data from EARS-NET (bacteremias) [54] and Tutone et al. (lower UTI) [55]

those for "tested" cystitis cases and bloodstream isolates and above the "true" rates for consecutive cystitis patients, whether sampled or not. Yet, as outlined, it is exceptionally rare to find any hospital that produces an antibiogram that distinguishes ascending and lower UTIs.

2.5 The Importance of Strains within Species

E. coli divides into four major phylogenetic groups: A, B1, B2, and D. Strains capable of causing extraintestinal infections, including UTIs, predominantly belong to phylogroup B2 and D, whereas group A strains are largely commensals. STs are defined within these phylogenetic groups, based upon the sequences of a panel of "housekeeping genes" responsible for core bacterial functions.

A few STs account for a large proportion of those UTIs that have microbiological investigation performed, and for an even larger proportion of bacteremias (Table 2.6). Thus, STs 69, 73, 95, 127, and 131 collectively accounted for 54% of cultured UTI isolates and for 62% of bloodstream isolates in the (UK) work of Ciesielczuk et al. [56] (Table 2.6), and are prominent in multiple further European and North American studies [57, 58]. Other types regularly encountered as uropathogens include STs 10, 12, 391, 405, and, historically, ST393 [57].

Numerous traits and products have been proposed to account for the success of particular lineages [59, 60], but true explanations are likely to be more complex, with different combinations of factors promoting success in different strains. Since UTIs are mostly endogenous in origin, involving the urinary spread of strains initially colonizing the gut, success requires the strain to be able to establish itself in the very different milieux of the colon/rectum and the urinary tract itself.

There is an association between clinical importance and chromosomal carriage of large "pathogenicity islands" encoding production of hemolysins, various secreted

Table 2.6 Phylogenetic groups and sequence type (STs) among *E. coli* from bacteremias and urinary tract infections, UK

		Urinary isolates (%)	Bloodstream isolates (%)
Phylogroup	A	54 (14)	22 (8)
	B1	24 (6)	7 (3)
	B2	215 (57)	202 (72)
	D	86 (23)	47 (17)
	NK	0	1 (<1)
Major ST	ST131	41 (11)	74 (27)
	ST127	16 (4)	12 (4)
	ST95	56 (15)	34 (12)
	ST73	40 (11)	39 (14)
	ST69	50 (13)	14 (5)
	Other	176 (46)	106 (38)

Data from Ciesielczuk et al. [56]

proteins, serotype determinants, iron acquisition systems, and fimbrial adhesins [61]. These are widely present, for example, in the ST73 and ST131 lineages [62].

Among the predominant uropathogenic lineages, only ST131 is notable for resistance to multiple antibiotics, frequently including fluoroquinolones and—owing to ESBL production—cephalosporins (above). The only resistances prevalent in the great majority of isolates of the other predominant lineages, at least in the West, are to older antibiotics, such as ampicillin and trimethoprim. ST73 (and ST69) isolates commonly lack resistance or resistance plasmids [62, 63]. This points to success as a uropathogen depending on a wider range of traits than resistance alone.

It should be cautioned here that little is known on the strain epidemiology of *E. coli* in UTIs outside Europe and North America. It may be that the especially high resistance rates in, for example, South and East Asia (Fig. 2.1), reflect (1) a particularly high prevalence of ST131, (2) that resistance has penetrated other lineages that are commonly susceptible in the West, (3) that resistant lineages uncommon in the West are widespread, or (4) some mixture of these scenarios, with their relative importance varying with time and place.

ST131 is the classic example of a global clone with a high rate of multiresistance [30, 64]. Its rise to prominence began late in the Twentieth Century, and putatively entailed either the acquisition of a pathogenicity island by a lineage that already had fluoroquinolone resistance mutations, or the acquisition of these mutations by a lineage that already hosted a pathogenicity island. Subsequently, ST131 has proved adept at acquiring IncFII plasmids encoding ESBLs, principally CTX-M-15, often together with the clavulanate- and tazobactam-resistant penicillinase, OXA-1 [11, 65]. Occasionally, ST131 isolates are found with other ESBLs including CTX-M-3 (a close relative of CTX-M-15) or CTX-M-9/14.

In the UK, ST131 accounted for 64% of ESBL-producing *E. coli* from bacteremias by 2013–2014 [65] - an even higher proportion than in the study shown in Table 2.6. The lineage's importance in this setting has been associated with an increased likelihood of treatment failure in prior UTIs [66], potentially explaining why the proportion of ST131 isolates is substantially greater in bacteremias than UTIs (Table 2.6).

2.6 Conclusion: Toward Better Surveillance of Resistance, or Alternative Futures?

This chapter has made five core points:

- Resistance has increased in UTIs. Once-good therapies, for example, trimethoprim, ampicillin, and fluoroquinolones, have been undermined or lost.
- For cystitis, growing resistance to once-standard treatments forces the use of agents with poor efficacy if the infection has begun, however insidiously, to ascend the urinary tract. For ascending infections, resistance drives hospitalization and carbapenem use.
- The probability of resistance reflects the type of UTI and the patient's risk factors, as well as the local prevalence of resistance.

- UTIs and contingent bacteremias are strongly associated with a few *E. coli* STs, but only one of the most prevalent lineages—ST131—clearly owes its success primarily to multiresistance.
- While these broad patterns are clear, measures of the prevalence of resistance remain inexact. This confounds comparison between sites, patient groups, and countries. It may drive inappropriate empirical therapy.

How might surveillance and the understanding of resistance rates be improved, to give both a truer epidemiological picture and better guide empirical therapy?

In the case of hospitalized patients, who mostly have urine culture performed, the key simply is better data linkage between the laboratory results and clinical information. This would allow "resistance prevalence rates" to be stratified according to the type of UTI and patient risk factors. Such data could then be used to produce a risk-based algorithm for empirical therapy until laboratory results become available.

The situation is more complex for community UTIs, since microbiological testing of every presenting case would add prohibitive cost for limited gain, given that empirical nitrofurantoin, mecillinam, or fosfomycin will prove effective in most cases [67]. Perhaps the most pragmatic approach would be to undertake microbiological testing on all consecutive cystitis patients presenting to a representative sample of GP practices and, for these patients, to record recent travel, antibiotics, and other risk factors. This would entail relatively little extra laboratory work and would generate useful epidemiological data. It would concentrate additional logistic work at particular GP practices, which would need to be remunerated.

Other and different ways of managing community UTIs are, however, being made possible by rapid testing, with implications for surveillance. One potential approach is rapid, low-cost multiplex PCR on collected urine to seek, say, (1) *E. coli* in general, (2) *E. coli* ST131 in particular, and (3) the prevalent *dfr* genes that account for most trimethoprim resistance [68]. These tests could be run, together with a phagocyte count, at a local clinic or pharmacy, with limited medical consultation to exclude ascending infection, and a turnaround of 30–90 min. The results would inform whether the patient had (1) a likely UTI, (2) the likeliest pathogen, (3) a strain likely to be multiresistant, and (4) whether trimethoprim—a drug likely to cover incipient ascending infection—should remain efficacious. Patients positive for non-ST131 *E. coli* but negative for *dfr* would receive trimethoprim; those with *E. coli* and/or a positive *dfr* test, or with *E. coli* ST131 would receive nitrofurantoin, fosfomycin, or mecillinam, as at present. Those with UTI symptoms, raised leukocytes, and entirely negative PCR would receive amoxicillin-clavulanate, as having broad coverage against other likely pathogens as diverse as *S. saprophyticus*, enterococci, and *Klebsiella* spp.

This approach would be better than present practice for patients and antibiotic stewardship, but would only deliver sketchy surveillance, with the hazard that new modes of resistance might spread unsuspected. Accordingly, culture-based testing on a representative sample of urines would need to be retained for surveillance purposes. Once again, this would best be delivered via selected GP practices.

A different agent of change lies in the development of vaccines directed against the predominant serotypes of *E. coli* [69], including ST131, which typically expresses O:25b antigens. After initial investigation on a 4-serotype vaccine, Johnson and Johnson now have a 9-serotype vaccine in phase 3 trials [70]. This has an endpoint of "prevention of invasive disease," but it may also have a wider effect on the types of *E. coli* prevalent in UTI, and therefore the prevalence of resistance, as with conjugate vaccines directed against particular (and often multiresistant) lineages of *Streptococcus pneumoniae*,. These were designed to prevent bacteremia, but also affect the serotypes prevalent in pneumonia, with some serotypes more associated with resistance than others. [71, 72]. If so, major shifts in the microbiology of UTIs may lie ahead.

Transparency Declaration Advisory Boards or ad hoc consultancy Accelerate, AdjuTec, Antabio, Centauri, GenPax, LipoVation, Meiji, Menarini, Mutabilis, Nordic, Paion, ParaPharm, Pfizer, Shionogi, Sumitovant, Summit, T.A.Z., Thermofisher, VenatoRx, Wockhardt, Zambon, Paid lectures—bioMérieux, GSK, Hikma, Merck/MSD, Menarini, Nordic, Pfizer, and Shionogi. Relevant shareholdings or options—Dechra, GSK, Merck, Oxford Nanopore and PerkinElmer, amounting to less than 10% of portfolio value. He also has nominated holdings in Arecor, Creo Medical, Genedrive, Poolbeg, Trellus and VericiD$_x$ (all with research/products pertinent to medicines or diagnostics) through Enterprise Investment Schemes, but has no authority to trade these shares directly.

References

1. Partridge SR. Analysis of antibiotic resistance regions in Gram-negative bacteria. FEMS Microbiol Rev. 2011;35(5):820–55.
2. Cantón R. Antibiotic resistance genes from the environment: a perspective through newly identified antibiotic resistance mechanisms in the clinical setting. Clin Microbiol Infect. 2009;15(Suppl 1):20–5.
3. Tacão M, Araújo S, Vendas M, Alves A, Henriques I. Shewanella species as the origin of blaOXA-48 genes: insights into gene diversity, associated phenotypes and possible transfer mechanisms. Int J Antimicrob Agents. 2018;51(3):340–8.
4. Antimicrobial Resistance Collaborators. Global burden of bacterial antimicrobial resistance in 2019: a systematic analysis. Lancet. 2022;399(10325):629–55.
5. Flores-Mireles AL, Walker JN, Caparon M, Hultgren SJ. Urinary tract infections: epidemiology, mechanisms of infection and treatment options. Nat Rev Microbiol. 2015;13(5):269–84.
6. Li XZ, Plésiat P, Nikaido H. The challenge of efflux-mediated antibiotic resistance in Gram-negative bacteria. Clin Microbiol Rev. 2015;28(2):337–418.
7. Bush K. Proliferation and significance of clinically relevant β-lactamases. Ann N Y Acad Sci. 2013;1277:84–90.
8. Giske CG. Contemporary resistance trends and mechanisms for the old antibiotics colistin, temocillin, fosfomycin, mecillinam and nitrofurantoin. Clin Microbiol Infect. 2015;21(10):899–905.
9. Livermore DM, Canton R, Gniadkowski M, Nordmann P, Rossolini GM, Arlet G, Ayala J, Coque TM, Kern-Zdanowicz I, Luzzaro F, Poirel L, Woodford N. CTX-M: changing the face of ESBLs in Europe. J Antimicrob Chemother. 2007;59(2):165–74.
10. Livermore DM. Determinants of the activity of beta-lactamase inhibitor combinations. J Antimicrob Chemother. 1993;31(Suppl A):9–21.
11. Livermore DM, Day M, Cleary P, Hopkins KL, Toleman MA, Wareham DW, Wiuff C, Doumith M, Woodford N. OXA-1 β-lactamase and non-susceptibility to penicillin/β-lactamase inhibitor combinations among ESBL-producing *Escherichia coli*. J Antimicrob Chemother. 2019;74(2):326–33.

12. Nordmann P, Poirel L. The difficult-to-control spread of carbapenemase producers among Enterobacteriaceae worldwide. Clin Microbiol Infect. 2014;20(9):821–30.
13. Livermore DM, Nicolau DP, Hopkins KL, Meunier D. Carbapenem-resistant enterobacterales, carbapenem resistant organisms, carbapenemase-producing enterobacterales, and carbapenemase-producing organisms: terminology past its "Sell-By Date" in an era of new antibiotics and regional carbapenemase epidemiology. Clin Infect Dis. 2020;71(7):1776–82.
14. Amyes SG. The success of plasmid-encoded resistance genes in clinical bacteria. An examination of plasmid-mediated ampicillin and trimethoprim resistance genes and their resistance mechanisms. J Med Microbiol. 1989;28(2):73–83.
15. Sköld O. Resistance to trimethoprim and sulfonamides. Vet Res. 2001;32(3–4):261–73.
16. Hooper DC, Jacoby GA. Topoisomerase inhibitors: fluoroquinolone mechanisms of action and resistance. Cold Spring Harb Perspect Med. 2016;6(9):a025320.
17. Shaw KJ, Rather PN, Hare RS, Miller GH. Molecular genetics of aminoglycoside resistance genes and familial relationships of the aminoglycoside-modifying enzymes. Microbiol Rev. 1993;57(1):138–63.
18. Wachino JI, Doi Y, Arakawa Y. Aminoglycoside resistance: updates with a focus on acquired 16S ribosomal RNA methyltransferases. Infect Dis Clin N Am. 2020;34(4):887–902.
19. Aghamali M, Sedighi M, Zahedi Bialvaei A, Mohammadzadeh N, Abbasian S, Ghafouri Z, Kouhsari E. Fosfomycin: mechanisms and the increasing prevalence of resistance. J Med Microbiol. 2019;68(1):11–25.
20. Wan Y, Mills E, Leung RCY, Vieira A, Zhi X, Croucher NJ, Woodford N, Jauneikaite E, Ellington MJ, Sriskandan S. Alterations in chromosomal genes *nfsA*, *nfsB*, and *ribE* are associated with nitrofurantoin resistance in *Escherichia coli* from the United Kingdom. Microb Genom. 2021;7(12):000702.
21. Jacoby GA. AmpC beta-lactamases. Clin Microbiol Rev. 2009;22(1):161–82.
22. https://www.eucast.org/expert_rules_and_expected_phenotypes/.
23. Leclercq R, Cantón R, Brown DF, Giske CG, Heisig P, MacGowan AP, Mouton JW, Nordmann P, Rodloff AC, Rossolini GM, Soussy CJ, Steinbakk M, Winstanley TG, Kahlmeter G. EUCAST expert rules in antimicrobial susceptibility testing. Clin Microbiol Infect. 2013;19(2):141–60.
24. Livermore DM. Multiple mechanisms of antimicrobial resistance in *Pseudomonas aeruginosa*: our worst nightmare? Clin Infect Dis. 2002;34(5):634–40.
25. Kennedy WP, Wallace AT, Murdoch JM. Ampicillin in treatment of certain Gram-negative bacterial infections. Br Med J. 1963;2(5363):962–5.
26. Darrell JH, Garrod LP, Waterworth PM. Trimethoprim: laboratory and clinical studies. J Clin Pathol. 1968;21(2):202–9.
27. Giamarellou H, Efstratiou A, Tsagarakis J, Petrikkos G, Daikos GK. Experience with ciprofloxacin in vitro and in vivo. Arzneimittelforschung. 1984;34(12):1775–8.
28. Tandogdu Z, Wagenlehner FM. Global epidemiology of urinary tract infections. Curr Opin Infect Dis. 2016;29(1):73–9.
29. Anderson ES, Datta N. Resistance to penicillins and its transfer in enterobacteriaceae. Lancet. 1965;1(7382):407–9.
30. Manges AR, Geum HM, Guo A, Edens TJ, Fibke CD, Pitout JDD. Global extraintestinal pathogenic *Escherichia coli* (ExPEC) lineages. Clin Microbiol Rev. 2019;32(3):e00135–18.
31. Castanheira M, Simner PJ, Bradford PA. Extended-spectrum β-lactamases: an update on their characteristics, epidemiology and detection. JAC Antimicrob Resist. 2021;3(3):dlab092.
32. Bevan ER, Jones AM, Hawkey PM. Global epidemiology of CTX-M β-lactamases: temporal and geographical shifts in genotype. J Antimicrob Chemother. 2017;72(8):2145–55.
33. Davies TJ, Stoesser N, Sheppard AE, Abuoun M, Fowler P, Swann J, Quan TP, Griffiths D, Vaughan A, Morgan M, Phan HTT, Jeffery KJ, Andersson M, Ellington MJ, Ekelund O, Woodford N, Mathers AJ, Bonomo RA, Crook DW, Peto TEA, Anjum MF, Walker AS. Reconciling the potentially irreconcilable? Genotypic and phenotypic amoxicillin-clavulanate resistance in *Escherichia coli*. Antimicrob Agents Chemother. 2020;64(6):e02026–19.

34. Cantón R, Morosini MI, de la Maza OM, de la Pedrosa EG. IRT and CMT beta-lactamases and inhibitor resistance. Clin Microbiol Infect. 2008;14(Suppl 1):53–62.
35. Walker AJ, Pretis F, Powell-Smith A, Goldacre B. Variation in responsiveness to warranted behaviour change among NHS clinicians: novel implementation of change detection methods in longitudinal prescribing data. BMJ. 2019;367:l5205.
36. Dos Santos C, Dos Santos LS, Franco OL. Fosfomycin and nitrofurantoin: classic antibiotics and perspectives. J Antibiot (Tokyo). 2021;74(9):547–58.
37. Syre H, Hetland MAK, Bernhoff E, Bollestad M, Grude N, Simonsen GS, Löhr IH. Microbial risk factors for treatment failure of pivmecillinam in community-acquired urinary tract infections caused by ESBL-producing *Escherichia coli*. APMIS. 2020;128(3):232–41.
38. Bollestad M, Grude N, Solhaug S, Raffelsberger N, Handal N, Nilsen HS, Romstad MR, Emmert A, Tveten Y, Søraas A, Jenum PA, Jenum S, Møller-Stray J, Weme ET, Lindbaek M, Simonsen GS; (The Norwegian ESBL UTI Study Group). Clinical and bacteriological efficacy of pivmecillinam treatment for uncomplicated urinary tract infections caused by ESBL-producing *Escherichia coli*: a prospective, multicentre, observational cohort study. J Antimicrob Chemother 2018;73(9):2503–2509
39. Miller GH, Sabatelli FJ, Hare RS, Glupczynski Y, Mackey P, Shlaes D, Shimizu K, Shaw KJ, The most frequent aminoglycoside resistance mechanisms—changes with time and geographic area: a reflection of aminoglycoside usage patterns? Aminoglycoside Resistance Study Groups. Clin Infect Dis. 1997;24(Suppl 1):S46–62.
40. Nordmann P, Poirel L. Epidemiology and diagnostics of carbapenem resistance in Gram-negative bacteria. Clin Infect Dis. 2019;69(Suppl 7):S521–8.
41. Zhanel GG, Pozdirca M, Golden AR, Lawrence CK, Zelenitsky S, Berry L, Schweizer F, Bay D, Adam H, Zhanel MA, Lagacé-Wiens P, Walkty A, Irfan N, Naber K, Lynch JP 3rd, Karlowsky JA. Sulopenem: an intravenous and oral Penem for the treatment of urinary tract infections due to multidrug-resistant bacteria. Drugs. 2022;82(5):533–57.
42. Sodhi V, Kronsberg KA, Clark M, Cho JC. Tebipenem pivoxil hydrobromide-No PICC, no problem! Pharmacotherapy. 2021;41(9):748–61.
43. Halaji M, Feizi A, Mirzaei A, Sedigh Ebrahim-Saraie H, Fayyazi A, Ashraf A, Havaei SA. The global prevalence of class 1 integron and associated antibiotic resistance in *Escherichia coli* from patients with urinary tract infections, a systematic review and meta-analysis. Microb Drug Resist. 2020;26(10):1208–18.
44. https://globalsmartsite.com.
45. Karlowsky JA, Lob SH, DeRyke CA, Siddiqui F, Young K, Motyl MR, Sahm DF. Prevalence of ESBL non-CRE *Escherichia coli* and *Klebsiella pneumoniae* among clinical isolates collected by the SMART global surveillance programme from 2015 to 2019. Int J Antimicrob Agents. 2022;59(3):106535.
46. Batista AD, Rodrigues DA, Figueiras A, Zapata-Cachafeiro M, Roque F, Herdeiro MT. Antibiotic dispensation without a prescription worldwide: a systematic review. Antibiotics (Basel). 2020;9(11):786.
47. https://www.urmc.rochester.edu/MediaLibraries/URMCMedia/urmc-labs/clinical/about-us/documents/Antibiogram-Community-Urine-Isolates-19-20.pdf.
48. McNulty CA, Richards J, Livermore DM, Little P, Charlett A, Freeman E, Harvey I, Thomas M. Clinical relevance of laboratory-reported antibiotic resistance in acute uncomplicated urinary tract infection in primary care. J Antimicrob Chemother. 2006;58(5):1000–8.
49. Boyd SE, Moore LSP, Gilchrist M, Costelloe C, Castro-Sánchez E, Franklin BD, Holmes AH. Obtaining antibiotics online from within the UK: a cross-sectional study. J Antimicrob Chemother. 2017;72(5):1521–8.
50. Borek AJ, Maitland K, McLeod M, Campbell A, Hayhoe B, Butler CC, Morrell L, Roope LSJ, Holmes A, Walker AS, Tonkin-Crine S, On Behalf of The Step-Up Study Team. Impact of the COVID-19 pandemic on community antibiotic prescribing and stewardship: a qualitative interview study with general practitioners in England. Antibiotics (Basel). 2021;10(12):1531.
51. Donnan PT, Wei L, Steinke DT, Phillips G, Clarke R, Noone A, Sullivan FM, MacDonald TM, Davey PG. Presence of bacteriuria caused by trimethoprim resistant bacteria in

patients prescribed antibiotics: multilevel model with practice and individual patient data. BMJ. 2004;328(7451):1297.

52. Tängdén T, Cars O, Melhus A, Löwdin E. Foreign travel is a major risk factor for colonization with *Escherichia coli* producing CTX-M-type extended-spectrum beta-lactamases: a prospective study with Swedish volunteers. Antimicrob Agents Chemother. 2010;54(9):3564–8.
53. Pitout JD, Campbell L, Church DL, Gregson DB, Laupland KB. Molecular characteristics of travel-related extended-spectrum-beta-lactamase-producing *Escherichia coli* isolates from the Calgary Health Region. Antimicrob Agents Chemother. 2009;53(6):2539–43.
54. https://www.ecdc.europa.eu/en/about-us/partnerships-and-networks/disease-and-laboratory-networks/ears-net.
55. Tutone M, Bjerklund Johansen TE, Cai T, Mushtaq S, Livermore DM. SUsceptibility and resistance to fosfomycin and other antimicrobial agents among pathogens causing lower urinary tract infections: findings of the SURF study. Int J Antimicrob Agents. 2022;59(5):106574.
56. Ciesielczuk H, Jenkins C, Chattaway M, Doumith M, Hope R, Woodford N, Wareham DW. Trends in ExPEC serogroups in the UK and their significance. Eur J Clin Microbiol Infect Dis. 2016;35(10):1661–6.
57. Riley LW. Pandemic lineages of extraintestinal pathogenic *Escherichia coli*. Clin Microbiol Infect. 2014;20(5):380–90.
58. Pitout JDD. Population dynamics of *Escherichia coli* causing bloodstream infections over extended time periods. mSphere. 2021;6(6):e0095621. https://doi.org/10.1128/msphere.00956-21.
59. Sora VM, Meroni G, Martino PA, Soggiu A, Bonizzi L, Zecconi A. Extraintestinal pathogenic *Escherichia coli*: virulence factors and antibiotic resistance. Pathogens. 2021;10(11):1355.
60. Sarowska J, Futoma-Koloch B, Jama-Kmiecik A, Frej-Madrzak M, Ksiazczyk M, Bugla-Ploskonska G, Choroszy-Krol I. Virulence factors, prevalence and potential transmission of extraintestinal pathogenic *Escherichia coli* isolated from different sources: recent reports. Gut Pathog. 2019;11:10.
61. Desvaux M, Dalmasso G, Beyrouthy R, Barnich N, Delmas J, Bonnet R. Pathogenicity factors of genomic islands in intestinal and extraintestinal *Escherichia coli*. Front Microbiol. 2020;11:2065.
62. da Cruz Campos AC, Couto N, Lucas da Silva Andrade N, Friedrich AW, de Paula Rosa AC, Vieira Damasco P, Chlebowicz-Fliss MA, Rossen JWA, SOLIDNESS Working Group. Virulence and resistance properties of *E. coli* isolated from urine samples of hospitalized patients in Rio de Janeiro, Brazil—the role of mobile genetic elements. Int J Med Microbiol. 2020;310(8):151453.
63. Bengtsson S, Naseer U, Sundsfjord A, Kahlmeter G, Sundqvist M. Sequence types and plasmid carriage of uropathogenic *Escherichia coli* devoid of phenotypically detectable resistance. J Antimicrob Chemother. 2012;67(1):69–73.
64. Mathers AJ, Peirano G, Pitout JD. *Escherichia coli* ST131: the quintessential example of an international multiresistant high-risk clone. Adv Appl Microbiol. 2015;90:109–54.
65. Day MJ, Hopkins KL, Wareham DW, Toleman MA, Elviss N, Randall L, Teale C, Cleary P, Wiuff C, Doumith M, Ellington MJ, Woodford N, Livermore DM. Extended-spectrum β-lactamase-producing *Escherichia coli* in human-derived and foodchain-derived samples from England, Wales, and Scotland: an epidemiological surveillance and typing study. Lancet Infect Dis. 2019;19(12):1325–35.
66. Can F, Azap OK, Seref C, Ispir P, Arslan H, Ergonul O. Emerging *Escherichia coli* O25b/ST131 clone predicts treatment failure in urinary tract infections. Clin Infect Dis. 2015;60(4):523–7.
67. Huttner A, Kowalczyk A, Turjeman A, Babich T, Brossier C, Eliakim-Raz N, Kosiek K, Martinez de Tejada B, Roux X, Shiber S, Theuretzbacher U, von Dach E, Yahav D, Leibovici L, Godycki-Cwirko M, Mouton JW, Harbarth S. Effect of 5-day nitrofurantoin vs single-dose fosfomycin on clinical resolution of uncomplicated lower urinary tract infection in women: a randomized clinical trial. JAMA. 2018;319(17):1781–9.
68. Schmidt K, Stanley KK, Hale R, Smith L, Wain J, O'Grady J, Livermore DM. Evaluation of multiplex tandem PCR (MT-PCR) assays for the detection of bacterial resistance genes among Enterobacteriaceae in clinical urines. J Antimicrob Chemother. 2019;74(2):349–56.

69. Magistro G, Stief CG. Vaccine development for urinary tract infections: where do we stand? Eur Urol Focus. 2019;5(1):39–41.
70. https://www.clinicaltrials.gov/ct2/show/NCT04899336.
71. Pick H, Daniel P, Rodrigo C, Bewick T, Ashton D, Lawrence H, Baskaran V, Edwards-Pritchard RC, Sheppard C, Eletu SD, Rose S, Litt D, Fry NK, Ladhani S, Chand M, Trotter C, McKeever TM, Lim WS. Pneumococcal serotype trends, surveillance and risk factors in UK adult pneumonia, 2013–2018. Thorax. 2020;75(1):38–49.
72. Briles DE, Paton JC, Mukerji R, Swiatlo E, Crain MJ. Pneumococcal vaccines. Microbiol Spectr. 2019;7(6):2018. https://doi.org/10.1128/microbiolspec.GPP3-0028-2018.

A Practical Guideline on Sampling and Analysis of Urine and Blood Specimens in Urinary Tract Infections

3

Tommaso Cai and Truls E. Bjerklund Johansen

3.1 Introduction

From the microbiologist's point of view, a urinary tract infection (UTI) is defined as the presence of bacteria in an individual with symptoms related to the urinary tract [1]. A correct approach to UTI starts from a correct microbiological diagnosis [2]. International guidelines suggest basing antimicrobial therapy on antibiograms [1]. The only clinical situation where an empirical approach is recommended without taking a urine culture is in case of acute uncomplicated urinary tract infection in women where antimicrobial therapy can be initiated based on symptoms only [1]. In all other cases of UTI, it is recommended to collect a urine specimen for culture prior to initiation of antimicrobial therapy. The collection method must minimize contamination; the urine sample must be forwarded promptly to the laboratory and processed according to appropriate standard procedures [1]. These methodological aspects are essential in order to avoid contamination and avoid wrong therapy with unwanted consequences on bacterial resistance and patient's outcome. A second urine sample is strongly recommended in the following situations: colony count lower than 10^5 CFU/mL, finding of Gram-positive organisms, and finding of

T. Cai (✉)
Department of Urology, Santa Chiara Regional Hospital, Trento, Italy

Institute of Clinical Medicine, University of Oslo, Oslo, Norway

Department of Urology, Oslo University Hospital, Oslo, Norway
e-mail: tommaso.cai@apss.tn.it

T. E. Bjerklund Johansen
Institute of Clinical Medicine, University of Oslo, Oslo, Norway

Department of Urology, Oslo University Hospital, Oslo, Norway

Institute of Clinical Medicine, University of Aarhus, Aarhus, Denmark
e-mail: tebj@uio.no

T. E. Bjerklund Johansen, T. Cai (eds.), *Guide to Antibiotics in Urology*,
https://doi.org/10.1007/978-3-319-92366-6_3

multiple organisms [3]. The quantitative diagnostic criterion for urinary tract infection in a voided urine specimen is $\geq 10^5$ CFU/mL of a single organism [1–3]. In this chapter we will discuss microbiological aspects related to UTI for use in everyday clinical practice.

3.2 Sample Collection and Isolation of Pathogens

The sample collection is an essential step in the management of UTI. All biological samples should be collected by method which minimizes contamination and forwarded promptly to the laboratory where appropriate methods are followed for isolation, identification, and quantification of organisms [4].

The types of biological samples to collect are related to the clinical type of infection. The types of samples for each type of UTI is given in cursive below.

- Uncomplicated UTI of the lower urinary tract: *Urine.*
- Complicated UTI of the lower urinary tract: *Urine, Meares and Stamey test, urine collection after catheter replacement.*
- Uncomplicated UTI of the upper urinary tract: *Urine.*
- Complicated UTI of the upper urinary tract and sepsis: *Blood and urine.*

Proper collection, transport, and storage of specimens are prerequisites for reliable culture results. The correct patient procedure for collection of urine for culture is described in Fig. 3.1.

Practical points for the nurse related to urine sampling are:

- Urine for culture should be collected in a sterile 90 mL container.
- Early morning urine specimens are preferred, although urine collected at other times of the day are acceptable.
- A "mid-stream clean catch" urine sample is necessary for culture so that any bacteria present around the urethra and on the hands do not contaminate the specimen.
- Wash and dry your hands thoroughly.
- Wash the patient's urogenital area.
- Collect the midstream of urine into the container. The container should only be 1/2–2/3 full.
- Immediately refrigerate the specimen, and submit to the laboratory within 24 h of collection (maintain sample at 2–8 °C during transportation).
- If a tuberculosis UTI is suspected, collect at least 40 mL midstream first morning urine specimen in a sterile container for three consecutive days. Store refrigerated at 2–8 °C and submit each specimen to the laboratory.

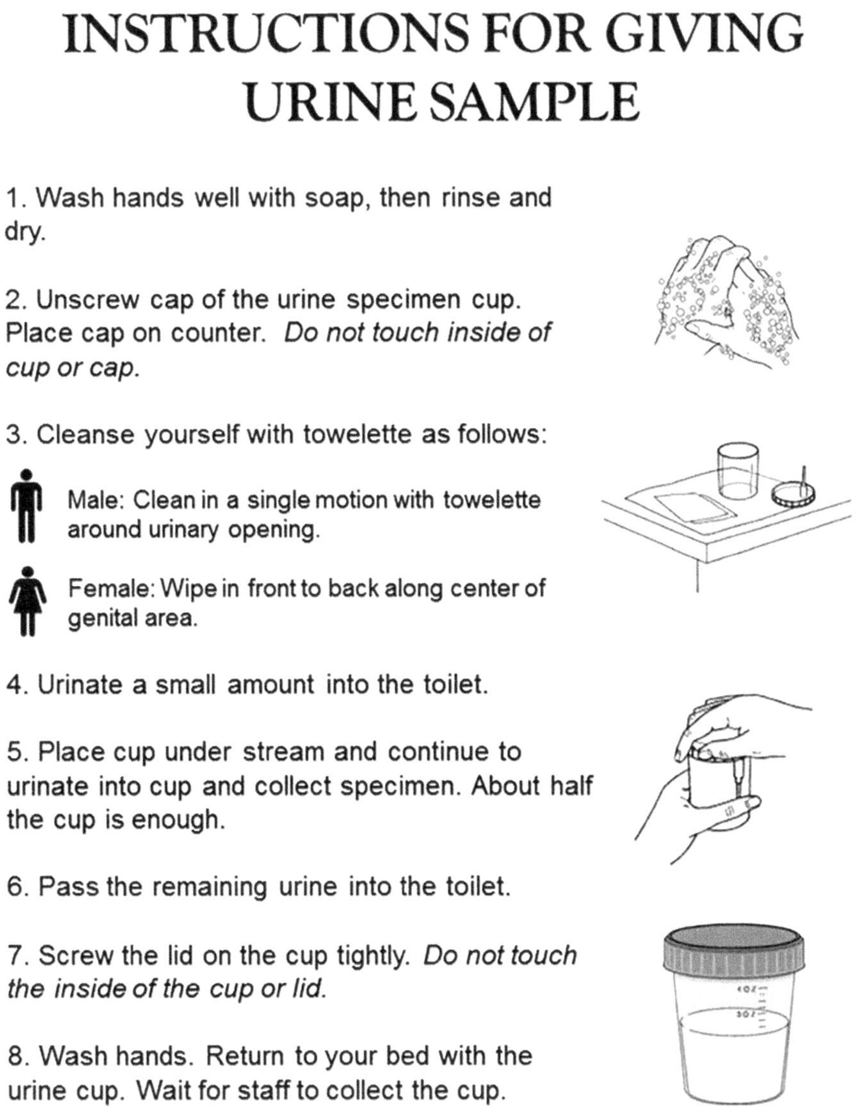

Fig. 3.1 The figure shows the correct urine collection procedure for urine culture. (Image taken from www.jem-journal.com/article/S0736-4679%2816%2930885-X/fulltext)

3.2.1 Urine Collection in Case of Uncomplicated UTI of the Lower Urinary Tract

A voided urine specimen collected from a woman will be contaminated with one or more organisms from the periurethral and vaginal flora, usually in counts of $\geq 10^2$ CFU/mL [5]. These organisms are predominantly Gram-positive bacteria which belong to the normal flora of the skin or mucous membranes. Kunin showed that 77% of asymptomatic women had a staphylococcal species other than *Staphylococcus saprophyticus* grown in counts of $\geq 10^2$ CFU/mL from voided urine specimens, while 51.8% of symptomatic women had the same finding [6]. Diphtheroids $\geq 10^2$ CFU/mL were isolated from 42% of asymptomatic women, and Gram-positive organisms isolated at $\geq 10^2$ CFU/mL included *Corynebacterium* spp., *Lactobacillus* spp. (55%), *Gardnerella* spp. (15%), and *Streptococcus* spp. (37.4%) [6]. Quantitative counts $\geq 10^5$ CFU/mL were isolated for *Corynebacterium* spp., *Lactobacillus* spp., *Gardnerella* spp., and *Streptococcus* spp. [6]. A more recent study of 120 young asymptomatic women showed the following isolated strains: *Enterococcus* spp., group B streptococci, and mixed Gram-positive organisms [7]. In this sense, all Gram-positive bacteria other than *Staphylococcus saprophyticus* isolated from otherwise healthy symptomatic or asymptomatic women should be interpreted as contaminants [2].

3.2.2 Urine Collection in Case of Complicated UTI of the Lower Urinary Tract: Urine, Meares and Stamey Test, and Urine Collection After Catheter Replacement

In case of complicated UTI of the lower urinary tract, biological samples should be chosen on the basis of the patient's clinical situation. In case of complicated cystitis in women, a single sample of urine is enough and should be collected following the guideline given above. In line with the definitions used in the European Association of Urology (EAU) guidelines on UTIs [1], catheter associated urinary tract infection (CAUTI) is defined as the presence of 10^5 CFU/mL in asymptomatic patients and 10^2.

CFU/mL in patients with symptoms related to the urinary tract. In these cases the following procedure steps are recommended:

- Remove the old catheter and insert a new one.
- Collect urine through the catheter.
- Deliver the urinary sample immediately to the laboratory.
- If a catheter replacement cannot be accomplished, urine for culture should be sampled by a direct needle puncture of the catheter with aseptic technique (Fig. 3.2).
- In all patients who have had a catheter removed, urine culture within 48 h is recommended regardless of subsequent symptoms.
- In all hospitalized patients with fever, a blood sample for culture is required.

Chronic bacterial prostatitis requires a specific biological sampling. The Meares and Stamey 4-glass test is the standard method of assessing inflammation and the presence of bacteria in the lower urinary tract in men presenting with the chronic prostatitis syndrome and should be done in all patients with prostatitis-like symptoms. This procedure is, however, not recommended in case of suspected acute

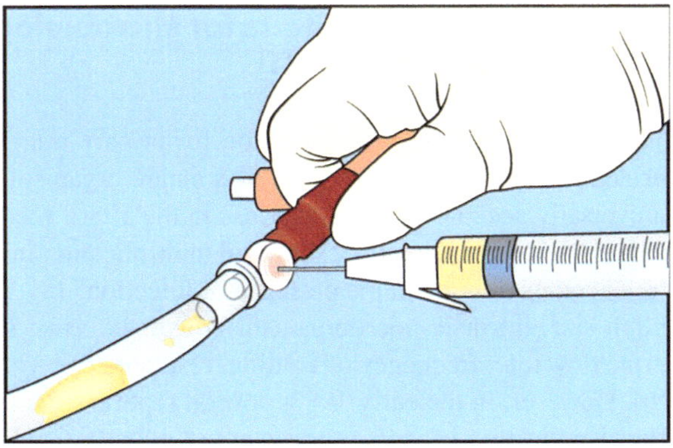

Fig. 3.2 Urine sample collection by aspiration from the collection port of catheter. (Image taken from https://slideplayer.com/slide/8291146/)

bacterial prostatitis. In this case urine sample and blood sample culture are recommended. The Meares and Stamey test includes (1) first voided urine (from urethra), (2) mid-stream urine (from the bladder), (3) expressed prostate secretion, if available, that is collected by prostatic massage after sampling bladder urine, and (4) the post-massage urine sample.

3.2.3 Urine Collection in Uncomplicated UTI of the Upper Urinary Tract

In case of patients with uncomplicated upper urinary tract infection (pyelonephritis), urine culture is recommended. Urinalysis is recommended too. Blood cultures should be obtained in patients with acute pyelonephritis only if there is diagnostic uncertainty and in all hospitalized patients with suspected pyelonephritis.

3.2.4 Blood and Urine Collection in Complicated UTI of the Upper Urinary Tract and Sepsis

In all cases of suspected complicated UTI of the upper urinary tract and/or sepsis, urinalysis and urine culture are recommended in order to guide the antimicrobial therapy. In all hospitalized patients and in all patients with suspected sepsis, a blood culture must be performed. Blood cultures are mandatory for the diagnosis of bacteremia.

Blood culture should be sampled in line with the following practical guidelines:

- Take a blood culture immediately after arrival in the hospital in case of fever.
- Do a repeat culture in case of negative results and new episode of fever.
- Consider testing for aerobic, facultative anaerobic microorganisms, and strict anaerobic bacteria.

3.3 Quantitative Criteria for Microbiological Confirmation of UTI

The quantitative diagnostic criterion for urinary tract infection based on a voided urine specimen is ≥10 CFU/mL of a single organism [2, 3], which has now been universally accepted. However, Kass in the 1980s recognized that "certain defined circumstances which inhibit bacterial multiplication in urine may lead to lower bacterial counts in urine in the presence of infection" [8]. These variables include inoculum size, intrinsic microorganism growth in urine, urine pH, urine constituents, urine flow rate, frequency of voiding, residual urine volume, and urinary antiseptics [6]. However, in the early 1980s several reports revisited the limitations of the uniform application of a quantitative count of $\geq 10^5$ CFU/mL for the diagnosis of urinary tract infection. In particular, the relatively high proportion of women with acute uncomplicated urinary tract infection from whom lower quantitative counts of uropathogens are isolated was recognized [9]. Subsequent guidelines for identification of urinary tract infection proposed variable quantitative criteria for bacterial growth depending on the clinical presentation, from $\geq 10^3$ to $\geq 10^5$ CFU/mL [10]. However, the present recommendation is to consider the following microbiological parameters for uncomplicated cystitis in women: clean-catch urine should have colony count more than 100,000 CFU/mL for a single organism [11]. 20–40% of women presenting with cystitis have 100–10,000 CFU/mL [11]. If associated with symptoms, the positive predictive value for a UTI with this range of colony counts is >90% [11].

In case of blood culture, it is very important to consider the risk of contamination. Contamination occurs when microbes that are not present in the bloodstream are introduced into the bottle during the blood sampling [11]. Even if blood cultures are drawn under aseptic conditions, contaminations are often due to organisms that are present in the environment and that can be part of the skin flora, such as coagulase-negative staphylococci, the third most prevalent microbe identified in blood cultures in our tertiary-care university hospital, and other organisms with low or absent virulence toward humans such as *Micrococcus* spp., *Propionibacterium acnes*, most *Bacillus* spp., and most *Corynebacterium* spp. [11]. The quantity of microbes present in the blood during bloodstream infections ranges from 1 to 10 CFU/mL to 1×10^3 and 1×10^4 CFU/mL. In case of positive bacterial growth, it is recommended to perform Gram staining on a sub-sample from the blood-culture bottle to confirm the presence of microbes and to determine the morphotype [11]. New microbiological methods such as PCR or FISH tests have been introduced in everyday clinical practice to make the process faster and improve the accuracy.

3.4 Urine Analysis

The convenience and cost-effectiveness of a urine dipstick test make it a common diagnostic tool [12]. It is an appropriate alternative to urinalysis and urine microscopy in the diagnoses of uncomplicated infections of the lower urinary tract. Urine analysis with dipstick test should be used as support to the diagnosis and for starting empiric antimicrobial treatment.

Nitrites Bacteria reduce nitrate to nitrite; typically Gram-negative organisms. Under normal circumstance, urine will have no nitrites. False positives can result from air exposure, and false negative can be the result of non-nitrite-producing organisms, low nitrate diet (decreased vegetables), vitamin C, concentrated urine, and low pH. The sensitivity ranges from 19 to 48%, and the specificity ranges from 92 to 100% [12].

Leukocyte Esterase This enzyme stems from presence of intact or broken-down neutrophils. False negatives can be the result of an early infection, vitamin C, concentrated urine, ketonuria, and proteinuria. False positives can be caused by contamination of the urine by skin flora. The sensitivity ranges from 62 to 98%, and the specificity ranges from 55 to 96% [12].

References

1. European Association of Urology Guidelines on urological infections. https://d56bochluxqnz.cloudfront.net/documents/full-guideline/EAU-Guidelines-on-Urological-Infections-2022.pdf.
2. ICUD book on urogenital infections. http://www.icud.info/urogenitalinfections.html.
3. Nicolle LE. Urinary tract infection. Crit Care Clin. 2013;29(3):699–715. https://doi.org/10.1016/j.ccc.2013.03.014.
4. McCarter YS, Sharp SE. Laboratory diagnosis of urinary tract infections. Washington, DC: ASM Press; 2009. p. 25.
5. Platt R. Quantitative definition of bacteriuria. Am J Med. 1983;75(1B):44–52.
6. Kunin CM. Bacteriuria, pyuria, proteinuria, hematuria, and pneumaturia. In: Kunin CM, editor. Urinary tract infections: detection, prevention, and management. Baltimore: Williams & Wilkins; 1997. p. 9.
7. Hooton TM, Stapleton AE, Roberts PL, and Stamm WE, Comparison of microbiologic findings in paired midstream and catheter urine specimens from women with acute uncomplicated cystitis. Abstract L 609 18th annual ICAAC, Washington DC, 2008
8. Kass EH. Chemotherapeutic and antibiotic drugs in the management of infections of the urinary tract. Am J Med. 1955;18(5):764–81.
9. Stamm WE, Counts GW, Running KR, Fihn S, Turck M, Holmes KK. Diagnosis of coliform infection in acutely dysuric women. N Engl J Med. 1982;307(8):463–8.
10. Rubin RH, Shapiro ED, Andriole VT, Davis RJ, Stamm WE. Evaluation of new anti-infective drugs for the treatment of urinary tract infection. Infectious Diseases Society of America and the Food and Drug Administration. Clin Infect Dis. 1992;15(Suppl 1):S216–27.
11. Opota O, Croxatto A, Prod'hom G, Greub G. Blood culture-based diagnosis of bacteraemia: state of the art. Clin Microbiol Infect. 2015;21(4):313–22. https://doi.org/10.1016/j.cmi.2015.01.003.
12. Lala V, Minter DA. Acute cystitis. In: StatPearls. Treasure Island (FL): StatPearls Publishing; 2022.

The Antibiogram: From MIC to Breakpoints

4

Carlo Tascini and Sozio Emanuela

4.1 The Antibiogram: From MIC to Breakpoints

Antimicrobial susceptibility testing (AST) or antibiogram is primarily performed to predict the outcome of antimicrobial therapy and to collect local data on susceptibility and resistance in order to create the basis for empiric antibiotic therapy.

Antibiogram can be made with:

- **Phenotypic methods**, based on antimicrobial activity and breakpoints.
- **Genotypic methods**, based on finding a known resistance (such as mecA, blaZ, vanA, vanB, PBP2a, β-lactamase, and so on).
- An **interpretative reading (expert rules)**, for example, if Staphylococci are mecA positive, report as resistant to all β-lactams except ceftaroline and ceftobiprole; if an *Enterobacteriaceae* is positive to ESBL, report as resistant to cephalosporins and aztreonam; if there is a *Streptococcus* spp. erythromycin-resistant, return as well as resistant to clarithromycin and azithromycin.

The adoption of antibiotic susceptibility guidelines in the USA is regulated by the Food and Drug Administration (FDA), and the most popular guidelines used are from the Clinical and Laboratory Standards Institute (CLSI). In 1997 the European Committee on Antimicrobial Susceptibility Testing (EUCAST) has unified the different standards for interpreting the antibiogram previously used in six European

C. Tascini (✉)
First Division of Infectious Diseases, Cotugno Hospital, Azienda Ospedaliera dei Colli, Naples, Italy
e-mail: carlo.tascini@uniud.it

S. Emanuela
Emergency Department, North-West District, Tuscany Health Care, Spedali Riuniti Livorno, Livorno, Italy
e-mail: emanuela.sozio@asufc.sanita.fvg.it

T. E. Bjerklund Johansen, T. Cai (eds.), *Guide to Antibiotics in Urology*,
https://doi.org/10.1007/978-3-319-92366-6_4

countries. The EUCAST is a committee jointly organized by ESCMID (European Society for Clinical Microbiology and Infectious Diseases), by ECDC (European Centre for Disease Prevention and Control), and by the six national committees previously active. At now, breakpoints defined by EUCAST are the only one officially recognized by the EMA (European Medicines Agency), a body authorizing the placing on the market of drugs in the countries of the European Union.

Italian microbiological laboratories have adopted EUCAST Guidelines since 2011 (previously US CLSI standards were adopted) [1, 2]. EUCAST documents are free and consultable on the web from www.eucast.org.

Genotypic methods can predict only the presence of resistance genes, and unless the phenotypic expression of the genes can be determined, this may be of uncertain clinical utility.

Susceptibility can be quantified using phenotypic methods, and isolates and species can be compared with each other. Categorization of minimum inhibitory concentrations (MIC) of various antibiotics in phenotypic AST depends on breakpoints. The phenotypic AST, as judged by minimal inhibitory concentration breakpoints, is the result of susceptibility tests in which the microorganism is in vitro essayed for its susceptibility to several antibiotics tested in different concentrations.

When the MIC (or a surrogate test value obtained through a disc diffusion test, a gradient test or an automated device) is known, the breakpoint is defined to predict the clinical outcome of therapy for the species in question.

These breakpoints define whether an antibiotic is reported as susceptible or not and are interpretive cut-offs for antibiotics based on MIC distributions and microbiological parameters, pharmacokinetic–pharmacodynamic (relationship between PK/PD index and response to treatment), clinical (best evidence from literature) properties, and the mechanisms of resistance [3].

Breakpoints are used to define the clinical category of susceptibility:

- **Susceptible**, if bacterial strain growth is inhibited in vitro by a concentration of the antibiotic that is associated with a high likelihood of therapeutic success.
- **Intermediate**, if there is uncertain probability of successful treatment.
- **Resistant**, if there is a high likelihood of therapeutic failure.

For each organism-antibiotic combination are set two breakpoints, and in this case there are three categories of interpretation (susceptible, intermediate, and resistant) or just a breakpoint, and so providing for two categories of interpretation (susceptible and resistant).

A clinical breakpoint is an MIC value that distinguishes between organisms where therapy is likely to succeed and fail: we talk about "clinical" breakpoint (BC) because the aim of these cut-offs is to use MIC values to separate strains where there is a high likelihood of treatment success using in vivo the given antibiotic from those whose treatment is more likely to fail due to a resistance mechanism.

The prediction can be strong, such as for high levels of ESBL and a cefotaxime MIC >1 mg/L in Enterobacteriaceae or vancomycin resistance in Enterococci. Conversely, the prediction may be weak, as for penicillin non-susceptibility in

Streptococcus pneumoniae, where the dosing and the clinical condition will determine the outcome [4].

EUCAST, different from the CLSI, has defined the epidemiological cut-off (ECOFF) [1]. ECOFF is the concentration value that divides wild-type isolates, which does not have any acquired and mutational resistance mechanisms, from the population of strains that have resistance mechanisms.

EUCAST also provides species-independent MIC breakpoints; however, species-independent breakpoints for the reading of disk diffusion tests are also available.

The MIC is the lowest concentration of antibiotic that is able to inhibit the in vitro growth of the microorganism after 18–24 h of incubation.

Since 2006, the International Organization for Standardization (ISO) described the standardized measurement of an MIC using the broth microdilution (BMD) technique [5]. All other phenotypic tests, including disc diffusion tests, gradient tests (E-test), and semi-automated susceptibility testing systems, are surrogate methods that must be calibrated to the ISO method to withstand modern requirements for performance.

Today, EUCAST breakpoints are available on semi-automated machines such as the Vitek2 (bioMerieux), the Phoenix (BD), and the MicroScan (Siemens) and can be used directly with any of three commercially available gradient tests (bioMerieux Thermofisher, Liofilchem).

E-test is a manual method, performed in agar, using paper strips with a gradient concentration of a given antibiotic, that is able to obtain MICs, and it is useful as a supplement to the other methods.

More frequently, BMD (method that can be automated) is used and represents the reference method.

Kirby–Bauer disk diffusion method provides for the evaluation of the diameters of the inhibition zones around the disks containing the antibiotic tested; Kirby–Bauer does not provide MIC values, but diameters of inhibition zones (Figs. 4.1, 4.2 and 4.3).

The diameters of inhibition zones and MICs must always be compared to clinical breakpoints standardized for different organism-antibiotic combinations.

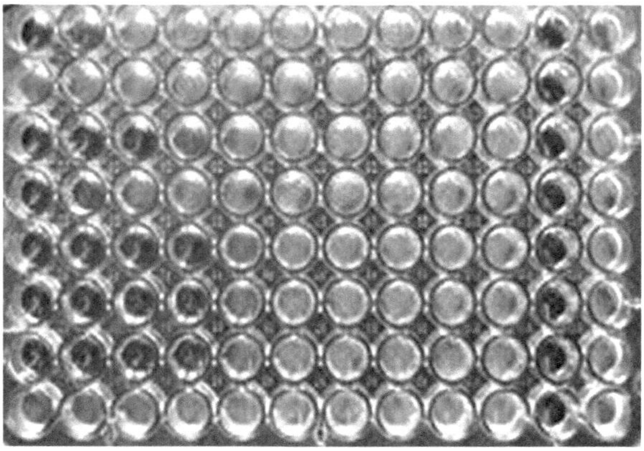

Fig. 4.1 BMD. Broth dilution is a technique in which containers holding identical volumes of broth with antimicrobial solution in incrementally (usually geometrically) increasing concentrations are inoculated with a known number of bacteria

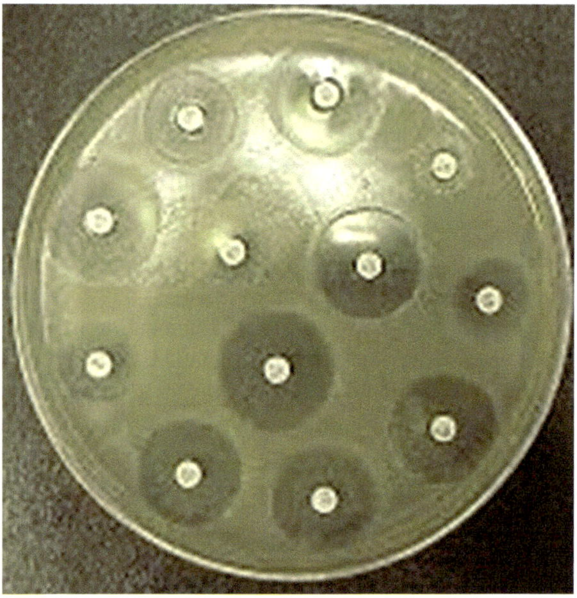

Fig. 4.2 Kirby–Bauer. The agar diffusion test (Kirby–Bauer antibiotic test) uses antibiotic discs to test the extent to which bacteria are affected by those antibiotics. If an antibiotic stops the bacteria from growing or kills the bacteria, there will be a zone of inhibition

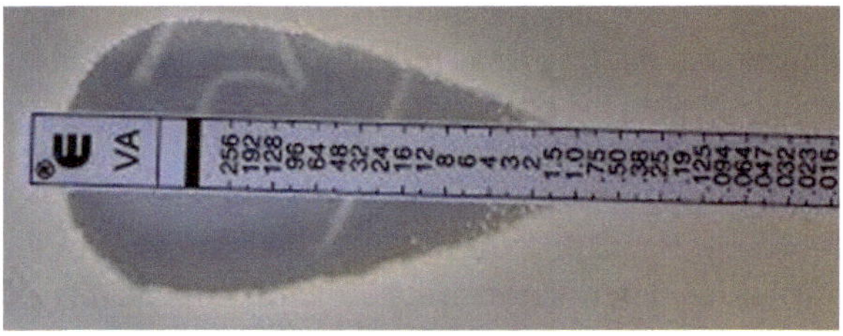

Fig. 4.3 E-test. It is a manual in vitro diagnostic device used by laboratories to determine the MIC. The MIC value can be read where the edge of the inhibition ellipse intersects the side of the strip

Summing up, MIC breakpoints are developed employing some combination of:

- MIC frequency distribution analysis
- Presence or not of known mechanisms of resistance
- Clinical correlation
- Evaluation of MICs based on drugs levels in patients (PK/PD)

Clinical breakpoint indicates likelihood of therapeutic success (susceptible) or failure (resistant) of antimicrobial treatment based on microbiological findings. Epidemiological cut-OFF values (ECOFF) separate microorganism without (wild type) and with acquired or mutational resistance (Fig. 4.4).

MIC value should also be assessed in relation to the distance from the breakpoint value of susceptibility, like summarized in Fig. 4.5.

Often in automated antibiograms MIC are reported ≤ at the minimum concentration tested regarding some antibiotics, but in some cases, for example, for Enterobacteria and quinolones, it is important to know the accurate MIC.

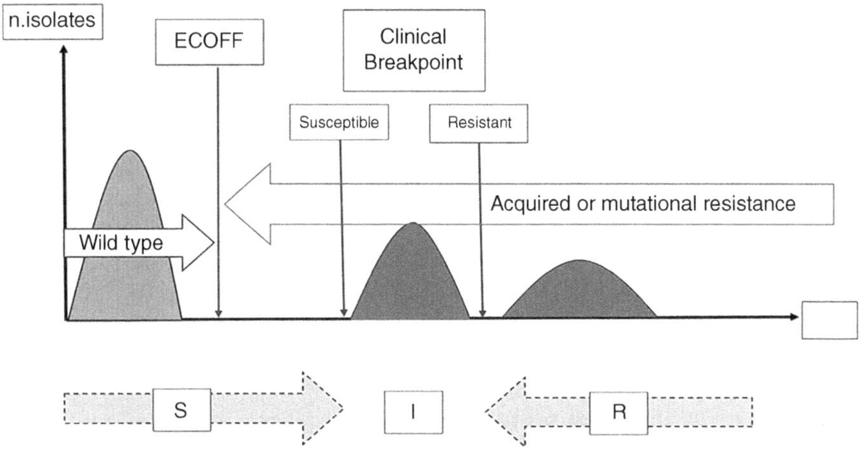

Fig. 4.4 Clinical breakpoints and epidemiological cut-off

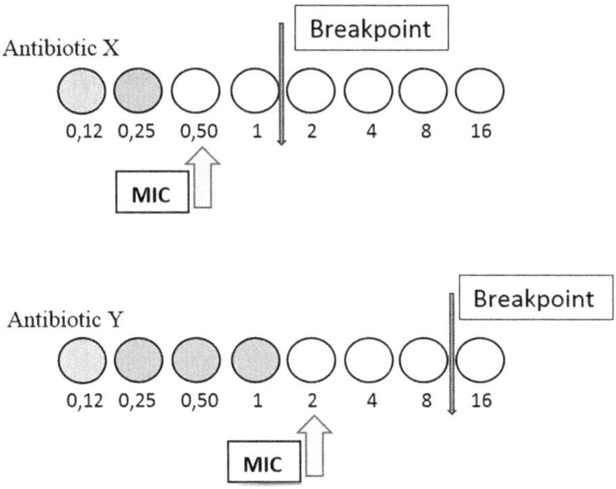

Fig. 4.5 The absolute value of the MICs reported on susceptibility testing must not be evaluated "vertically" between the different drugs tested. For example, if there is an antibiotic X with a MIC of 0.5 mg/L and breakpoint 2 mg/L, and an antibiotic Y with a MIC of 2 mg/L but breakpoints of 16 mg/L, the drug with a MIC more favorable is the antibiotic Y. This ratio is named MIC Breakpoint Quotient (MBQ). Therefore, should be useful to have the values of clinical breakpoints on the antibiograms

In those cases where the epidemiological cut-off is different from the clinical breakpoints: to know with accuracy the MIC allows to understand if the germ has already developed some mutation that could let failure with mono-therapy.

The clinician must also consider the potential to induce resistance in selecting the appropriate antibiotic therapy. For example, mono-therapy with certain molecules can select resistance during the treatment: Staphylococci may develop resistance with mono-therapy with rifampicin or quinolones (these drugs should be considered partners of another antibiotic); all strains of gram-negative rods that are inducible AmpC chromosomal carriers can develop resistance to third-generation cephalosporins after induction and derepression of the enzyme; *Enterobacteriaceae* have the ability to select for resistant strains during mono-therapy with fosfomycin; *Pseudomonas aeruginosa* has the ability to develop resistance against all molecules of antibiotics except polymyxins.

Furthermore, it is very important to know the bacteriostatic activity (antibiotics that only inhibit the growth) and bactericidal activity (antibiotics that kill), since the mechanisms that allow the bacteriostasis can be different from those of the bactericidal, either to the same drug or for the same bacterial species (penicillins are bactericidal against pneumococci but bacteriostatic against enterococci).

Antibiograms should be read with attention to recognize unusual results and drugs best prevented owing to their risk of selecting resistance and using "indicator drugs." An "indicator drug" is used to detect the presence of resistance also to the related agents, and it is chosen as the member of the drug family to which the mechanism gives the most obvious resistance. An indicator drug is chosen as the member of the drug family to which the mechanism gives the most obvious resistance, and it is used to detect the presence of mechanism that gives resistance not only to the indicator, but also to related agents. Table 4.1 illustrates indicator drugs more used.

We must know that the reporting rules of the antibiograms are not immutable over time, but may change in relation, for example, to the need to put in place new strategies for limiting the spread of resistance or based on new evidence in the literature.

Since 2010, some changes were made in the interpretation of susceptibility, especially for gram-negative rods.

In addition to lowering of the breakpoint for some specific microorganism-antibiotic combinations, will be deleted from reporting some combinations as they are considered inadequate in the therapeutic area, or the microorganism is naturally resistant to the drug, or because there is no clinical evidence.

Both CLSI and EUCAST decided in separate process to modify breakpoints for oxymino-cephalosporins and Enterobacteria [1, 2].

EUCAST breakpoints are often lower than those of the CLSI [1, 2], with more restrictive interpretation of susceptibility, except for those related to carbapenems and *Enterobacteriaceae*.

The expert rules dictated by EUCAST, which are based on current clinical breakpoints and knowledge of resistance mechanisms, describe the actions to be taken on the basis of specific results with the aim to help the clinician, and the microbiologist, in an interpretative reading on an antibiogram [1, 6].

Moreover, the new rule recommended, for some combination microorganism-antibiotic, such as *Enterobacteriaceae* and cephalosporins or carbapenems,

Table 4.1 Useful indicator antibiotic drugs and interpretative rules [6]

Organism	Agents tested	Action or inference
Staphylococcus spp.	Oxacillin or methicillin, cefoxitin	Resistance to all β-lactam except ceftobiprole and ceftaroline
Staphylococcus spp.	Erythromycin and clindamycin	If resistance to macrolides but susceptible to clindamycin: test for constitutive MLS_B resistance. Quinupristin/dalfopristin likely to be bacteriostatic, not bactericidal
Staphylococcus spp.	Gentamicin	Resistance to gentamicin is generally caused by a production of enzyme that determines loss of synergism of all aminoglycosides (except streptomycin) with β-lactam agents and glycopeptides irrespective of MIC value
Staphylococcus spp.	Levofloxacin and moxifloxacin	Acquisition of combined mutation that leads to complete or partial cross-resistance to all fluoroquinolones
Streptococcus pneumoniae	Oxacillin	If resistant by screening, determine MIC of benzylpenicillins and other β-lactam agents and report as interpreted for each of the drug: Production of mosaic leads to various patterns of β-lactam resistance
Viridans groups of streptococci	Benzylpenicillin	If resistant by screening, determine MIC of amoxicillin or ampicillin and cefotaxime or ceftriaxone and report as interpreted for each of the drug: Production of mosaic leads to various patterns of β-lactam resistance
Streptococcus spp.	Erythromycin and clindamycin	If resistance to erythromycin but susceptible to clindamycin then test for inducible MLBs resistance. Streptococci may be resistant to macrolides by production of MLBs phenotype or by production of an efflux pump
Streptococcus pneumoniae	Levofloxacin and moxifloxacin	Acquisition of combined mutation that leads to complete or partial cross-resistance to all fluoroquinolones
Enterococcus spp.	Ampicillin	Resistance to ureidopenicillins and carbapenems
Enterococcus faecalis	Ampicillin	It is probably *E. faecium*, but may be less frequent species or may have acquired resistance: check speciation
Enterococcus spp.	Gentamicin	Resistance to gentamicin is generally caused by a production of enzyme that determines loss of synergism of all aminoglycosides (except streptomycin) with β-lactam agents and glycopeptides irrespective of MIC value

(continued)

Table 4.1 (continued)

Organism	Agents tested	Action or inference
Enterobacteriaceae	Cefotaxime, ceftriaxone, ceftazidime, cefepime, amoxicillin-clavulanate, ampicillin-sulbactam, and piperacillin-tazobactam	If intermediate or resistant to any third-generation or fourth generation oxyimino-cephalosporin and susceptible to combination of penicillin and a β-lactamase inhibitor, they are often ESBL; then report as tested
Enterobacter spp. *Citrobacter freundii* *Serratia* spp. *Morganella morganii*	Cefotaxime, ceftriaxone, and ceftazidime	Selection of AmpC-derepressed cephalosporin-resistant mutants may occur during therapy. Third-generation cephalosporin in combination with quinolones may also lead selection of resistant mutant. The selection risk is diminished for cefepime and cefpirome
Enterobacteriaceae	Ciprofloxacin	Resistant to all fluoroquinolones
Klebsiella spp. *Escherichia coli*	Ceftazidime	Likely ESBL producer. Resistant to all cephalosporin except cephamycins (cefoxitin, cefotetan)
Klebsiella spp.	Ertapenem	Probably KPC, carbapenemase producers

MLS_B macrolide–lincosamide–streptogramin B, *MIC* minimum inhibitory concentration, *ESBL* extended-spectrum β-lactamases

reporting MIC results "as found," regardless of resistance mechanisms and do not search anymore the mechanism of resistance, such as ESBL or carbapenemases, except for epidemiological purposes and for infection control.

ESBL-producing enterobacteria then will be reported as "susceptible" to some cephalosporins (instead as "resistant"), and the interpretation will be based on clinical breakpoints and is no longer required to test for ESBL and consequently change the result, as in the past. This is mainly created to limit the irresponsible use of carbapenems made in clinical practice in the past decades.

In conclusion, the interpretation of AST is much more than the categorization of susceptibility and represents an attempt of phenotypic interpretation of the resistance mechanisms exhibited by the microorganisms that are isolate in clinical practice.

To properly use antibiotics, the characteristics of microbiological activity (susceptibility of the microorganism) should be considered as well as the pharmacokinetic and pharmacodynamics characteristics, even simply the penetration of the antibiotic at the site of infection.

Interpretation of antibiogram is based on the recognition of the possible mechanism at the base of resistance, which can be extended to non-tested drugs or that lead the change of category obtained in vitro (as, e.g., the presence of oxacillin-resistant Staphylococci determines resistance to all beta-lactams, except ceftaroline and ceftobiprole).

The basic concept is that you cannot think of reading an antibiogram if you do not know previously the main potential characteristics of resistance of the microorganism tested.

References

1. European Committee for Antimicrobial Susceptibility Testing (EUCAST). Breakpoint table for interpretation of MICs and zone diameters. Version 6.0. 2016. http://www.eucast.org.
2. Clinical and Laboratory Standards Institute. Performance standards for antimicrobial susceptibility testing: nineteenth informational supplement. Document M-100-S19. Wayne: CLSI; 2010.
3. Marchese A, Esposito S, Barbieri R, Bassetti M, Debbia E. Does the adoption of EUCAST susceptibility breakpoints affect the selection of antimicrobials to treat acute community-acquired respiratory tract infections? BMC Infect Dis. 2012;12(1):181.
4. Kahlmeter G. The 2014 Garrod lecture: EUCAST—are we heading towards international agreement? J Antimicrob Chemother. 2015;70:2427–39. https://doi.org/10.1093/jac/dkv145.
5. International Organization for Standardization (ISO). Clinical laboratory testing and in vitro diagnostic test systems. Susceptibility.
6. Leclercq R, Cantón R, Brown DF, et al. EUCAST expert rules in antimicrobial susceptibility testing. Clin Microbiol Infect. 2011;19:141–60.

Classification of Urinary Tract Infections: A Contemporary Guide for Clinical Practice and Research

5

Truls E. Bjerklund Johansen, Zafer Tandogdu, Tommaso Cai, and Kurt G. Naber

5.1 Introduction

Classifications in clinical medicine guide diagnostics, treatment, research, and teaching. Classifications are based on available information from patients' history, symptoms, clinical findings, biochemistry, imaging techniques, and pathology. Variables that are being included in a classification should give the most valuable information about severity and prognosis.

The information that is available about a disease increases over time as new diagnostic methods and biomarkers appear. Therefore, classifications need to be updated too. At any given time, there might be external factors that modify a classification. For example, when the concept of complicated and uncomplicated UTI was developed, new antibiotics were introduced almost every year, and the main objective of the classification was to facilitate the design of research protocols to study the effect of new antibiotics and decide the dosing and duration of treatment. Today, the situation is different. New antibiotics are only rarely being introduced, and collateral

T. E. Bjerklund Johansen (✉)
Department of Urology, Oslo University Hospital, Oslo, Norway

Institute of Clinical Medicine, University of Oslo, Oslo, Norway

Institute of Clinical Medicine, University of Aarhus, Aarhus, Denmark
e-mail: tebj@uio.no

Z. Tandogdu
University College London Hospital, London, UK

T. Cai
Institute of Clinical Medicine, University of Oslo, Oslo, Norway

Department of Urology, Santa Chiara Regional Hospital, Trento, Italy

K. G. Naber
Technical University of Munich, Munich, Germany
e-mail: kurt@nabers.de

T. E. Bjerklund Johansen, T. Cai (eds.), *Guide to Antibiotics in Urology*,
https://doi.org/10.1007/978-3-319-92366-6_5

effects of antibiotics and antibiotic resistance of common pathogens have become major issues. According to antibiotic stewardship, physicians shall now avoid prescribing antibiotics whenever possible and use narrow-spectrum antibiotics for as short periods as possible. The situation calls for a more differentiated assessment of patients and tailoring the treatment according to the concept of personalized medicine.

The aim of this chapter is to introduce the reader to classifications of urinary tract infections (UTI) as a guide for diagnostics, treatment, and research in an era of antimicrobial stewardship.

5.2 Current Classifications of UTI

5.2.1 Uncomplicated and Complicated

The most widely used classifications of UTI are those developed by the Centers for Disease Control and Prevention in USA (CDC) in 1988 [1] and updated in 2008 [2], IDSA in 1992 [3], and ESCMID in 1993 [4].

In the 1988 edition, UTI comprised symptomatic UTI, asymptomatic bacteriuria (ASB), and other infections of the urinary tract. Diagnosis of symptomatic UTI was based on symptoms and evidence for the presence of a pathogen. The definition provided several possible types of evidence such as culture, dipstick, microscopy, physician's diagnosis, or appropriate antibiotic therapy. Repeated cultures were needed when the urinary culture revealed colony-forming units (CFU) $<10^2$/mL. Likewise, two cultures were needed for diagnosing ASB in patients without an indwelling catheter for the last 7 days before culture was taken.

The purpose of the CDC definitions was to define and report health care-associated UTI (HA-UTI). In the 2008 update, the concept of HA-UTI was broadened, and nosocomially acquired UTI (NA-UTI) became a subtype of HA-UTI [5]. In both editions, it was not made quite clear, however, whether ASB was considered an infection or probably only a risk factor under certain circumstances.

The IDSA [3] and ESCMID [4] guidelines were mainly developed for the evaluation of new anti-infective drugs in clinical studies. IDSA introduced the concept of complicated and uncomplicated UTI in order to obtain more homogeneous study groups. In "uncomplicated" UTI mainly UTI due to *Escherichia coli* and in "complicated" UTI also UTI caused by other pathogens than *E. coli* could be studied. The term "uncomplicated" means that the patient has no known factors that will render him or her more susceptible to develop UTI. Complicated is defined as the presence of these factors, but the understanding of "complicating factors" is not always clear. Some factors are related to the urinary tract like obstruction, stones, diversion, and catheters. Other factors relate to kidney diseases or comorbidities like diabetes mellitus, malignancies, or immune competence (e.g., immune-compromised patients). In these guidelines, "complicated" also means a higher risk for clinical complications if the UTI is not properly treated as in pregnancy and childhood. The investigations needed to diagnose or exclude all the risk factors are not clearly described. IDSA also introduced graded criteria for the amount of bacteria in urine, as expressed by colony-forming units per mL (CFU/mL), in the diagnosis of UTI in different groups of patients and situations.

Most current UTI guidelines and study protocols are based on the IDSA [3] and ESCMID [4] guidelines using the concept of uncomplicated and complicated UTI with some modifications. However, the term "complicated" sometimes means an increased risk of getting UTI, sometimes it refers to an increased risk of treatment failure, and sometimes an increased risk of losing nephrons or even the patient's life. In complicated UTI other pathogens than *E. coli*, other antimicrobials and longer treatment duration must be considered as well.

5.2.2 ESIU-ORENUC Classification I

The mixed understanding of "complicated" made the group of complicated UTI very heterogeneous, and results of a clinical study on patients with one criterion defining "complicated" could not be transferred to other patients with complicated UTI where the diagnosis was based on different criteria. Therefore, more than two categories were needed for a comprehensive description of patients' risk factors related to UTI. In an attempt to meet this need, the ORENUC classification was introduced by the European Section of Infections in Urology in 2010 [6].

5.2.2.1 Criteria for Classification of UTI

The information required for assessment of a patient suspected of having a UTI is presented in Table 5.1. The criteria are organized into five main categories. Not all criteria are equally relevant for classification of UTI per se, but in a clinical situation, all criteria have to be considered. Categories I–III and V are important for diagnosis and treatment, while category IV is important for surveillance of treatment quality and the environment. The comprehensive table illustrates the complexity of clinical decision-making in the treatment of UTI. In research projects even a more detailed assessment of certain criteria may be relevant.

5.2.2.2 Definition of Symptomatic UTI

A patient has a symptomatic UTI if there are clinical symptoms indicative of UTI and if presence of pathogens can be verified or suspected by culture, microscopy, dipstick, or PCR-techniques, or if the diagnosis is made or an appropriate therapy of symptomatic UTI is prescribed by a physician upon clinical evaluation. This is consistent with the CDC definitions. For acute uncomplicated cystitis in women, a questionnaire, the Acute Cystitis Symptom Score (ACSS), has been developed, translated, and validated in many languages to increase the specificity and sensitive of the diagnosis just by scoring the severity of clinical symptoms [7, 8]. The same questionnaire in reverse can then be used as a patient-reported outcome (PRO) measure [9].

Table 5.1 The most important criteria for patient assessment in UTI

I. Clinical criteria
1. Clinical presentation
(a) Urethritis* (UR)
(b) Cystitis (CY)
(c) Pyelonephritis (PY)
(d) Urosepsis (US)
(e) Male accessory gland infection ("male adnexitis") (MA) (prostatitis, vesiculitis, epididymitis, orchitis) *need to be considered separately, because the clinical presentations show great diversity
2. Specificity of symptoms
(a) UTI specific
1. For lower UTI (cystitis), e.g., dysuria, frequency, urgency, suprapubic pain
2. For upper UTI (pyelonephritis), e.g., fever, flank pain, CVA tenderness
(b) UTI non-specific symptoms, but relevant in specific clinical situations
1. For catheter associated UTI, e.g., bladder spasm, fever not explained otherwise
2. For newborn and young children (see section #8 on UTI in children)
3. For elderly patients, e.g., fever not explained otherwise, confusion
4. For patients with neurogenic disorders, e.g., incontinence, vegetative disorders
3. Severity of symptoms
(a) Mild
(b) Moderate
(c) Severe
(d) Septic
4. Pattern of infection
(a) Isolated or sporadic
(b) Recurrent
1. Relapse
2. Reinfection
(c) Unresolved or chronic
II. Risk factors
1. Patient's characteristics
(a) Gender (male, female)
(b) Prematurity, newborn, young child, adolescent
(c) Premenopause
(d) Pregnancy
(e) Postmenopause
(f) Elderly (geriatric: physically and/or mentally handicapped)
2. Relevant* diseases outside the urinary tract (*needs to be verified in clinical studies)
(a) Immunosuppression (not clear at which state it is relevant for which kind of UTI)
1. Innate
2. Acquired, e.g., AIDS
(b) Diabetes mellitus (not clear at which state it is relevant for which kind of UTI)
(c) Other diseases (?) (not clear which ones are relevant and for which kind of UTI)
3. Nephrological risk factors—status of the kidneys
(a) Impaired kidney function (not clear which degree of renal insufficiency is relevant for which kind of UTI)
(b) Kidney abscess
(c) Polycystic renal disease

Table 5.1 (continued)

4. Urological risk factors (functional or morphological disorders (impaired urodynamics) within the urinary tract. (The degree of impairment is not well defined)
(a) Functional disorders, e.g., reflux, neurogenic bladder disturbances
(b) Obstruction without infectious nidus, e.g., tumor, non-infected stone
(c) Obstruction with infectious nidus, e.g., infective stones, necrotizing tumor, stent
(d) Others
5. External catheter
(a) Urethral
(b) Suprapubic
(c) Nephrostomy
(d) Others
6. Asymptomatic bacteriuria (ASB): ASB is not considered an infection and is usually not relevant, but in some situations ASB may be a risk factor, e.g., in pregnancy and before traumatizing interventions of the urinary tract. In some situations differentiation between asymptomatic and symptomatic bacteriuria is difficult, e.g., young children, elderly patients, patients, with spinal cord injury
III. Pathogen/etiological agent
1. Bacterial load (colony counts)
2. Pathogens (type, species)
3. Antimicrobial susceptibility/resistance
4. Virulence, etc.
IV. Situation—circumstances under which UTI was acquired
1. Community
2. Outpatient service
(a) Hospital setting
(b) Private practice
3. Inpatient service (hospital)
4. Long-term residential accommodation, nursing home
5. Health care associated [2–4]
V. Therapeutic options
1. Pathogen(s) is (are) susceptible against commonly used antimicrobials
(a) Which are available
(b) Which are not easily available
2. Pathogen(s) has (have) limited susceptibility against commonly used antimicrobials
(a) But alternative antimicrobials are available
(b) But alternative antimicrobials are not easily available
3. Pathogen(s) is (are) multidrug-resistant (MDR) or extended drug-resistant (EDR) [6, 7] and appropriate antimicrobials are not (or not easily) available

5.2.2.3 Clinical Presentation

The clinical situation is classified as cystitis (CY), pyelonephritis (PY), and urosepsis (US) as in the CDC definitions [2, 6]. Asymptomatic bacteriuria (ASB) is considered not as infection, but as a risk factor for UTI in certain circumstances. The clinical presentation of the three UTI entities discussed here (CY, PN, US) is used to create overall severity grades considering that a PN is always more severe than a CY and a US always more severe than the two former ones. In addition, PN can present as a mild or severe infection, which usually can be treated by oral antimicrobials in an outpatient setting, or as a severe infection with systemic reactions like nausea and vomiting, which usually needs initial parenteral therapy and hospitalization may be recommended. For urosepsis the severity grading of sepsis in general use can be adapted: sepsis, severe sepsis, septic shock [10, 11].

5.2.2.4 Risk Factors

Ideally, all five main categories as outlined in Table 5.1 should be weighted and graded according to their impact on prognosis. Unfortunately, our knowledge about their relative impact is scarce, and therefore they cannot just be added together. Furthermore, some criteria are numerical, like number of CFU. Some are dichotomous variables like gender. Others are categorical, like names of pathogens, and types of accommodation. We therefore recommended to apply the principle of phenotyping.

Risk factors may affect the patient in different ways and may be grouped according to existing knowledge of their importance. Some risk factors, for example, pregnancy, prematurity, newborns, and immune deficiency, mean an increased risk of a serious outcome like abortion, loss of nephrons, or even the patient's life. Others mean that a more elaborate treatment regimen is needed, for example, obstruction of the urinary tract and kidney abscess. Some risk factors increase the risk that a UTI will recur, for example, incomplete bladder emptying and indwelling catheter. In recognition of the characteristics of risk factors relevant for the three infections (CY, PN, US), we organized the risk factors into six groups and proposed the **ORENUC** system for phenotyping:

O **NO** known risk factor, ***R*** risk for **R**ecurrent UTI, but without risk of more severe outcome, ***E*** **E**xtraurogenital risk factors, ***N*** relevant **N**ephropathic diseases, ***U*** **U**rological resolvable (transient) risk factors, ***C*** permanent external urinary **C**atheter and non-resolved urological risk factors (see also Chap. 19 by Qvigstad et al. on antibiotic prophylaxis).

5.2.2.5 Antimicrobial Treatment Options

Antibiotics are cornerstones in the treatment of UTI. Without antibiotics (as in some developing countries) or without effective antibiotics (as already in some developed countries today), the prognosis may be very serious. For assessment of prognosis and severity of UTI, we suggested that the availability of effective antimicrobial treatment is included in the overall assessment of severity in a patient with UTI. We suggested a grading with small letters a–c based on the susceptibility of the causative pathogen(s) and the availability of effective antimicrobials and acknowledged that an updating of this part of the classification had to be made as further knowledge was acquired.

5.2.2.6 Severity Assessment

When assessing a patient with suspected UTI, the severity of the situation always has to be considered. The clinical presentation outweighs all other categories of information from the diagnostic workup as regards prognosis and treatment. Assessment of severity always starts with the clinical presentation and the treatment needed. The evaluation of underlying risk factors is descriptive and may modify the severity of the clinical presentation. For example, a cystitis (CY) combined with a risk factor of category "E" or "U" is usually more severe than of category "O" or "R." Therefore, the severity category for CY could be modified accordingly. The same applies for pyelonephritis (PN) and urosepsis (US). In addition, the availability of an appropriate antimicrobial therapy modifies also the risk of a more severe outcome in any of the clinical presentations.

5.3 Clinical Practice

When a patient presents with symptoms and signs suspicious of UTI, the clinician has to consider:

- The clinical presentation or type of infection according to the organs affected; lower tract, upper tract, or systemic.
- The severity of the situation by differentiating cystitis, mild or severe type of pyelonephritis, and the three presentations or forms of urosepsis according to SIRS criteria and SOFA score.
- The presence of risk factors or disease modifiers, for example, obstruction in the urinary tract.
- The most likely pathogen and its susceptibility to available antibiotics.

The ESIU-ORENUC classification can guide the clinician in the initial considerations (Fig. 5.1). Usually, patients with severity grade 3 and higher (Fig. 5.1) will need hospitalization and intravenous administration of antibiotics. The ORENUC

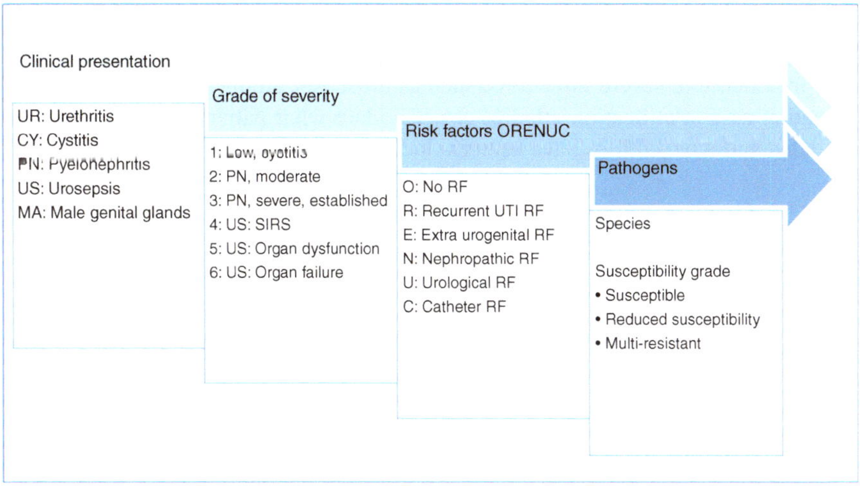

Fig. 5.1 Flow chart for assessment of patients with suspected UTI (modified from [12]). *RF* risk factor. Other acronyms are explained in Sect. II.b.3. There are two types of pyelonephritis, one with mild symptoms and no fever, and one with more severe symptoms and fever [5]

phenotyping can be a checklist for questions to ask the patient, to identify factors that need to be eliminated in the acute phase and factors that can be modified to prevent recurrences. The circumstances under which the UTI was acquired will influence the evaluation of the most likely pathogen, its susceptibility, and the necessary duration of antibiotic treatment.

The differentiation of UTIs into uncomplicated and complicated UTI is still useful and valid, but the borders that separate the two entities are not always clear and the dichotomous classification does not always provide clear guidance for diagnostic work-up and prevention of recurrences in a very heterogeneous patient population.

5.4 Research

5.4.1 Complicated UTI/Pyelonephritis as a Model Population

Patients with cUTI/pyelonephritis have been an interesting group for treatment studies of new antibiotics in patients expected to have severe infections with Gram-negative pathogens. The reasons are that pathogens can be easily identified and their eradication from the urinary tract can be easily confirmed. According to a recent review by Wagenlehner et al. [13], the populations selected for the evaluation of the primary outcome criteria varied in the studies reviewed. Most patients were enrolled on an empirical basis, due to the fact that treatment of cUTI/pyelonephritis needs to be started empirically. Non-evaluable patients were therefore excluded post-hoc, and the primary evaluable population often became substantially smaller than the intention to treat population. For example, in some studies, only patients with infections due to Gram-negative organisms were included. In other studies only patients with causative organisms that tested susceptible to the study drugs were included.

The authors recommended that future studies should include extended patient populations that better reflect the everyday clinical situation. Future studies should also include more severe infections, such as urosepsis. Adding the ORENUC classification as a stratification attempt can elucidate what patient entities have been included and what entities have been excluded in a given study.

5.4.2 Moving Toward Personalized Medicine

UTIs are infections of the urothelium that might progress to parenchymal infection as in pyelonephritis, provoke systemic reaction as in SIRS, and progress to systemic disease as in sepsis. The development of an infection is the result of a battle between the patient and microorganisms where the course of the disease depends on host and pathogen factors alike.

We can describe pathogen factors in terms of genetic changes. As regards host factors, we have limited knowledge about genetic changes that increase the risk of UTI. The clinical risk factors included in the ORENUC classification obviously have corresponding genetic alterations.

Oncological patients are now undergoing gene sequencing in order to differentiate prevention and treatment according to their genetic profile. This approach should be copied in the field of UTI. Ultimately, the virulence factors of the pathogen and the resistance mechanisms of the host determine the UTI, and the genes of the pathogen and the host, respectively, determine the virulence factors and resistance mechanisms.

In oncology, the concept of neo-adjuvant, adjuvant, and combination treatment is well established. In UTI, we have just started to look into this by using antibiotic peptides as adjuvant treatment [14]. A further exploration of this concept in UTI will require a careful differentiation of patient groups, and the ORENUC classification seems to be a reasonable platform to develop further.

5.4.3 Adherence to Antimicrobial Stewardship Principles

Avoidance of antibiotics is an alternative in case of cystitis and asymptomatic bacteriuria, and elimination or modification of risk factors is a valid alternative in recurrent cystitis. Both approaches are consistent with the principles of antibiotic stewardship, and both approaches have to be based on a differentiated assessment of patients where the ESIU-ORENUC classification is most relevant.

5.5 Do We Need an Update of the ESIU-ORENUC Classification?

The CDC, IDSA, and ESCMID classification focused on development of research protocols in an era when many new antibiotics were introduced and when resistance was not an issue. The ESIU-ORENUC classification focused on severity assessment and identification of risk factors that can be eliminated to modify disease course, prevent recurrences, and reduce the need for antibiotics. Since the ESIU-ORENUC classification was presented in 2010, we have witnessed a significant increase in available information in the field of UTI.

The most significant feature is the increase in antimicrobial resistance and the frightening prospects for the coming decades as outlined by the O'Neill report [15]. The scientific community has responded by defining the concept of antimicrobial stewardship. International bodies like EMA and FDA have posed restrictions on the use of certain antibiotics, and international scientific communities and national health departments have adjusted their guidelines recommendations accordingly [16].

In recognition of the threat from increasing resistance, we have seen numerous research reports in the field of UTI about measures to improve empirical treatment, tailor antibiotic treatment, and even avoid use of antibiotics. As in other fields of medicine, recent studies increasingly use big data in modeling and statistical analyses to support and guide clinical decisions (Table 5.2).

Table 5.2 Recent developments that might help to update the ESIU-ORENUC classification

Publ. year	Authors	References*	Main findings
2012	Hebert et al.	[17]	The authors developed a novel method of displaying microbiology data called the weighted-incidence syndromic combination antibiogram (WISCA) for UTI by combining simple diagnosis and microbiology data. This allows data to be presented so that clinicians can see the probability that a particular regimen will cover a particular infection rather than the probability that a single drug will cover a single organism. WISCA can overcome limitations to the utility of the traditional antibiogram in helping providers choose empiric antibiotics
2013	Cai et al.	[18]	Cai and co-workers presented a validated nomogram to predict recurrence in women with symptomatic urinary tract infections. They concluded that the nomogram accurately predicts the recurrence risk within 1 year and that the nomogram is suitable in identifying women that might benefit from a prophylactic strategy
2013	Tandogdu et al.	[19]	Based on 8-year data from the GPIU study, Tandogdu et al. demonstrated that Asia had the highest rates of resistance, and the only antibiotic worldwide with an overall resistance rate below 10% was imipenem. They concluded that knowledge of regional and local resistance data and prudent use of antibiotics is necessary to optimize antibiotic therapy in urological patients with NAUTI
2015	Cai et al.	[20]	Cai et al. showed that adherence to EAU guidelines on antibiotic prophylaxis is an important step in antimicrobial stewardship
2016	Tandogdu et al.	[21]	Tandogdu and co-workers showed that it is not appropriate to use pathogen spectrum and resistance rates of other HAUTIS to decide on empirical treatment of sepsis. The authors warned of increasing resistance rates in patients with urosepsis and argued that precautions must be made to avoid further increase
2016	Cai et al.	[22]	Cai et al. demonstrated that a restricted use of antibiotic prophylaxis in line with EAU guidelines was not associated with a higher incidence of postoperative infections
2016	Wagen-lehner et al.	[23]	Wagenlehner et al. published data from the GPIU study based on surveillance data from 27,542 patients in 70 countries. Resistance rates of most uropathogens against antibiotics were high, and the severity of HAUTI was increasing with 25% being urosepsis
2017	Cai et al.	[24]	Cai and co-workers demonstrated that increasing leukocyturia might detect the transition from asymptomatic bacteriuria to symptomatic infection. This simple measure may help in reducing unnecessary antibiotic treatment of asymptomatic bacteriuria and thereby improve antibiotic stewardship

Table 5.2 (continued)

Publ. year	Authors	References*	Main findings
2018	Cai et al.	[25]	Cai et al. demonstrated that phytotherapy was not inferior to antibiotics to obtain symptom relief in patients with recurrent urinary tract infections, a finding of great interest in an antibiotic stewardship perspective
2019	Dixon et al.	[26]	This paper explored the limitations of traditional methods of culture and sensitivity and delves into recent studies involving new high-throughput genomic technologies in urological research, demonstrating the advances made in the role of urinary microbiome in a whole spectrum of pathologies from urinary tract infection, to prostate cancer. Authors discuss the challenges that must be overcome for such technology to become widely used in clinical practice
2019	Tandogdu et al.	[27]	Tandogdu et al. showed that most single agent antibiotic choices had limited coverage for HAUTI and combination choices had improved chance of coverage. Urology departments that adhere to infection control policies have more antibiotic choices. Over a 10-year time period in the GPIU study, there was no clear time trend in the chances of coverage of antibiotics as estimated by Bayesian WISCA
2019	Tandogdu et al.	[28]	Tandogdu et al. analyzed 10 years findings from the GPIU study by means of mathematical modeling with Bayesian WISCA and the Bayesian factor. They demonstrated that antibiotic choices can be different between HAUTI conditions, and empirical antibiotic selection can be improved by means of mathematical modeling. Including local resistance data and the clinical type of infection in the modeling will further improve antibiotic selection toward a personalized approach
2020	Tandogdu et al.	[29]	Tandogdu et al. performed a mathematical modeling study of severe urinary tract infections in adults in 17 countries to analyze the impact of different antibiotic stewardship scenarios. They could show that a substantial improvement in the empirical treatment of severe UTIs would be achieved by excluding certain classes of antibiotics. Each country needs to adopt its own antibiotic armamentarium for empirical antibiotics, and in most countries, a suspension of quinolones can be useful
2022	Cai et al.	[30]	Cai et al. adopted artificial intelligence to guide antibiotic choice in recurrent UTI and showed a sensitivity of 87.8% and specificity of 97.3% in predicting clinical efficacy of the prescribed antimicrobial drug. Previous isolation of *E. coli*, historic antibiotic usage, and resistance data predict the subsequent treatment failure to other antibiotics. Their findings represent a new way for improving antimicrobial stewardship

As metagenomic sequencing provides more information about the presence of microbial DNA, there is increased risk of overtreatment with antibiotics [25]. We need clear classification criteria to decide if microbial DNA stems from dead or living, and clinically relevant, microorganisms. New criteria should also include collateral effects of antibiotics on other microbiomes in the patient's body such as the intestine as well as on the environment. FDA and EMA have already adopted these concerns [16, 31].

New clinical diagnostic criteria should also include the work of Alidjanov et al. [8, 9] using the ACSS questionnaire as a diagnostic tool. The ACSS as a validated diagnostic measure may help to define better the need for patients to visit a GP.

Criteria and risk factors in the ESIU-ORENUC classification might be reorganized and further differentiated according to influence of diagnostic work-up, host response, spectrum of pathogens, and resistance. For example, we should elaborate on the importance of diagnostic work-up of ORENUC categories such as extraurogenital disease and nephrological and urological risk factors. We should be more specific as regards the impact of recurrent UTI, traveling, clinical condition, urological risk factors, and catheters on the spectrum of pathogens and resistance.

The studies by Cai et al. [17–25, 27–30] demonstrate that sophisticated mathematical analyses of carefully registered patient data improve empirical treatment and enhance antibiotic stewardship. Modeling and artificial intelligence give new information that even the brightest minds can retrieve through cognitive exercises. One can easily imagine a situation where clinicians receive recommendations on antibiotic choices through a smart phone upon entry of key patient and situation criteria in a bedside situation.

We can expect that instant identification of pathogens and resistance will become available within short. This will change the concept of empirical treatment and strengthen the argument for including pathogen identity in the classification of UTI. Likewise, the O'Neill report [15] underlines the importance of availability of effective antibiotics as a classification criterion. A revision of the ORENUC classification should also include bacterial virulence factors, which unfortunately are usually not available at point of care.

Contemporary available information relevant for classification of UTI is taking us away from a simple dichotomous classification of uncomplicated and complicated infections toward an even more differentiated classification than is used in the present ESIU-ORENUC.

5.6 Conclusions

Everyone working with UTI in clinical practice, quality registration, and research should keep in mind the importance of a good classification and a precise terminology, and remember to:

- Take a careful history to identify risk factors that need further work-up.
- Identify risk factors that must be eliminated immediately.
- Identify risk factor that may be eliminated to prevent recurrences.

- Know the characteristics of severe UTI and sepsis and when immediate combination antibiotic regimens are required.
- Be familiar with local resistance rates.
- Be aware of the need for antibiotic stewardship and when antibiotic treatment and prophylaxis can be avoided, reduced, or amended.
- Engage in research to improve patient care.

It is time for an ESIU-ORENUC II classification that:

- Includes metagenomics and collateral effects of antibiotics.
- Includes mathematical modeling, artificial intelligence, and modern communication technology to facilitate bedside decision-making.
- Includes new information about host-pathogen interaction that can facilitate development of personalized prophylaxis and treatment.
- Acknowledges the importance of availability of effective antibiotics and antibiotic stewardship.

References

1. Garner JS, Jarvis WR, Emori TG, Horan TC, Hughes JM. CDC definitions for nosocomial infections, 1988. Am J Infect Control. 1988;16(3):128–40.
2. Horan TC, Andrus M, Dudeck MA. CDC/NHSN surveillance definition of health care-associated infection and criteria for specific types of infections in the acute care setting. Am J Infect Control. 2008;36(5):309–32.
3. Rubin RH, Shapiro ED, Andriole VT, Davis RJ, Stamm WE. Evaluation of new anti-infective drugs for the treatment of UTI. Clin Infect Dis. 1992;15:216.
4. Rubin RH, Shapiro ED, Andriole VT, Davis RJ, Stamm WE, with a Modification by a European Working Party (Norrby SR). General guidelines for the evaluation of new anti-infective drugs for the treatment of urinary tract infection. Taukirchen: The European Society of Clinical Microbiology and Infectious diseases; 1993. p. 240–310.
5. https://www.reliasmedia.com/articles/9959-cdc-is-on-the-fast-track-with-new-uti-prevention-guidelines.
6. Johansen TEB, Botto H, Cek M, Grabe M, Tenke P, Wagenlehner FME, Naber KG. Critical review of current definitions of urinary tract infections and proposal of an EAU/ESIU classification system, pp 979–93, Chapter 16: Classification of urinary tract infections. In: Naber KG, Scaeffer AJ, Heyns CF, Matsumoto T, Shoskes DA, Johansen TEB, editors. Urogenital infections (Textbook 1182 pp). Arnheim: International Consultation on Urological Diseases (ICUD) and European Association of Urology; 2010.
7. Alidjanov JF, Overesch A, Abramov-Sommariva D, Hoeller M, Steindl H, Wagenlehner FM, Naber KG. Acute cystitis symptom score questionnaire for measuring patient-reported outcomes in women with acute uncomplicated cystitis: clinical validation as part of a phase III trial comparing antibiotic and nonantibiotic therapy. Investig Clin Urol. 2020;61(5):498–507. https://doi.org/10.4111/icu.20200060.
8. Alidjanov JF, Khudaybergenov UA, Ayubov BA, Pilatz A, Mohr S, Münst JC, Ziviello ON, Yuen SP, Christmann C, Dittmar F, Mirsaidov NM, Buch-Heberling M, Naber KG, Johansen TEB, Wagenlehner FME. Linguistic and clinical validation of the acute cystitis symptom score in German-speaking Swiss women with acute cystitis. Int Urogynecol. 2021;32:3275–86.
9. Weldring T, Smith SMS. Patient-reported outcomes (PROs) and patient-reported outcome measures (PROMs). Health Serv Insights. 2013;6:61–8. https://doi.org/10.4137/HSI.S11093.

10. Bone RC, Balk RA, Cerra FB, Dellinger RP, Fein AM, Knaus WA, Schein RM, Sibbald WJ. Definitions for sepsis and organ failure and guidelines for the use of innovative therapies in sepsis. The ACCP/SCCM consensus conference committee. American College of Chest Physicians/Society of Critical Care Medicine. Chest. 1992;101(6):1644–55.
11. Levy MM, Fink MP, Marshall JC, Abraham E, Angus D, Cook D, Cohen J, Opal SM, Vincent JL, Ramsay G. 2001 SCCM/ESICM/ACCP/ATS/SIS international sepsis definitions conference. Crit Care Med. 2003;31(4):1250–6.
12. Grabe M, Bartoletti R, Johansen TEB, Cai T, Cek M, Köves B, Naber KG, Pickard RS, Tenke P, Wagenlehner F, Wullt B. Guidelines on urinary tract infections. Eur Assoc Urol. 2015:1–86.
13. Wagenlehner FME, Johansen TEB, Cai T, Koves B, Kranz J, Pilatz A, Tandogdu Z. Epidemiology, definition and treatment of complicated urinary tract infections. Nat Rev Urol. 2020;17(10):586–600. https://doi.org/10.1038/s41585-020-0362-4. Epub 2020 Aug 25.
14. Panjla A, Kaul G, Chopra S, Titz A, Verma S. Short peptides and their mimetics as potent antibacterial agents and antibiotic adjuvants. ACS Chem Biol. 2021;16(12):2731–45. https://doi.org/10.1021/acschembio.1c00626. Epub 2021 Nov 15.
15. O'Neill J. Antimicrobial resistance: tackling a crisis for the health and wealth of nations. The Review on Antimicrobial Resistance Chaired by Jim O'Neill. 2014. 1.pdf (amr-review.org).
16. https://www.ema.europa.eu/en/documents/referral/quinolone-fluoroquinolone-article-31-referral-disabling-potentially-permanent-side-effects-lead_en.pdf.
17. Hebert C, Ridgway J, Vekhter B, Brown EC, Weber SG, Robicsek A. Demonstration of the weighted-incidence syndromic combination antibiogram: an empiric prescribing decision aid. Infect Control Hosp Epidemiol. 2012;33(4):381–8.
18. Cai T, Mazzoli S, Migno S, Malossini G, Lanzafame P, Mereu L, Tateo S, Wagenlehner FM, Pickard RS, Bartoletti R. Development and validation of a nomogram predicting recurrence risk in women with symptomatic urinary tract infection. Int J Urol. 2014;21(9):929–34. https://doi.org/10.1111/iju.12453.
19. Tandogdu Z, Cek M, Wagenlehner F, Naber K, Tenke P, Ostrum E, Johansen TEB. Resistance patterns of nosocomial urinary tract infections in urology departments: 8-year results of the global prevalence of infections in urology study. World J Urol. 2014;32(3):791–801. https://doi.org/10.1007/s00345-013-1154-8.
20. Cai T, Verze P, Brugnolli A, Tiscione D, Luciani LG, Eccher C, Lanzafame P, Malossini G, Wagenlehner FM, Mirone V, Johansen TEB, Pickard R, Bartoletti R. Adherence to European Association of Urology guidelines on prophylactic antibiotics: an important step in antimicrobial stewardship. Eur Urol. 2016;69(2):276–83. https://doi.org/10.1016/j.eururo.2015.05.010.
21. Tandogdu Z, Bartoletti R, Cai T, Cek M, Grabe M, Kulchavenya E, Koves B, Menon V, Naber K, Perepanova T, Tenke P, Wult B, Johansen TEB, Wagenlehner F. Antimicrobial resistance in urosepsis: outcomes from the multinational, multicenter global prevalence of infections in urology study (2003–2013). World J Urol. 2016;34:1193–200. https://doi.org/10.1007/s00345-015-1722-1.
22. Cai T, Bonkat G, Tandogdu Z, Bartoletti R, Wagenlehner FME, Grabe M, Johansen TEB. How to use antimicrobial prophylaxis in urological procedures. Eur Urol Focus. 2016;2(4):348–50.
23. Wagenlehner F, Tandogdu Z, Bartoletti R, Cai T, Cek M, Kulchavenya E, Koves B, Naber K, Perepanova T, Tenke P, Wult B, Bogenhard F, Johansen TEB. The global prevalence of infections in urology study: a long-term, worldwide surveillance study on urological infections. Pathogens. 2016;5(1):10. https://doi.org/10.3390/pathogens5010010.
24. Cai T, Lanzafame P, Caciagli P, Migno S, Mereu L, Mattevi D, Luciani LG, Tateo S, Malossini G, Johansen TEB. Role of increasing leukocyturia for detecting the transition from asymptomatic bacteriuria to symptomatic infection in women with recurrent urinary tract infections: a new tool for improving antibiotic stewardship. Int J Urol. 2018;25(9):800–6. https://doi.org/10.1111/iju.13723.
25. Cai T, Cocci A, Tiscione D, Puglisi M, Di Maida F, Malossini G, Verze P, Palmieri A, Mirone V, Johansen TEB. L-Methionine associated with *Hibiscus sabdariffa* and *Boswellia serrata* extracts are not inferior to antibiotic treatment for symptoms relief in patients affected by recurrent uncomplicated urinary tract infections: focus on antibiotic-sparing approach. Arch Ital Urol Androl. 2018;90(2):97–100. https://doi.org/10.4081/aiua.2018.2.97.

26. Dixon M, Stefil M, McDonald M, Johansen TEB, Naber K, Wagenlehner F, Mouraviev V. Metagenomics in diagnosis and improved targeted treatment of UTI. World J Urol. 2020;38(1):35–43.
27. Tandogdu Z, Kakariadis ETA, Naber K, Wagenlehner F, Johansen TEB. Appropriate empiric antibiotic choices in health care associated urinary tract infections in urology departments in Europe from 2006 to 2015: a Bayesian analytical approach applied in a surveillance study. PLoS One. 2019;14(4):e0214710.
28. Tandogdu Z, Koves B, Cai T, Cek M, Tenke P, Naber K, Wagenlehner F, Johansen TEB. Condition-specific surveillance in health care-associated urinary tract infections as a strategy to improve empirical antibiotic treatment: an epidemiological modelling study. World J Urol. 2019;38:27–34. https://doi.org/10.1007/s00345-019-02963-9.
29. Tandogdu Z, Naber K, Kakaridas E, Wagenlehner F, Johansen TEB. The Bayesian WISCA to optimize antibiotic selection: a novel decision-making tool applied in urosepsis. (Wellcome Trust Award 2019). https://www.synapse.org/#!Synapse:syn18377564/wiki/588796.
30. Cai T, Anceschi U, Prata F, Collini L, Brugnolli A, Migno S, Rizzo M, Liguori G, Gallelli L, Wagenlehner FME, Johansen TEB, Montanari L, Tascini C, Palmieri A. Artificial intelligence can guide antibiotic choice in recurrent UTI and become an important aid to improve antimicrobial stewardship. Antibiotics. 2022;12(2):375.
31. https://www.fda.gov/news-events/press-announcements/fda-updates-warnings-fluoroquinolone-antibiotics.

Novel Antibiotics in Urology

6

Kurt G. Naber, Truls E. Bjerklund Johansen, and Florian M. E. Wagenlehner

6.1 Antibiotic Resistance of Uropathogens

Antibiotic resistance in Gram-negative uropathogens is increasing worldwide and is surveilled in distinct local and multinational studies. A compilation of worldwide studies, for example, showed resistance rates of Gram-negative uropathogens against fluoroquinolones in 10–80%, against cephalosporins in 5–70%, and against carbapenems in 0–35% [1]. A specific surveillance study in urology represents the Global Prevalence of Infections in Urology (GPIU) study, which is a worldwide point prevalence study, performed each November since 2003. This study is intended to create surveillance data in patients at urological departments with health-care associated urinary tract infections (HAUTI) [2]. Resistance rates of most uropathogens against all tested antibiotics were high, especially with note of multidrug resistance (Fig. 6.1). In many countries the resistance rate of Gram-negative uropathogens only against carbapenems is below 10%, a threshold used for empiric therapy of severe infections, such as urosepsis. A worrying finding in the GPIU study was also that the severity of HAUTI is also increasing, 25% being urosepsis in recent years.

K. G. Naber (✉)
Department of Urology, Technical University of Munich, Munich, Germany
e-mail: kurt@nabers.de

T. E. Bjerklund Johansen
Urology Department, Oslo University Hospital, Oslo, Norway

Institute of Clinical Medicine, University of Oslo, Oslo, Norway

Institute of Clinical Medicine, University of Aarhus, Aarhus, Denmark
e-mail: t.e.b.johansen@medisin.uio.no

F. M. E. Wagenlehner
Clinic for Urology, Pediatric Urology and Andrology, Justus Liebig University, Giessen, Germany
e-mail: Florian.Wagenlehner@chiru.med.uni-giessen.de

T. E. Bjerklund Johansen, T. Cai (eds.), *Guide to Antibiotics in Urology*,
https://doi.org/10.1007/978-3-319-92366-6_6

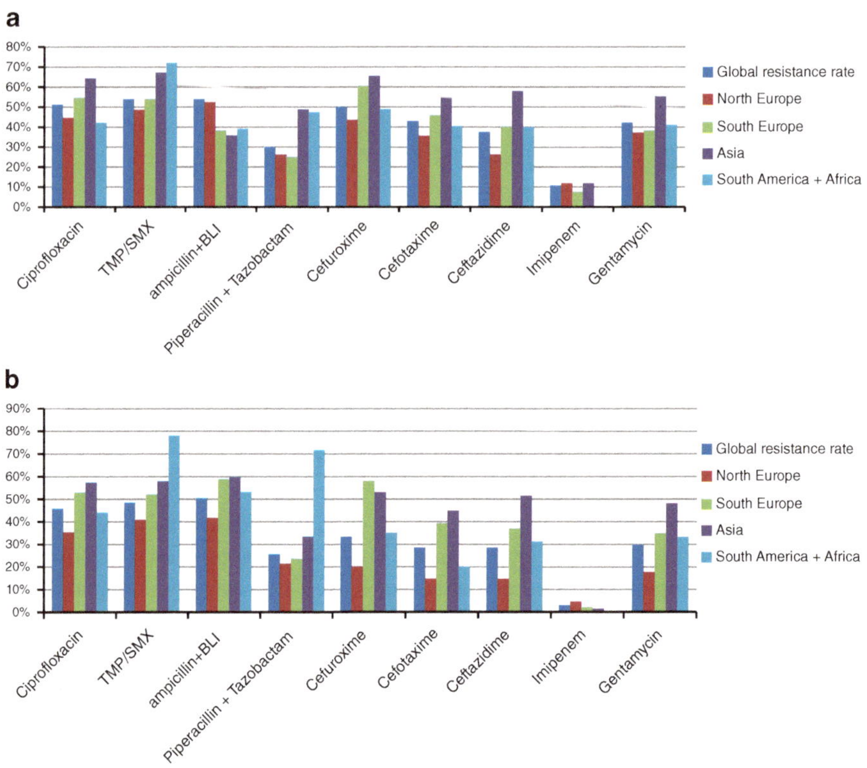

Fig. 6.1 Global and regional resistance rates of uropathogens in health-care associated urinary tract infections (HAUTI). (**a**) Total bacterial spectrum of uropathogens. (**b**) *Escherichia coli*. Data taken from Tandogdu Z, Cek M, Wagenlehner F, Naber K, Tenke P, van Ostrum E, Bjerklund Johansen T. Resistance patterns of nosocomial urinary tract infections in urology departments: 8-year results of the global prevalence of infections in urology study. World J Urol 2014;32:791–801 [2]

6.2 Need for Novel Antibiotics

Although for uncomplicated cystitis still old antibiotics, such as fosfomycin trometamol, nitrofurantoin, nitroxoline, and pivmecillinam, are recommended as first line [3, 4], for complicated and especially HAUTI novel antibiotics need to be developed. Several novel antibiotics or antibiotic combinations are recently approved or in clinical studies for the treatment of complicated UTI (cUTI).

Several strategies are currently employed in the development of novel antibiotics:

Beta-lactam/beta-lactamase inhibitor combinations are extended to cephalosporins and also carbapenems. A so-called siderophore antibiotic (cephalosporin) was introduced, and novel aminoglycoside, fluoroquinolone, and tetracycline are also in clinical development phases (Table 6.1).

Table 6.1 Novel antibiotics approved or in clinical studies tested vs. standard antibiotics in the treatment of complicated UTI incl. Acute uncomplicated pyelonephritis

	Novel antibiotic/combination vs. standard antibiotic—Phase	Company
1.1	Ceftolozane/tazobactam vs. levofloxacin—Approved and listed	Merck Sharp & Dohme
1.2	Ceftazidime/avibactam vs. doripenem—Approved and listed	Pfizer
1.3	Cefepime/enmetazobactam vs. piperacillin/tazobactam—Phase 3	Allecra Therapeutics
1.4	Cefiderocol (S-649266) vs. imipenem—Phase 2, 3	Shionogi
2.1	Meropenem/vaborbactam vs. piperacillin/tazobactam—Approved	The Medicines Company
2.2	Imipenem/relebactam vs. colistin—Phase 3	Merck Sharp & Dohme
2.3	Tebipenem pivoxil hydrobromide oral vs. ertapenem iv—Phase 3	Spero Therapeutics
2.4	Sulopenem iv-oral vs ertapenem iv—Oral ciprofloxacin or amoxicillin-clavulanate—Phase 3	Iterum Therapeutics
3	Plazomicin vs. levofloxacin—Phase 3	Achaogen
4.1	Finafloxacin vs. ciprofloxacin—Phase 2	Merlion
4.2	Sitafloxacin oral vs. ertapenem iv and levofloxacin oral—Phase 2	Daiichi Sankyo
5	Eravacycline vs. levofloxacin—Phase 3 (unpublished)	Tetraphase Pharm
6	Fosfomycin disodium vs. ceftriaxone or meropenem—Phase 3	Study Funded by Grants

Within the novel antibiotics, there are two novel cephalosporins, ceftolozane and cefiderocol, and one new carbapenem. Three of the cephalosporins and two of the carbapenems are combined with a beta-lactamase inhibitor (BLI), of which four of the BLI are novel: avibactam, enmetazobactam, vaborbactam, and relebactam. In addition there is one new aminoglycoside, plazomicin, one new fluoroquinolone, finafloxacin, and fosfomycin sodium (as a revival) in the last few years also evaluated in the treatment of complicated UTI, including pyelonephritis.

6.2.1 Ceftolozane/Tazobactam

Ceftolozane-tazobactam is a novel cephalosporin combined with an established beta-lactamase inhibitor that was developed to address the rising rates of antimicrobial resistance in Gram-negative pathogens. This drug has potent in vitro activity against multidrug-resistant strains of *Pseudomonas aeruginosa* and other common Gram-negative pathogens, including most ESBL-producing Enterobacteriaceae spp.

In the Assessment of the Safety Profile and Efficacy of Ceftolozane/Tazobactam in Complicated Urinary Tract Infections (ASPECT-cUTI) clinical program, the efficacy and safety of ceftolozane-tazobactam were compared with those of levofloxacin, a widely used antibacterial, in hospital inpatients with complicated lower-urinary-tract infections or pyelonephritis. Patients were randomly assigned in a 1:1 ratio to receive 1.5 g intravenous (IV) ceftolozane-tazobactam every 8 h or 750 mg IV levofloxacin once daily, both for 7 days.

Of 1083 patients enrolled, 800 (73.9%), of whom 656 (82.0%) had pyelonephritis, were included in the microbiological MITT population. Ceftolozane-tazobactam was non-inferior to levofloxacin for composite (microbiological and clinical) cure (306 [76.9%] of 398 vs. 275 [68.4%] of 402, 95% CI: 2.3–14.6) and, as the lower bound of the two-sided 95% CI around the treatment difference was positive and greater than zero, superiority was indicated. Adverse event profiles were similar in the two treatment groups and were mainly non-serious. It was concluded that treatment with ceftolozane-tazobactam led to better responses than high-dose levofloxacin in patients with complicated lower-urinary-tract infections or pyelonephritis [5].

6.2.2 Ceftazidime/Avibactam

Ceftazidime-avibactam combines ceftazidime and avibactam, a first-in-class non–beta-lactam beta-lactamase inhibitor which restores the in vitro activity of ceftazidime against Ambler class A (e.g., ESBL and *K. pneumoniae* carbapenemase), class C (e.g., AmpC), and some class D β-lactamase–producing bacteria. It is not active against metallo-β-lactamases. Ceftazidime-avibactam (2000/500 mg every 8 h) was approved by the US Food and Drug Administration (FDA) based on phase 2 data (including a phase 2 cUTI trial [NCT00690378] evaluating efficacy and safety of ceftazidime-avibactam 500/125 mg every 8 h) for the treatment of cUTI, including acute pyelonephritis, and complicated intra-abdominal infections (in combination with metronidazole) in adults with limited/no alternative treatment options [6, 7].

RECAPTURE 1 and 2 comprised 2 identical phase 3, randomized, multicenter, double-blind, double-dummy, parallel-group trials designed incorporating FDA and EMA guidance. Eligible patients were randomized 1:1 to IV ceftazidime-avibactam 2000/500 mg every 8 h or IV doripenem 500 mg every 8 h. Of 1033 randomized patients, 393 and 417 treated with IV ceftazidime-avibactam and IV doripenem, respectively, were eligible for the primary efficacy analyses; 19.6% had ceftazidime-nonsusceptible baseline pathogens. Noninferiority of ceftazidime-avibactam vs. doripenem was demonstrated for the FDA co-primary endpoints of (1) patient-reported symptomatic resolution at day 5: 276 of 393 (70.2%) vs. 276 of 417 (66.2%) patients (difference, 4.0% [95% confidence interval {CI}: −2.4 to 10.4%]); and (2) combined symptomatic resolution/microbiological eradication at test of cure (TOC): 280 of 393 (71.2%) vs. 269 of 417 (64.5%) patients (difference, 6.7% [95% CI: 0.3–13.1%]). Microbiological eradication at TOC (EMA primary endpoint) occurred in 304 of 393 (77.4%) ceftazidime-avibactam vs. 296 of 417 (71.0%) doripenem patients (difference, 6.4% [95% CI: 0.3–12.4%]), demonstrating superiority at the 5% significance level. Both treatments showed similar.

efficacy against ceftazidime-nonsusceptible pathogens. Ceftazidime-avibactam had a safety profile consistent with that of ceftazidime alone. It was concluded that ceftazidime-avibactam was highly effective for the empiric treatment of cUTI (including acute pyelonephritis) and may offer an alternative to carbapenems in this setting [8].

6.2.3 Cefepime/Enmetazobactam

In vitro, the activity of cefepime against β-lactamase–producing Gram-negative pathogens was restored if combined with the novel β-lactamase inhibitor enmetazobactam (formerly AAI101). This combination was more potent than piperacillin/tazobactam against extended-spectrum β-lactamase producers [9]. In a phase 2 study, it was shown that cefepime and enmetazobactam had similar pharmacokinetic profiles, with urinary excretion and similar half-lives of 2.3 h [10].

A randomized, phase 3 clinical trial was conducted to establish whether cefepime/enmetazobactam was noninferior to piperacillin/tazobactam with respect to efficacy in adult patients with complicated UTI or acute pyelonephritis [11]. Patients received a 2-h infusion of either cefepime 2 g/enmetazobactam 0.5 g, or piperacillin 4 g/tazobactam 0.5 g, every 8 h for 7 days (up to 14 days in patients with a positive blood culture at baseline). Patients with moderate kidney impairment at baseline received a dose of cefepime 1 g/enmetazobactam 0.25 g, by 2-h infusion every 8 h starting at day 1. Piperacillin/tazobactam did not require dose adjustment. The primary analysis set included 678 patients who received at least 1 dose of treatment and had a Gram-negative bacterium that was not resistant to either treatment in urine at more than 10^5CFU/mL or the same Gram-negative pathogen in both urine and blood. The most common pathogen at baseline was *Escherichia coli* (76.4%;

518/678), followed by *Klebsiella pneumoniae* (9.7%; 66/678), *Proteus mirabilis* (5.6%; 38/678), *Pseudomonas aeruginosa* (3.5%; 24/678), and *Enterobacter cloacae* (1.5%; 10/678).

The primary outcome was the proportion of patients in the primary analysis set who achieved a composite outcome of complete resolution of the baseline signs and symptoms present at screening (clinical cure) and reduction of qualifying baseline pathogen to less than 10^3 CFU/mL in urine (microbiological eradication) at day 14.

The primary outcome at day 14 showing a composite of complete resolution of the baseline signs and symptoms present at screening (clinical cure) and reduction of the qualifying baseline pathogen to less than 10^3 CFU/mL in urine (microbiological eradication) occurred in 273 of 345 patients (79.1%) in the cefepime/enmetazobactam group and 196 of 333 patients (58.9%) in the piperacillin/tazobactam group (difference, 21.2% [95% CI: 14.3–27.9%], indicating that cefepime/enmetazobactam was not only noninferior, but also met the criterion for superiority compared with piperacillin/tazobactam. Rates of drug-related treatment-emergent adverse events were 19.8% and 14.5%, respectively, and treatment-emergent serious adverse events were 4.3% and 3.7%, respectively. The most common treatment-emergent adverse events were elevations of liver function parameters: alanine aminotransferase (11.4 vs. 11.6%), aspartate aminotransferase (9.1 vs. 8.9%), and blood bilirubin (5.8 vs. 3.9%) [11].

6.2.4 Cefiderocol

Cefiderocol (S-649266) is a novel parenteral siderophore cephalosporin conjugated with a catechol moiety at the third-position side chain. Cefiderocol utilizes a novel mechanism of entry into the periplasmic space of Gram-negative bacteria and is broadly stable to ESBLs and carbapenemases. The in vitro activity of cefiderocol against *Pseudomonas aeruginosa* was enhanced under iron-depleted conditions, whereas that of ceftazidime was not affected. Cefiderocol was shown to have potent chelating activity with ferric iron, and extracellular iron was efficiently transported into *P. aeruginosa* cells in the presence of cefiderocol as well as siderophores, while enhanced transport of extracellular ferric iron was not observed when one of the hydroxyl groups of the catechol moiety of cefiderocol was replaced with a methoxy group. The authors conclude that cefiderocol forms a chelating complex with iron, which is actively transported into *P. aeruginosa* cells via iron transporters, resulting in potent antibacterial activity of cefiderocol against *P. aeruginosa* [12].

In total 189 non-fermentative Gram-negative bacteria (107 *Acinetobacter baumannii* and 82 *Pseudomonas aeruginosa*) and 282 Enterobacteriaceae (including 244 *Klebsiella pneumoniae*, 14 *Enterobacter cloacae*, and 11 *Providencia stuartii*) were studied. For both *A. baumannii* and *P. aeruginosa* the MIC 90 of cefiderocol was 0.5 mg/L. For *K. pneumoniae*, *E. cloacae*, and *P. stuartii* the MIC 90 of cefiderocol was 1, 1, and 0.5 mg/L, respectively. Cefiderocol exhibited greater antimicrobial activity in vitro against carbapenem-resistant Gram-negative bacteria than several comparator antibiotics. Tigecycline was the second most active antibiotic, followed by colistin [13].

In a phase 2 study the efficacy and safety of IV cefiderocol vs. IV IMP/CS was tested in hospitalized adults with complicated urinary tract infections with or without pyelonephritis or acute uncomplicated pyelonephritis caused by Gram-negative pathogens. Patients with Gram-negative pathogens were randomized on a 2:1 basis to receive cefiderocol (2 g) administered intravenously every 8 h, or high-dose IMP/CS (1/1 g) administered intravenously every 8 h, for 7–14 days in hospital. Of the 452 patients randomized, 448 were treated, and 371 met the definition of the micro-ITT population and were assessed for efficacy. All treated subjects were assessed for safety. The median duration of treatment was 9 days for both cefiderocol and IMP/CS for all populations [14].

Cefiderocol met the FDA primary efficacy endpoint of composite of clinical cure and microbiologic eradication at test of cure (TOC) in 72.6% of patients ($n = 252$) which was superior to IMP/CS at 54.6% ($n = 119$), a weighted difference of 18.58% (95% CI: 8.23, 28.92). Cefiderocol was well tolerated in the study, with 40% of patients experiencing an adverse event in the cefiderocol arm vs. 50% of patients in the IMP/CS arm. Serious adverse events (SAEs) occurred in 14 patients (4.7%) who received cefiderocol and 12 patients (8.1%) who received IMP/CS [15].

A randomized, open-label, multicenter, parallel-group, pathogen-focused, descriptive, phase 3 study was performed in 95 hospitals in 16 countries in North America, South America, Europe, and Asia in hospitalized patients with nosocomial pneumonia, bloodstream infections or sepsis, or complicated urinary tract infections (UTI), and evidence of a carbapenem-resistant Gram-negative pathogen. For patients with complicated UTI, the primary endpoint was microbiological eradication at test of cure in the carbapenem-resistant microbiological ITT population, which was achieved by nine (53%) of 17 patients in the cefiderocol group and one (20%) of five patients in the best available therapy group. In the safety population, treatment-emergent adverse events were noted for 91% (92 patients of 101) of the cefiderocol group and 96% (47 patients of 49) of the best available therapy group [15].

6.2.5 Meropenem/Vaborbactam

Vaborbactam is a novel cyclic boronic acid inhibitor of many class A and class C enzymes. It was designed and synthesized to be a potent inhibitor of serine carbapenemases, and KPC in particular. In vitro data suggest that meropenem-vaborbactam (M-V) is highly active against KPC-producing Enterobacteriaceae (*K. pneumoniae*: MIC_{50} [M-V] = 0.06–4 and 0.03–8 mg/mL; MIC_{90} = 2/4 and 0.5/8 mg/mL). Little effect on *A. baumannii* containing OXA-type carbapenemases was observed [7, 16].

A phase 3, multicenter, randomized, double-blind, double-dummy study (TANGO I) to evaluate the efficacy, safety, and tolerability of M-V (Vabomere®) compared to piperacillin/tazobactam (P-T) in the treatment of complicated urinary tract infections, including acute pyelonephritis, in adults was completed in April 28, 2016. M-V (meropenem 2 g plus vaborbactam 2 g), administered intravenously (IV) every 8 h (q8h) vs. P-T (piperacillin 4 g plus tazobactam 0.5 g), q8h. After a minimum of 15 IV doses levofloxacin 500 mg could be administered orally every 24 h (q24h), if clinically indicated. Total treatment was 10 days, unless a participant had baseline bacteremia where up to 14 days of therapy could be administered IV (https://clinicaltrials.gov/ct2/show/NCT02166476).

Of 550 subjects randomized, 374 (68.0%) were included in m-MITT (165/192 [85.9%] in M-V and 154/182 [84.6%] in P-T groups had baseline Enterobacteriaceae). Mean duration of IV therapy was 8 days. At the end of intravenous treatment, clinical cure was observed with M-V in 162/165 = 98.2% and with P-T in 147/154 = 95.5% of the patients. Microbiological eradication was found in 161/165 = 97.6% with M-V and 142/154 = 92.2% with P-T. Clinical outcomes were > 90% across all MICs. Although 19.5% of baseline Enterobacteriaceae isolates were non-susceptible to P-T, clinical and microbiologic outcomes were similar for subjects with susceptible and non-susceptible isolates ($p > 0.1$) [17–19].

Approximately 7 days after completing treatment, 77% of patients treated with M-V compared with 73% of patients treated with piperacillin/tazobactam had resolved symptoms and a negative urine culture. The most common adverse reactions in patients taking M-V were headache, infusion site reactions, and diarrhea. M-V is associated with serious risks including allergic reactions and seizures. M-V should not be used in patients with a history of anaphylaxis, a type of severe allergic reaction to products in the class of drugs called beta-lactams [17–19].

TANGO-2 is a multicenter, randomized, open-label phase III clinical trial of M-V vs. "best available therapy (BAT)" in patients with serious infections (cUTI, bacteremia, hospital-acquired or ventilator-associated bacterial pneumonia, and complicated intraabdominal infections) suspected or documented to be caused by carbapenem-resistant Enterobacteriaceae (CRE). Patients with CRE were randomized to receive either meropenem-vaborbactam monotherapy or the best available therapy for up to 14 days. Patients randomized to the BAT arm of the trial were given antimicrobial therapy selected for each patient by the investigator based on laboratory and other patient data, and thus represents the current standard of care used for the treatment of CRE infections.

The TANGO-2 trial was stopped early, based on an analysis of 72 patients, including 43 patients with microbiologically evaluable CRE of blood, lung, urinary tract, and abdominal organs, because M-V demonstrated improved clinical cure rates across all infection types and reduced rate of renal adverse events compared to BAT and the risk-benefit analysis of available data no longer supported randomization of additional patients to the BAT comparator arm [20].

6.2.6 Imipenem/Relebactam

Relebactam is a non-β-lactam serine β-lactamase inhibitor, similar to avibactam, that was designed to have inhibitory activity against class A and C β-lactamases. In vitro assays with carbapenem-resistant Enterobacteriaceae isolates demonstrated that MICs were significantly lowered when imipenem was tested with relebactam against KPC-producing *K. pneumoniae* (MIC_{50} = 0.25/4 mg/mL; MIC_{90} = 1/4 mg/mL). Compared to imipenem alone, little reduction in imipenem-relebactam MICs was noted in OXA-48-producing *K. pneumoniae* or OXA-23-producing *A. baumannii*, suggesting that relebactam, unlike avibactam, does not have significant activity against the class D enzymes [13, 14]. Clinical trials have used imipenem-cilastatin (IMP/CS) combined with relebactam in phase 2 and phase 3 clinical trials. Phase 2 clinical trials investigating the safety, tolerability, and efficacy of IMP/CS-relebactam in treating complicated urinary tract infections and complicated intra-abdominal infections have been completed [7].

To explore relebactam's safety, tolerability, and efficacy, a randomized (1:1:1), controlled, Phase 2 trial was conducted comparing IMP/CS (500/500 mg) + relebactam 250 mg, IMP/CS (500/500 mg) + relebactam 125 mg, and IMP/CS (500/500 mg) alone in adults with complicated urinary tract infections (cUTI) or acute pyelonephritis, regardless of baseline pathogen susceptibility. Treatment was administered intravenously every 6 h for 4–14 days, with optional step-down to oral ciprofloxacin. The primary endpoint was favorable microbiological response rate (pathogen eradication) at discontinuation of intravenous therapy (DCIV) in the microbiologically evaluable (ME) population.

At DCIV, 71 patients in the IMP/CS + 250 mg relebactam, 79 in the IMP/CS + 125 mg relebactam, and 80 in the IMP/CS-only group were ME; 51.7% had cUTI, and 48.3% acute pyelonephritis. Microbiological response rates were 95.5%, 98.6%, and 98.7%, respectively, confirming noninferiority of both IMO/CS + relebactam doses to IMP/CS alone. Clinical response rates were 97.1%, 98.7%, and 98.8%, respectively. All 23 ME patients with IMP non-susceptible pathogens had favorable DCIV microbiological responses (100% in each group). Among all 298 patients treated, 28.3%, 29.3%, and 30.0% of patients, respectively, had treatment-emergent adverse events. The most common treatment-related adverse events across groups (1.0–4.0%) were diarrhea, nausea, and headache. It was concluded that IMP/CS + relebactam (250 or 125 mg) was as effective as IMP/CS alone for treatment of cUTI. Both relebactam-containing regimens were well tolerated [21].

A phase 3 trial—RESTORE-IMI 1—is underway investigating efficacy and safety of IMP/CS + relebactam vs. colistin + IMP/CS for cUTI due to IMP-resistant pathogens.

Group 1: IMP/CS—relebactam at (200/100 mg–500/250 mg depending on renal function) IV once every 6 h and placebo for colistimethate sodium (CMS) IV infusion once every 12 h. Group 2: CMS [colistimethate base activity 300 mg (~720 mg CMS)] IV loading dose, followed by colistimethate base activity 75–150 mg (~180–360 mg CMS) depending on renal function IV infusion once every 12 h and IMP/CS (200–500 mg depending on renal function) IV infusion once every 6 h. Group 3: participants with documented IMP-resistant and colistin-resistant bacterial infections will receive open-label IMP/CS—relebactam (200/100–500/250 mg depending on renal function) IV infusion once every 6 h. Treatment duration: 5–21 days (https://clinicaltrials.gov/ct2/show/NCT02452047).

6.2.7 Tebipenem Pivoxil Hydrobromide

Tebipenem pivoxil hydrobromide, a prodrug of tebipenem, is the first orally available carbapenem antibiotic. It has shown potent antimicrobial activity in vitro against clinical isolates of Enterobacterales species from patients with UTI, including those producing extended-spectrum β-lactamases (ESBLs) and/or AmpC β-lactamase. Similar to other carbapenems, tebipenem was resistant to hydrolysis by TEM-1, CTX-M, and AmpC β-lactamases but was susceptible to hydrolysis by KPC, OXA-48, and NDM-1 enzymes as the other carbapenems [22].

The antimicrobial activity of tebipenem and other carbapenem agents was also tested in vitro against a set of clinical uropathogens, including *Escherichia coli* (101 isolates), *Klebsiella pneumoniae* (208 isolates), and *Proteus mirabilis* (103 isolates) species [23]. Within each species tested, tebipenem showed equivalent $MIC_{50/90}$ values to those of meropenem and consistently displayed MIC90 values eightfold lower than imipenem. All carbapenem agents, however, were less active (MIC_{50}, ≥8 mg/L) against isolates carrying carbapenemase genes. In a pharmacokinetic study it was shown, that approximately 55–60% of tebipenem is recovered in the urine [24]. Overall, the microbiological and pharmacokinetic data support its utility as an oral therapy for adult complicated UTI.

In a phase 3 study including patients with complicated UTI or acute pyelonephritis, oral tebipenem pivoxil hydrobromide (600 mg t.i.d.) was not inferior to IV ertapenem (ig once daily) for 7–10 days (or up to 14 days in patients with bacteremia) and had a similar safety profile as well. Tebipenem pivoxil hydrobromide may provide an option for the treatment of complicated UTI and acute pyelonephritis due to antibiotic-resistant uropathogens [25].

6.2.8 Sulopenem

Sulopenem, a broad-spectrum thiopenem β–lactam antibiotic being developed for treatment of infections caused by multidrug-resistant bacteria, is active against species of Enterobacterales that encode ESBLs or AmpC–type β–lactamases that confer resistance to third-generation cephalosporins, similar to ertapenem [26]. The availability of both intravenous (IV) and oral formulations will facilitate earlier hospital discharge. Sulopenem etzadroxil, the prodrug of intravenous sulopenem, is an oral thiopenem. If combined with probenecid to extend its half-life in plasma, it obtains high concentrations in urine. The oral form was evaluated for treatment of uncomplicated UTI in women [27] and the intravenous (IV) and oral formulation as step down therapy for complicated UTI including pyelonephritis in hospitalized patients [28]. Of 1392 treated patients with complicated UTI, 444 and 440 treated with sulopenem and ertapenem, respectively, had a positive baseline urine culture and were eligible for the primary efficacy analyses. Eligible patients were randomized 1:1 to receive either IV sulopenem 1000 mg once daily followed by sulopenem etzadroxil 500 mg/probenecid 500 mg (referred to as oral sulopenem) twice daily or IV ertapenem 1000 mg once daily followed by oral ciprofloxacin 500 mg or amoxicillin–clavulanate 875 mg twice daily; duration of treatment was to be 7–10 days. Treatment could be extended to 14 days for patients with bacteremia at baseline. After at least 5 days of IV therapy, patients could be switched to oral therapy if they could tolerate oral medications, if signs and symptoms of infection were improving, and if the baseline pathogen was susceptible to the oral study drugs. Study drug doses could be adjusted for patients with severe renal impairment (creatinine clearance <30 mL/min) who were not on regular hemodialysis.

Extended-spectrum β-lactamase-producing organisms were identified in 26.6% of patients and fluoroquinolone-nonsusceptible pathogens in 38.6%. For the primary end point, noninferiority of sulopenem to the comparator regimen was not demonstrated, 67.8 vs. 73.9% (difference, −6.1%; 95% confidence interval, −12.0 to −0.1%). The difference was driven by a lower rate of asymptomatic bacteriuria in the subgroup of ertapenem-treated patients who stepped down to ciprofloxacin. No substantial difference in overall response was observed at any other time point. Both IV and oral formulations of sulopenem were well-tolerated and compared favorably to the comparator [28].

6.3 Plazomicin

Plazomicin (PLZ) is a novel aminoglycoside that was synthetically derived from sisomicin. Like other aminoglycosides, it is a bactericidal agent that works primarily through inhibition of protein synthesis. PLZ is structurally similar to the traditional aminoglycosides (amikacin, gentamicin, tobramycin), though was modified to resist aminoglycoside-modifying enzymes that are often present in CRE. PLZ is not affected by carbapenemase production and has demonstrated good in vitro activity against carbapenem-resistant isolates of *K. pneumoniae*, *E. coli*, and *Enterobacter* species producing a variety of carbapenemases and ESBLs. Of note, in one study PLZ was less active vs. isolates producing NDM-1 enzymes due to the co-existence of ArmA and RmtC 16S rRNA methyltransferases. The presence of 16S rRNA methyltransferase in Enterobacteriaceae, which modifies the ribosomal site that binds PLZ, leads to plazomicin resistance. PLZ has been demonstrated to be more potent than other aminoglycosides in treating Enterobacteriaceae [7, 29, 30]. The in vitro activity of PLZ was evaluated against 300 multidrug-resistant (MDR) (carbapenemase and/or ESBL-producing) isolates from four hospitals in Athens, an area where carbapenemase-producing organisms are endemic. PLZ retained activity (MICs ≤4 μg/mL) against all isolates of *Klebsiella pneumoniae*, *Escherichia coli*, and *Enterobacter* spp. tested with MIC_{50} and MIC_{90} of 1 and 2 μg/mL, respectively, irrespective of their MDR phenotype, and it represents a promising alternative for the treatment of the most problematic Gram-negative pathogens [7, 29, 30].

Safety and efficacy of PLZ were evaluated in a double-blind, randomized, comparator-controlled phase 2 study in patients with cUTI or AP. Patients were randomized 2:1 to IV PLZ (10 or 15 mg/kg) or IV levofloxacin (LVX, 750 mg), administered once daily for 5 days. Co-primary efficacy endpoints were microbiological eradication (MBE) at test-of-cure (TOC) 7 ± 2 days after the last treatment in patients with 1 or 2 causative pathogens in urine at baseline (MITT population) and in patients who were microbiologically evaluable (ME). In the MITT population, MBE rates at TOC were 37/63 = 58.7% (95% CI: 45.6, 71.0) and 17/29 = 58.6% (95% CI: 38.9, 76.5). MBE rates in the ME population were 37/42 = 88.1% (95% CI: 74.4, 96.0) and 17/21 = 81.0% (95% CI: 58.1, 94.6). At TOC, 69.8% and 65.5% in MITT and 76.2% and 76.2% in ME were assessed as clinically cured by the investigator. *E. coli* was the most common pathogen. Adverse events (AEs) considered related to study treatment occurred in 17.7% and 27.3% of patients and were typically mild or moderate. Serious AEs occurred in 1 PLZ (unrelated) and 2 LVX patients (1 related; 1 unrelated). It was concluded that PLZ was well tolerated with no unexpected toxicities. The efficacy of PLZ was similar to LVX as determined by microbiological and clinical outcomes [31].

In a phase 3, randomized, multicenter, double-blind study (EPIC), the Efficacy and Safety of PLZ was compared with meropenem followed by optional oral therapy for the treatment of cUTI and acute pyelonephritis (AP) in adults (https://clinicaltrials.gov/ct2/show/NCT02486627). Hospitalized patients with cUTI or AP received IV PLZ (15 mg/kg q24h) or IV meropenem (1 g q8h) for 4–7 days, followed by optional oral therapy, for a total of 7–10 days of therapy. Microbiological eradication (reduction of baseline pathogen to <10^4 CFU/mL), clinical cure (based on baseline symptoms), and composite cure (combined microbiological eradication and clinical cure) rates at the end-of-IV therapy (EOIV) and test-of-cure (TOC; Day 15–19) visits in the microbiological modified intent-to-treat (mMITT) population were analyzed for cUTI and AP subgroups. At TOC, PLZ achieved higher composite cure rates than meropenem in cUTI (84/107 = 78.5% vs. 82/119 = 68.9%; difference 9.6 (95% CI: −2.6 to 21.3) and AP (72/84 = 85.7% vs. 56/78 = 71.8%; difference 13.9 (95% CI: 0.4 to 27.1), driven by higher microbiological eradication rates in each subgroup. The incidence of AEs, including serious AEs and AEs leading to discontinuation of IV study drug, was low and comparable between treatment arms [32].

6.3.1 Finafloxacin

Finafloxacin, an investigational fluoroquinolone, suitable for intravenous and oral administration, is being developed as sequential therapy of bacterial infections including the treatment of UTIs [33–36]. The compound exhibits essential features required to successfully treat such infections: good activity against Gram-positive, Gram-negative, and anaerobic pathogens with a bactericidal mechanism of action, a high level of excretion in the urine, and increased potency at acidic pH. Fluoroquinolones inhibit the activity of bacterial type II topoisomerases, i.e., DNA-gyrase and topoisomerase IV. Despite an affinity of most second- and third-generation fluoroquinolones to both targets, they usually inhibit one enzyme preferentially facilitating development of bacterial resistance. Methoxy-quinolones, however, inhibit both enzymes at almost the same concentrations which may potentially limit emergence of resistance [36].

In a phase II, multicenter, double-blind, double-dummy, active-control, randomized clinical trial, finafloxacin (IV and oral) was examined for a total of 5 days (FINA05) or for a total of 10 days (FINA10) vs. ciprofloxacin (IV and oral) for a total of 10 days (CIPRO10) for the treatment of cUTI and/or acute pyelonephritis. Patients were randomized 1:1:1 into one of the three treatment arms. Physicians could switch from the initial IV to oral dosing after day 3. The study lasted 24 ± 2 days with examinations on day 3, on day 10 + 2 days and on day 17 ± 2 days (TOC).

The treatment success (combined clinical and microbiological response, primary endpoint) for the mITT population at test of cure (TOC) visit on day 17 was 70.3% (95% CI: 57.6–81.1%) in the FINA05 group, 67.6% (55.2–78.5%) in the FINA10 group, and 57.4% (44.1–70.0%) in the CIPRO10 group. Finafloxacin dosed for 5 or 10 days showed higher treatment success rates than ciprofloxacin dosed for 10 days. The microbiological eradication rate of ciprofloxacin was lower in the patient group with an acidic urine pH as compared to those with an alkaline urine-pH, while finafloxacin's microbiological eradication rate was equally high at either pH range as determined by the microbiological response on day 3. The safety profiles of the 3 treatment groups were equivalent, and the majority of the AEs were mild to moderate in severity and regarded to be unrelated to study medication [36].

6.3.2 Sitafloxacin

Sitafloxacin, a new oral fluoroquinolone, is more active than levofloxacin, ciprofloxacin, and moxifloxacin against isolated bacteria from Thai patients with UTI and lower respiratory infections including antibiotic-resistant bacteria, such as MRSA, ESBL-producing Gram-negatives, and carbapenem-resistant *A. baumannii* [37], and against clinical isolates of less common nonfermenting Gram-negative bacteria, such as *Stenotrophomonas maltophilia* (0.25/1 mg/L), *Burkholderia cepacia* complex (0.25/2 mg/L), *Achromobacter xylosoxidans* (0.25/1 mg/L), and *Chryseobacterium gleum* (1/2 mg/L), but less active for *Elizabethkingia* (1/8 mg/L) and *Chryseobacterium indologenes* (16/32 mg/L) [38].

In a pilot study oral sitafloxacin (19 patients) and IV ertapenem (17 patients) were compared in the treatment of non-bacteremic acute pyelonephritis caused by *E. coli* (ESBL-EC). At day 10, all but one patient in the ertapenem group had clinical cure. Microbiological eradication was comparable between the sitafloxacin and ertapenem groups (84.2 vs. 75%, $p = 0.677$). There were no significant adverse effects [39].

In a randomized, active-controlled clinical trial, patients with complicated UTI were randomized to receive sitafloxacin 100-mg twice daily or levofloxacin 500-mg qd orally for 10–14 days. The clinical cure rate was 81.8% (27/33) in the sitafloxacin group and 76.9% (20/26) in the levofloxacin group corresponding to the bacterial eradication rate of 93.3% (14/15) and 63.6% (7/11) (all $p > 0.05$), respectively.

Sitafloxacin and levofloxacin showed similar incidence of drug-related adverse events [40].

6.4 Eravacycline

Eravacycline is a novel synthetic fluorocycline that is active against most Gram-negative species. In vitro assays have demonstrated that eravacycline is two- to four-fold more potent than tigecycline against CRE [13]. A phase 2, randomized, double-blind study was done to evaluate the efficacy and safety of eravacycline compared with ertapenem in adult hospitalized patients with complicated intra-abdominal infections (cIAIs) [41].

A phase 3, randomized, multicenter, double-blind study to evaluate the efficacy and safety of eravacycline 1.5 mg/kg vs. 750 mg levofloxacin for the treatment of cUTI or acute pyelonephritis (IGNITE2) with an oral step-down did not achieve noninferiority. These data remain unpublished to date, and thus further studies are needed to establish the role of eravacycline in treating CRE [42]. Eravacycline may have advantages over tigecycline due to its improved in vitro activity against CRE isolates, higher serum levels, and better tolerability, though further investigation is needed [7].

6.5 Fosfomycin Disodium

The oral form, fosfomycin trometamol, is well known for many years and included in several guidelines for treatment of uncomplicated cystitis in women [3, 4]. The parenteral form, fosfomycin disodium, for treatment of complicated UTI incl. Pyelonephritis and also sepsis has recently experienced a revival [43, 44]. In this clinical trial including 143 adults with multidrug-resistant bacteremic urinary tract infections due to *E. coli* patients were randomized 1–1 to receive intravenous fosfomycin disodium at 4 g every 6 h (70 participants) or a comparator (ceftriaxone or meropenem if resistant; 73 participants) with the option to switch to oral fosfomycin trometamol for the fosfomycin group or an active oral drug or parenteral ertapenem for the comparator group after 4 days. Clinical and microbiological cure was achieved by 68.6% of patients treated with fosfomycin and 78.1% of patients treated with comparators, with fosfomycin not reaching noninferiority. This was due to an increased rate of adverse event–related discontinuations with fosfomycin (8.5 vs. 0%). While fosfomycin did not demonstrate noninferiority, the findings of this study suggest that it may still be considered among selected patients [44].

6.6 Conclusion

Thus, several antibiotic substances are currently upon marketing, or in the late clinical phase of development. Nevertheless, unique novel substances are rare; therefore, antimicrobial stewardship plays a more and more important role to preserve the antibiotic substances available.

References

1. Zowawi HM, Harris PNA, Roberts MJ, Tambyah PA, Schembri MA, Pezzani MD, Williamson DA, Paterson DL. The emerging threat of multidrug-resistant gram-negative bacteria in urology. Nat Rev Urol. 2015;12:570–84.
2. Tandogdu Z, Cek M, Wagenlehner F, Naber K, Tenke P, van Ostrum E, Bjerklund JT. Resistance patterns of nosocomial urinary tract infections in urology departments: 8-year results of the global prevalence of infections in urology study. World J Urol. 2014;32:791–801.
3. Bonkat G, Pickard R, Bartoletti R, Bruyère F, Geerlings SE, Wagenlehner F, Wullt B, Cai T, Köves B, Pilatz A, Pradere B, Veeratterapillay R. EAU guidelines on urological infections. Arnhem: European Association of Urology; 2017. http://uroweb.org/guideline/urological-infections/. Accessed 31 Jan 2018.
4. Kranz J, Schmidt S, Lebert C, Schneidewind L, Mandraka F, Kunze M, Helbig S, Vahlensieck W, Naber K, Schmiemann G, Wagenlehner FM. The 2017 update of the German clinical guideline on epidemiology, diagnostics, therapy, prevention and management of uncomplicated urinary tract infections in adult patients. Part II: therapy and prevention. Urol Int. 2018;100(3):271–8. https://doi.org/10.1159/000487645.
5. Wagenlehner FM, Umeh O, Steenbergen J, Yuan G, Darouiche RO. Ceftolozane-tazobactam compared with levofloxacin in the treatment of complicated urinary-tract infections, including pyelonephritis: a randomised, double-blind, phase 3 trial (ASPECT-cUTI). Lancet. 2015;385:1949–56.
6. Zhanel GG, Lawson CD, Adam H, Schweizer F, Zelenitsky S, Lagacé-Wiens PR, Denisuik A, Rubinstein E, Gin AS, Hoban DJ, Lynch JP 3rd, Karlowsky JA. Ceftazidime-avibactam: a novel cephalosporin/β-lactamase inhibitor combination. Drugs. 2013;73:159–77.
7. Thaden JT, Pogue JM, Kaye KS. Role of newer and re-emerging older agents in the treatment of infections caused by carbapenem-resistant Enterobacteriaceae. Virilence. 2017;8:403–16.
8. Wagenlehner FM, Sobel JD, Newell P, Armstrong J, Huang X, Stone GG, Yates K, Gasink LB. Ceftazidime-avibactam versus doripenem for the treatment of complicated urinary tract infections, including acute pyelonephritis: RECAPTURE, a phase 3 randomized trial program. Clin Infect Dis. 2016;63:754–62.
9. Belley A, Morrissey I, Hawser S, Kothari N, Knechtle P. Third-generation cephalosporin resistance in clinical isolates of enterobacterales collected between 2016–2018 from USA and Europe: genotypic analysis of β-lactamases and comparative in vitro activity of cefepime/enmetazobactam. J Glob Antimicrob Resist. 2021;25:93–101. https://doi.org/10.1016/j.jgar.2021.02.031.
10. Carmeli Y, Knechtle P, Hardenberg J, Knecht M. Randomized phase 2 study of cefepime combined with the novel extended Spectrum β-lactamase inhibitor enmetazobactam in hospitalized adults with complicated urinary tract infections (cUTI) including acute pyelonephritis (AP). Poster Abstracts OFID. 2019;6(Suppl 2):S539.
11. Kaye KS, Belley A, Barth P, Lahlou O, Knechtle P, Motta P, Velicitat P. Effect of cefepime/enmetazobactam vs piperacillin/tazobactam on clinical cure and microbiological eradication in patients with complicated urinary tract infection or acute pyelonephritis. A randomized clinical trial. JAMA. 2022;328(13):1304–14. https://doi.org/10.1001/jama.2022.17034.

12. Ito A, Nishikawa T, Matsumoto S, Yoshizawa H, Sato T, Nakamura R, Tsuji M, Yamano Y. Siderophore cephalosporin Cefiderocol utilizes ferric iron transporter systems for antibacterial activity against Pseudomonas aeruginosa. Antimicrob Agents Chemother. 2016;60:7396–401.
13. Falagas ME, Skalidis T, Vardakas KZ, Legakis NJ, Hellenic Cefiderocol Study Group. Activity of cefiderocol (S-649266) against carbapenem-resistant gram-negative bacteria collected from inpatients in Greek hospitals. J Antimicrob Chemother. 2017;72:1704–8.
14. Portsmouth S, van Veenhuyzen D, Echols R, Machida M, Ferreira JCA, Ariyasu M, Tenke P, Den Nagata T. Cefiderocol versus imipenem-cilastatin for the treatment of complicated urinary tract infections caused by gram-negative uropathogens: a phase 2, randomised, double-blind, non-inferiority trial. Lancet Infect Dis. 2018;18(12):1319–28. https://doi.org/10.1016/S1473-3099(18)30554-1.
15. Bassetti M, Echols R, Matsunaga Y, Ariyasu M, Doi Y, Ferrer R, Lodise TP, Naas T, Niki Y, Paterson DL, Portsmouth S, Torre-Cisneros J, Toyoizumi K, Wunderink RG, Nagata TD. Efficacy and safety of cefiderocol or best available therapy for the treatment of serious infections caused by carbapenem-resistant gram-negative bacteria (CREDIBLE-CR): a randomised, open-label, multicentre, pathogen-focused, descriptive, phase 3 trial. Lancet Infect Dis. 2021;21(2):226–40. https://doi.org/10.1016/S1473-3099(20)30796-9.
16. Zhanel GG, Lawrence CK, Adam H, Schweizer F, Zelenitsky S, Zhanel M, Lagacé-Wiens PRS, Walkty A, Denisuik A, Golden A, Gin AS, Hoban DJ, Lynch JP 3rd, Karlowsky JA. Imipenem-relebactam and meropenem-vaborbactam: two novel carbapenem-β-lactamase inhibitor combinations. Drugs. 2018;78(1):65–98. https://doi.org/10.1007/s40265-017-0851-9.
17. Walsh TJ, Tanaya Bhowmick T, Darouiche R, Zaitsev V, Giamarellos-Bourboulis E, Shorr AF, Fedosiuk E, File TM Jr, Loutit JS, Lomovskaya O, Dudley MN, Perlin D. Meropenem-vaborbactam vs. piperacillin-tazobactam in TANGO I (a Phase 3 randomized, double-blind trial): outcomes by baseline MIC in adults with complicated urinary tract infections or acute pyelonephritis. Open Forum Infect Dis. 2017;4(suppl.1):S536. https://doi.org/10.1093/ofid/ofx163.1396.
18. Kaye KS, Bhowmick T, Metallidis S, Bleasdale SC, Sagan OS, Stus V, Vazquez J, Zaitsev V, Bidair M, Chorvat E, Dragoescu PO, Fedosiuk E, Horcajada JP, Murta C, Sarychev Y, Stoev V, Morgan E, Fusaro K, Griffith D, Lomovskaya O, Alexander EL, Loutit J, Dudley MN, Giamarellos-Bourboulis EJ. Effect of meropenem-vaborbactam vs piperacillin-tazobactam on clinical cure or improvement and microbial rradication in complicated urinary tract iInfection: the TANGO I randomized clinical trial. JAMA. 2018;319(8):788–99. https://doi.org/10.1001/jama.2018.0438.
19. Dhillon S. Meropenem/vaborbactam: a review in complicated urinary tract infections. Drugs. 2018;78:1259–70. https://doi.org/10.1007/s40265-018-0966-7.
20. Wunderink RG, Giamarellos-Bourboulis EJ, Rahav G, Mathers AJ, Bassetti M, Vazquez J, Cornely OA, Solomkin J, Bhowmick T, Bishara J, Daikos GL, Felton T, Lopez Furst MJ, Kwak EJ, Menichetti F, Oren I, Alexander EL, Griffith D, Lomovskaya O, Loutit J, Zhang S, Dudley MN, Kaye KS. Effect and safety of meropenem–vaborbactam versus best-available therapy in patients with carbapenem-resistant Enterobacteriaceae infections: the TANGO II randomized clinical trial. Infect Dis Ther. 2018;7(4):439–55. https://doi.org/10.1007/s40121-018-0214-1.
21. Sims M, Mariyanovski V, McLeroth P, Akers W, Lee YC, Brown ML, Du J, Pedley A, Kartsonis NA, Paschke A. Prospective, randomized, double-blind, phase 2 dose-ranging study comparing efficacy and safety of imipenem/cilastatin plus relebactam with imipenem/cilastatin alone in patients with complicated urinary tract infections. J Antimicrob Chemother. 2017;72:2616–26.
22. Sun Z, Su L, Cotroneo N, Critchley I, Pucci M, Jain A, Palzkill T. Evaluation of tebipenem hydrolysis by β-lactamases prevalent in complicated urinary tract infections. Antimicrob Agents Chemother. 2022;66(5):e0239621. https://doi.org/10.1128/aac.02396-21.
23. Arends SJR, Rhomberg PR, Cotroneo N, Rubio A, Flamm RK, Mendes RE. Antimicrobial activity evaluation of tebipenem (SPR859), an orally available carbapenem, against a global set of Enterobacteriaceae isolates, including a challenge set of organisms. Antimicrob Agents Chemother. 2019;63(6):e02618. https://doi.org/10.1128/AAC.02618-18.

24. Eckburg PB, Jain A, Walpole S, Moore G, Utley L, Manyak E, Dane A, Melnick D. Safety, pharmacokinetics, and food effect of tebipenem pivoxil hydrobromide after single and multiple ascending oral doses in healthy adult subjects. Antimicrob Agents Chemother. 2019;63(9):e00618–9. https://doi.org/10.1128/AAC.00618-19.
25. Eckburg PB, Muir L, Critchley IA, Walpole S, Kwak H, Phelan AM, Moore G, Jain A, Keutzer T, Dane A, Melnick D, Talley AK. Oral tebipenem pivoxil hydrobromide in complicated urinary tract infection. N Engl JMed. 2022;386(14):1327–38.
26. Karlowsky JA, Adam HJ, Baxter MR, et al. In vitro activity of sulopenem, an oral penem, against urinary isolates of Escherichia coli. Antimicrob Agents Chemother. 2018;63:e01832–18.
27. Dunne MW, Aronin SI, Das AF, Akinapelli K, Zelasky MT, Puttagunta S, Boucher HW. Sulopenem or ciprofloxacin for the treatment of uncomplicated urinary tract iInfections in women: a phase 3, randomized trial. Clin Infect Dis. 2023;76(1):66–77. https://doi.org/10.1093/cid/ciac738.
28. Dunne MW, Aronin SI, Das AF, Akinapelli K, Breen J, Zelasky MT, Puttagunta S. Sulopenem for the treatment of complicated urinary tract infections including pyelonephritis: a phase 3, randomized trial. Clin Infect Dis. 2023;76(1):78–88. https://doi.org/10.1093/cid/ciac704.
29. Galani I, Souli M, Daikos GL, Chrysouli Z, Poulakou G, Psichogiou M, Panagea T, Argyropoulou A, Stefanou I, Plakias G, Giamarellou H, Petrikkos G. Activity of plazomicin (ACHN-490) against MDR clinical isolates of Klebsiella pneumoniae, Escherichia coli, and Enterobacter spp. from Athens, Greece. J Chemother. 2012;24:191–4.
30. Zhanel GG, Lawson CD, Zelenitsky S, Findlay B, Schweizer F, Adam H, Walkty A, Rubinstein E, Gin AS, Hoban DJ, Lynch JP, Karlowsky JA. Comparison of the next-generation aminoglycoside plazomicin to gentamicin, tobramycin and amikacin. Expert Rev Anti-Infect Ther. 2012;10:459–73.
31. Riddle VD, Cebrik DS, Armstrong ES, Cass RT, Clobes TC, Hillan KJ. Plazomicin safety and efficacy in patients with complicated urinary tract infection (cUTI) or acute pyelonephritis (AP) (Poster L2-2118a). 52nd Interscience Conference on Antimicrobial Agents and Chemotherapy (ICAAC), San Francisco, USA, Sept 9–12, 2012. https://static1.squarespace.com/static/51199d96e4b084d1d0b105c3/t/51f97f11e4b022983127d741/1375305489164/ICAAC2012_Poster_L2-2118a.pdf. Accessed 31 Jan 2018.
32. Cloutier DJ, Miller LG, Komirenko AS, Cebrik DS, Krause KM, Keepers TR, Connolly LE, Wagenlehner FME. Plazomicin versus meropenem for the treatment of complicated urinary tract infection and acute pyelonephritis: results of the EPIC Study. Poster 1855. 27th European Congress of Clinical Microbiology and Infectious Diseases (ECCMID), Vienna, Austria, April 22-25, 2017. https://static1.squarespace.com/static/51199d96e4b084d1d0b105c3/t/58fb6714b8a79b0b91ba96a6/1492870939778/ECCMID+17-EPIC_Final.pdf; Accessed 31 Jan 2018; https://idsa.confex.com/idsa/2017/webprogram/Paper65235.html. Accessed 31 Jan 2018.
33. Wagenlehner FM, Wagenlehner CM, Blenk B, Blenk H, Schubert S, Dalhoff A, Naber KG. Urinary pharmacokinetics and bactericidal activity of finafloxacin (200 and 800 mg) in healthy volunteers receiving a single oral dose. Chemotherapy. 2011;57(2):97–107. https://doi.org/10.1159/000321028.
34. Bartoletti R, Cai T, Perletti G, ME Wagenlehner F, Bjerklund Johansen TE. Finafloxacin for the treatment of urinary tract infections. Expert Opin Investig Drugs. 2015;24(7):957–63. https://doi.org/10.1517/13543784.2015.1052401.
35. Taubert M, Lückermann M, Vente A, Dalhoff A, Fuhr U. Population pharmacokinetics of finafloxacin in healthy volunteers and patients with complicated urinary tract infections. Antimicrob Agents Chemother. 2018;62(4):e02328–17. https://doi.org/10.1128/AAC.02328-17.
36. Wagenlehner F, Nowicki M, Bentley C, Lückermann M, Wohlert S, Fischer C, Vente A, Naber K, Dalhoff A. Explorative randomized phase II clinical study of the efficacy and safety of finafloxacin versus ciprofloxacin for treatment of complicated urinary tract infections. Antimicrob Agents Chemother. 2018;62(4):e02317. https://doi.org/10.1128/AAC.02317-17.
37. Tiengrim S, Phiboonbanakit D, Thunyaharn S, Tantisiriwat W, Santiwatanakul S, Susaengrat W, Srisurat N, Malithong A, Srisangchan P, Thamlikitkul V. Comparative in vitro activity of

sitafloxacin against bacteria isolated from Thai patients with urinary tract infections and lower respiratory tract infections. J Med Assoc Thail. 2012;95(Suppl 2):S6–17.
38. Zhou X, Wang L, Wu S, Yang Y, Guo Y, Shen S, Hu F, Yang F. Antimicrobial activities of sitafloxacin and comparators against the clinical isolates of less common nonfermenting gram-negative bacteria. J Glob Antimicrob Resist. 2022;30:123–6. https://doi.org/10.1016/j.jgar.2022.06.003.
39. Malaisri C, Phuphuakrat A, Wibulpolprasert A, Santanirand P, Kiertiburanakul S. A randomized controlled trial of sitafloxacin vs. ertapenem as a switch therapy after treatment for acute pyelonephritis caused by extended-spectrum beta-lactamase-producing Escherichia coli: A pilot study. J Infect Chemother. 2017;23(8):556–62.
40. Li Y, Yin Y, Peng X, Zheng H, Fu F, Liu Z, Wu X, Wu X, Zheng S, Chen N, He L, Ren L, Ni Z, Li D, Liang P, Lv X, Zhang Y. A randomized, active-controlled, multicentre clinical trial to evaluate the efficacy and safety of oral sitafloxacin versus levofloxacin in Chinese adults with acute uncomplicated or complicated urinary tract infection. Ann Med. 2021;53(1):217–26. https://doi.org/10.1080/07853890.2020.1861322.
41. Solomkin JS, Ramesh MK, Cesnauskas G, Novikovs N, Stefanova P, Sutcliffe JA, Walpole SM, Horn PT. Phase 2, randomized, double-blind study of the efficacy and safety of two dose regimens of eravacycline versus ertapenem for adult community-acquired complicated intra-abdominal infections. Antimicrob Agents Chemother. 2014;58:1847–54.
42. Zhanel GG, Cheung D, Adam H, Zelenitsky S, Golden A, Schweizer F, Gorityala B, Lagacé-Wiens PRS, Walkty A, Gin AS, Hoban DJ, Karlowsky JA. Review of eravacycline, a novel fluorocycline antibacterial agent. Drugs. 2016;76(5):567–88.
43. Rosso-Fernández C, Sojo-Dorado J, Barriga A, Lavín-Alconero L, Palacios Z, López-Hernández I, Merino V, Camean M, Pascual A, Rodríguez-Baño J, and the FOREST Study Group. Fosfomycin versus meropenem in bacteraemic urinary tract infections caused by extended-spectrum β-lactamase-producing Escherichia coli (FOREST): study protocol for an investigator-driven randomised controlled trial. BMJ Open. 2015;5:e007363. https://doi.org/10.1136/bmjopen-2014-007363.
44. Sojo-Dorado J, López-Hernández I, Rosso-Fernandez C, Morales IM, Palacios-Baena ZR, Hernández-Torres A, de Lucas EM, Escolà-Vergé L, Bereciartua E, García-Vázquez E, Pintado V, Boix-Palop L, Natera-Kindelán C, Sorlí L, Borrell N, Giner-Oncina L, Amador-Prous C, Shaw E, Jover-Saenz A, Molina J, Martínez-Alvarez RM, Dueñas CJ, Calvo-Montes J, Silva JT, Cárdenes MA, Lecuona M, Pomar V, de Santis LV, Yagüe-Guirao G, Angeles Lobo-Acosta M, Merino-Bohórquez V, Pascual A, Rodríguez-Baño J, REIPI-GEIRAS-FOREST group. Effectiveness of fosfomycin for the treatment of multidrug-resistant Escherichia coli bacteremic urinary tract infections. A randomized clinical trial. JAMA Netw Open. 2022;5(1):e2137277. https://doi.org/10.1001/jamanetworkopen.2021.37277.

Part II

Treatment of Low Severity Urinary Tract Infections Without Risk Factors

Acute Uncomplicated and Complicated Cystitis: From Empiric Treatment to Antibiogram-Based Tailored Treatment

7

Michael McDonald, Darien Kameh, Mark E. Johnson, Truls E. Bjerklund Johansen, and Vladimir Mouraviev

Abbreviations

C&S	Culture and sensitivity
CFU	Colony forming units

Vladimir Mouraviev was deceased at the time of publication.
This chapter is an edited version of an original paper in "Reviews in Urology", 2017: Michael McDonald, Darien Kameh, Mark E. Johnson, Truls E. Bjerklund Johansen, and Vladimir Mouraviev. "A Head-to-Head Comparative Phase II Study of Standard Urine Culture and Sensitivity Versus DNA Next-generation Sequencing Testing for Urinary Tract Infections," *Reviews in Urology*, 19(4), 213–220.

M. McDonald
Department of Urology, AdventHealth Celebration Hospital, Celebration, FL, USA
e-mail: Michael.Mcdonald.MD@AdventHealth.com

D. Kameh
Department of Pathology, Florida Hospital Celebration Health, Celebration, Kissimmee, FL, USA
e-mail: Darian.Kameh.MD@AdventHealth.com

M. E. Johnson (✉)
Department of Statistics, University of Central Florida, Orlando, FL, USA
e-mail: mark.johnson@ucf.edu

T. E. Bjerklund Johansen
Department of Urology, Oslo University Hospital and University of Oslo, Oslo, Norway

Institute of Clinical Medicine, University of Aarhus, Aarhus, Denmark
e-mail: t.e.b.johansen@medisin.uio.no

V. Mouraviev (Deceased)
Central Florida Cancer Institute, Davenport, FL, USA

T. E. Bjerklund Johansen, T. Cai (eds.), *Guide to Antibiotics in Urology*,
https://doi.org/10.1007/978-3-319-92366-6_7

DNA	Deoxyribonucleic acid
IRB	Institutional review board
NGS	Next generation sequencing.
RNA	Ribonucleic acid
UTI	Urinary tract infection
UTISA	The UTI Symptoms Assessment

7.1 Introduction

Urinary tract infections (UTIs) are the most common type of infection among urology diseases, accounting for approximately eight million visits to health care providers in 2015 and over one million hospital admissions in the United States each year [1–4]. Worldwide the estimated number of yearly UTIs treated is 150 million, and the financial costs of treatment are over 6 billion US dollars [1, 5]. Advances in the treatment of UTIs can come from improved diagnosis. This can be accomplished by increasing the speed and accuracy of detection that ultimately decrease patient morbidity and improve patient satisfaction.

Various institutions and associations have developed clinical practice guidelines for the treatment of cystitis and pyelonephritis [5–7]. Generally, many cases of uncomplicated UTI treatment can be based on empiric antibiotic therapy. On the contrary, for complicated or recurrent UTIs, therapy can be tailored or targeted to the pathogen(s) based on laboratory identification of organisms growing on culture and suggested sensitivity (C&S) to certain antibiotics [5, 8]. The limitation of diagnosis of UTI by clinical criteria alone can lead to misdiagnosis in up to 33% of cases [9]. The routine laboratory culture errors may be as high as 50% due to low sensitivity especially in cases with low bacterial loads present in the urine specimen with colony counts of less or equal than 10^5 CFU/L [10, 11].

The proper identification of the causal agents in the urine of those who suffer from infections is a prerogative for successful UTI treatment that can significantly decrease medical expenditures. Therefore, there is an obvious unmet need of a new technology to decrease health care costs by a more efficient and rapid treatment, and restoring patients' well-being and faster return to work. In this light, an introduction of deoxyribonucleic acid (DNA) next generation sequencing is very appealing to test its clinical feasibility and validity. This may help to improve the accuracy of testing and determine which antibacterial therapy can help to decrease patient's urinary tract symptoms faster. The improved diagnosis of UTIs with precise targeting of pathogens may also help in facilitating the prevention of resistance of many strains of bacteria and fungi, which is as high as 34% in certain areas of the USA [6]. National and international recommendations warn against the broad use of fluoroquinolones for uncomplicated UTIs and the increasing rates of bacterial resistance worldwide [12–14]. In this context it is now more important than ever that antibiotic therapy is used rationally and specifically in the treatment of UTIs.

The introduction of a new diagnostic modality requires the test to be efficient (high sensitivity and specificity) more than the currently existing tests based on results of phase I–III studies with sufficient internal and external validation. Regarding urine diagnostics of a UTI, it should serve to accurately detect bacterial species, establish the bacterial load present, and improve the speed of diagnosis. The clinical outcomes for each patient based on objective scoring by a validated instrument should be evaluated. The purpose of our study was to conduct a head-to-head comparative phase II trial of standard urine culture and sensitivity versus DNA next generation sequencing testing for diagnosis and treatment efficacy in patients with acute cystitis based on short-term outcomes.

7.2 Material and Methods

7.2.1 Study Design and Participants

The trial was created to conduct a standard prospective randomized open label controlled repeated measures design study. The study cohort represents patients with acute either complicated or uncomplicated cystitis.

In total, 56 patients were enrolled into this study with symptoms of a UTI between January 2016 and December 2016. Six patients did not meet entry criteria according to the IRB approved protocol. Another 6 patients did not complete the follow-up symptom score review and therefore were removed from the study. This left 44 patients that completed the study. The control group included twenty-two volunteers who did not have symptoms of a urinary tract infection. The study schema is presented in Fig. 7.1.

The randomization was conducted by enrollment of patients into Arm A-treatment based on C&S results and Arm B-treatment based on DNA next generation sequencing results. In the case of a negative C&S in Arm A, treatment could be initiated on day 8 depending on DNA sequencing results. In the case of negative DNA sequencing in Arm B, treatment could again be initiated on day 8 depending on C&S results. Treatment was tailored taking into consideration sensitivity reports as determined on routine culture results or antibiograms in the case of DNA sequencing. The duration of antibacterial therapy was 7 days only.

We used a validated instrument specifically the UTI Symptoms Assessment (UTISA) questionnaire which is a self-administered, assessment tool used to ascertain the effect of UTIs on the individual's quality of life [15]. Specifically focusing on the severity and "bothersomeness" (causing annoyance) of several key symptoms, extensive testing conducted in 2005 confirmed excellent predictive validity and reliability of this instrument. Three domains of urinary frequency, problems with urination, and pain are captured by the seven key symptoms that comprise the UTISA. Each symptom has a Likert-type response scale. The "severity" item response options are scored from 0 to 3: "did not have," "mild," "moderate," "severe"; the bothersomeness symptom response options are scored from 0 to 3: "not at all," "a little," "moderately," and "a lot." This survey was administered to

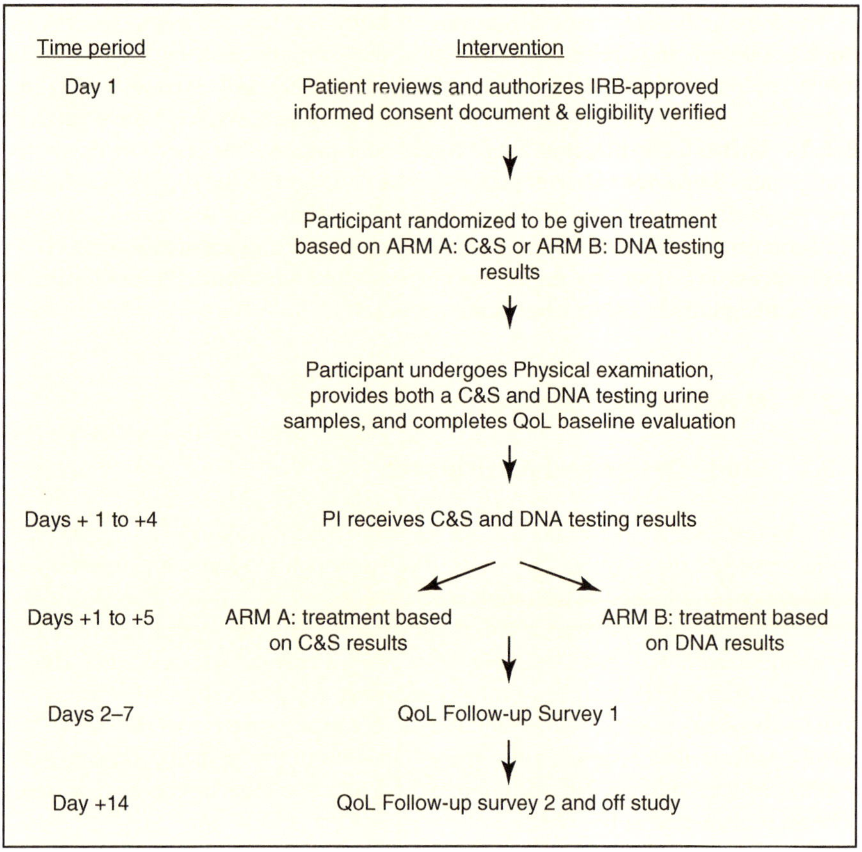

Fig. 7.1 Study schema

participants within three intervals during the research process: after consent but prior to leaving the clinic, daily from days 2 to 7, and on day 14 after completion of antibiotic therapy. Follow-up surveys were done through telephone or email contact. The 22 asymptomatic volunteers underwent the same steps as symptomatic patients with the exception of completing the questionnaire on days 1, 7, and 14 only.

Each patient's urine samples were obtained from standard, mid-stream clean catch urine. The clinic nursing staff provided participants with the routine instructions on how to obtain their urine specimen. All participants provided two urine samples, one for C&S and a second for DNA testing. A total of approximately 20 mL of urine was needed for both tests. For those with an indwelling catheter, a catheter sample aspiration was done with the assistance of the nursing staff.

The metagenomic evaluation was performed using two sequential levels. In both types of analysis, the microbial DNA was extracted from the patient's urine sample. The microbial DNA was then analyzed using molecular diagnostic methods. The patient report contained information about the pathogenic organisms detected. Once the bacteria had been identified, antibiotic recommendations were made based on research confirming the effectiveness of treatment. The reference used for antibiotic treatment in the MicrogenDX (former Pathogenius) laboratory is the Johns Hopkins antimicrobial guidelines reference 2015–2016.

7.2.1.1 Level 1: Rapid Screen Using qPCR Methods

The Level 1 Panel consisted of a quantitative real-time polymerase chain reaction (PCR) test for bacteria and fungi. This also included a qualitative real-time PCR test to detect genetic resistance to bacteria. The eight main groups of antibiotics tested for resistance genes included fluoroquinolones, vancomycin, methicillin, beta-lactams, carbapenems, macrolides, aminoglycosides, and tetracyclines which were reported as present or absent. Level 1 test for quinolone resistance was a real-time qualitative PCR assay utilizing the Roche LightCycler 480. This TaqMan assay used dye labeled hydrolysis probes to detect the presence of a unique sequence in the qnr and gyrA gene specific to quinolone resistance. Quinolone antibiotics inhibit bacterial replication by the stabilizing the complex between DNA and DNA gyrase or topoisomerase and blocking the polymerase from binding during replication. Quinolone resistance occurred when the DNA gyrase or topoisomerase was protected against the cleaving caused by quinolone antibiotics. Qnr was a common quinolone resistance gene that blocks the quinolone antibiotics from inhibiting the DNA gyrase activity. A mutation in the DNA gyrase subunit A, gyrA, caused the quinolone antibiotics to become ineffective at stopping the DNA gyrase replication. The accuracy, sensitivity, and specificity of the qPCR assay were 100%. The limit of detection was 0.001 ng/μL.

The panel utilized the unique genes present in each organism to identify how much of that organism was present in each patient sample that was reported as an individual bacterial association. This quantification was achieved in a multistep process. First, each gene was specifically chosen for its ability to distinguish the bacterial or fungal targets from their closely related species and its abundance in the cells themselves (1 gene per bacterial or fungal cell). Each target was then measured to get an initial concentration (CFU/mg or mL and DNA concentration ng/μL after DNA extraction is performed). The initial concentration of CFU/mg or mL is also used to evaluate and calculate the extraction efficiency of each bacteria and fungi. The extraction efficiency percentage is taken into account when calculating the target analytes' concentration in order to negate the slight loss of cells during the extraction process. Next, each initial target bacteria or fungi DNA, whose concentration was measured to obtain an initial concentration ng/μL, was diluted to obtain a six to eight 1:10 dilution series and run on the quantitative PCR (qPCR) panel assay on the Roche LightCycler 480 II instrument. The dilution series was designed to span the entire analytic range (very high to very low concentrations). The dilution series' concentration and cycle threshold generated a standard curve for each target. Based on this standard curve, the concentration for each target can be calculated.

The main uropathogens tested in Level 1 were for *Escherichia coli*, *Enterococcus faecalis*, *Enterococcus faecium*, *Klebsiella pneumoniae*, Group Beta *Streptococcus*

(*S. agalactiae*), Group A *Streptococcus* (*S. pyogenes*), *Candida albicans*, *Pseudomonas aeruginosa*, *Staphylococcus aureus*, and *Serratia marcescens*. The above organisms, except for mecA, vanA, and 16S, were run on a quantitative assay, which reported out the organisms as copy per mL or mg. The 16S universal bacteria are a semi-quantitative assay, which reports the total bacteria load as low, ($<10^5$ copy number/mL, medium (10^5–10^7), and $>10^7$(high) load, respectively.

The sensitivity and specificity were 100% on *Enterococcus faecalis*, *Enterococcus faecium*, *Klebsiella pneumoniae*, *Pseudomonas aeruginosa*, *Staph. aureus*, *Staph. pyogenes*, vanA, *C. albicans*, *Escherichia coli*, *Proteus mirabilis*, and *Strep. pneumoniae*. The sensitivity and specificity for *Strep. agalactiae* were 100% and 99.4%. The sensitivity and specificity for mecA were 100% and 95.2% and for 16S were 100% and 97.1%.

7.2.1.2 Level 2: DecodEX™ DNA Pyrosequencing Method

The Level 2 test defined virtually a complete genetic profile of all microbial organisms and fungal pathogens that could be present in-patient specimens. Microbial DNA in each sample was sequenced using the Ion Torrent PGM sequencer in order to establish what type of bacterial and fungal species are present. Forward and reverse primers were used to detect and amplify the target sequence in each sample. The samples were differentiated from each other when run on the PGM sequencer by a "tag," a unique identifying sequence attached to the forward primer implemented when the targeted sequence was amplified using polymerase chain reaction or PCR. The PCR contains a 5-min denaturation step at 95 °C, 35 cycles of 94 °C for 30 s, 52 °C for 40 s, and 72 °C for 60 s, and a final extension step of 72 °C for 10 min. After the sample DNA had been amplified and each sample had its own unique sequence tag, the sample DNA could be pooled together based on amplification strength for downstream applications. Purification of the pooled DNA was done by removing small fragments using both Agencourt AMpure beads and Qiagen MinElute Kit. The DNA added to the emulsion PCR, which attached one DNA strand to one Ion Sphere Particle. The DNA was amplified, and the one Ion Sphere Particle or ISP contained numerous copies of the one DNA strand. The DNA ISPs were recovered, enriched, and prepared for sequencing. Finally, the beads were run on the PGM sequencer.

The Ion Torrent PGM sequencer uses DNA polymerase to incorporate phosphorylated dNTPs into the DNA strand. When each dNTP was incorporated, a Hydrogen Ion or Hydron was released. The Hydron caused a change in pH proportional to the number of nucleotides incorporated in the DNA strand and was captured by sequencer's sensing layer inside the chip.

The sequencing reads were analyzed for quality and length. Any reads that fell below the quality score or appropriate length were discarded due to the poor quality. Only the high-quality reads were interpreted and reported to physicians. Data for each detected bacterial or fungal species were reported as Relative Percent of total instrument reads. This assay was capable of detecting the organisms listed here from as little as 100 ng of patient specimen. Every species could be accurately detected with as little as 10 ng/μL of extracted DNA with at least 1000 copies of each species. Each organism was reported as a relative abundance in the sample.

180 ATCC species were run on bacteria and fungi sequencing assays to confirm accuracy, sensitivity, and specificity. All ATCC species matched their intended targets. 10 fungi samples were detected on the bacterial assay; however, the cultures were confirmed contaminated using an alternate sequencing platform (Roche 454 sequencer). Both assays produced 100% accuracy, sensitivity, and specificity. 83 patient samples were run on both assays twice on two different sequencers to test the precision of the Ion Torrent PGMs. All patient samples were compared for read count and species identification using an analysis of variance. In addition to these measures of quality, both assays' sensitivity/limit of detection was verified every 6 months using a dilutions series of common bacteria and fungi. Also, the specificity was verified every 6 months using BEI standards containing multiple species of bacteria. The BEI standards contained equal concentrations and varying concentrations of bacteria species. These identified compositions on the sequencer were compared to the BEI givens to ensure accuracy. The uneven concentration specimen was compared to the previous sequence run of the BEI standard to verify the same organisms were in abundance and other organisms were in minor amounts.

7.2.1.3 Antibiotic Susceptibility

Molecular testing of clinical specimens for microbial species detection and identification is performed by (a) extraction of the microbial DNA from the specimen, (b) amplification of the DNA using a polymerase chain reaction (PCR), and subsequently (c) analysis and comparison of the amplified targets to known DNA references to unambiguously determine the microbial census of the specimen. The Ion Torrent sequencing platform was used to get the longest read lengths possible in order to maximize the number of uniquely identifiable amplicons. The database used for comparison of DNA amplicon from 16S analysis has been curated to eliminate incomplete entries and known mistakes in entry. Comparisons are against the entire 16S database. The laboratory has used the information gained from the analysis of over 100,000 samples to understand the circumstances from which we could get multiple potential species identified as probable results (ties) and have used multiple techniques to help us determine the most probable result in these circumstances.

The determination of the bacterial species, including genetic resistance targets, provides for a susceptibility determination that clinicians can base upon local antibiograms and/or clinical references.

The laboratory employed the antibiotic susceptibility database from the Johns Hopkins Antimicrobial Guideline database. This database is compiled from current best practice literature references to identify the most common antibiotics to treat the identified microbes. The laboratory deliberately recommended antibiotics that were not subject to mobile genetic element issues (e.g., mec A cassette, ESBL, van) and that were as specific to each patient as possible.

7.2.1.4 Culture and Sensitivity (C&S) Testing

Processing of urine specimens for C&S was performed according to the protocol of the Florida Hospital pathology laboratory. Mid-stream urine collection was submitted in the BD Vacutainer C&S Preservative Tube. The preservative was used to protect the level of bacteria present at collection. Urine collected in preservative and stored at room temperature was acceptable for culture up to 48 h after collection.

Urine specimens collected in a sterile container without preservative had the time of collection written on the label and were processed for culture in the microbiology laboratory within 2 h of collection. After 18–24 h of incubation, urine results are reported. Negative urine reports are resulted at less than or equal to 21 h. Positive urine reports are attempted to be resulted at less than or equal to 35 h.

Antibiotic susceptibility testing was provided when the most aggressive bacteria were present in significant amounts: for example, Gram-negative rods (*E. coli*, *Klebsiella pneumoniae*, *Pseudomonas aeruginosa*, etc.), *Staphylococcus* spp., yeasts, beta-hemolytic *Streptococcus* spp., *Enterococcus* spp., *Aerococcus urinae*, and *Corynebacterium urealyticum*. Susceptibility testing was performed using the Vitek 2/Biomerieux instrument. Four different antibiotic cards are utilized which test numerous Gram-positive and Gram-negative bacteria. Etest was also utilized for numerous Gram-negative bacteria.

7.2.1.5 Statistical Evaluation

The one-way Student-t test was used to calculate difference between groups. All statistical results presented in this paper used the statistical software package JMP® Pro 12.

7.3 Results

There were 44 patients and 22 controls who completed the study, over a 14-day duration. Twenty-two patients were randomly selected to each treatment arm, A and B (Table 7.1). The distribution by gender was as follows:

Group A: 14 females, 8 males (treatment based on C&S).
Group B: 15 females, 7 males (treatment based on DNA NGS).

Table 7.1 Designations based on treatment and by result

Group A	**Subset 1**	**Subset 2**
22 Patients Treatment based on C&S results	(+C&S, +DNA 7/22)	(−C&S, +DNA 15/22) patients were treated Day 8 based on DNA NGS results
Group B	**Subset 3**	**Subset 4**
22 Patients Treatment based on DNA NGS results	(+DNA, +C&S 6/22)	(+DNA, −C&S 16/22)

The 13/44 patients had positive urine cultures while all 44/44 patients had positive DNA NGS results. All 15 males and 4 females with positive laboratory findings were diagnosed with a complicated UTI. In total 19/44 patients were diagnosed with complicated UTIs.

The validated patient symptom severity (SS) score was documented at entry as a baseline for a viable comparison of C&S to DNA-based treatment. Symptom scores measured a scale from 0 to 21 with 21 demonstrating the worst score scenario. At baseline the difference between Arm A and Arm B was not significant with the mean score for Arm A being 9.00 and for Arm B 10.22.

In Arm A 7 of the 22 patients had a positive culture (Subset 1). The 15/22 patients in Arm A (Subset 2) had negative cultures and positive DNA results. This subset of patients started treatment on day 8 based on DNA NGS results. On the contrary, all 22 patients in Arm B had positive DNA NGS test. The distribution of patients in Arm B showed a positive urine culture test in 6 of the 22 patients (Subset 3) while the remaining 16 revealed no growth in their urine cultures (Subset 4).

The results of C&S versus DNA NGS were compared based on the change in symptom severity scale from baseline to 14 days completion. The change in average improvement of 8.5 score in Arm B was highly significant, as demonstrated in Fig. 7.2. The average scores decreased in Arm A from 9.0 down to 5.3; Arm B, subset 3, from 11.2 down to 4.3; and in subset 4, from 11.6 down to 3.7.

The real value of DNA NGS performance as a diagnostic test can be seen in the Arm A, Subset 2 in patients, whose cultures were negative. Subset 2 had the benefit of a DNA diagnostics to suggest a treatment protocol that was initiated on day 8 of the study. The 15 patients from this Subset showed an average improvement score of 7.4 that was considered as an intermediate increment to the score changes in Arm B, Subsets 3 and 4 (6.67 and 10.56, respectively) and significantly better than Arm A, Subset 1.

The DNA NGS test was sensitive enough to detect on average 3 pathogens in each sample (each one with quantitative dominance more than 2%). Moreover, the DNA testing results revealed 34/44 patients with association of 2 or more bacterial

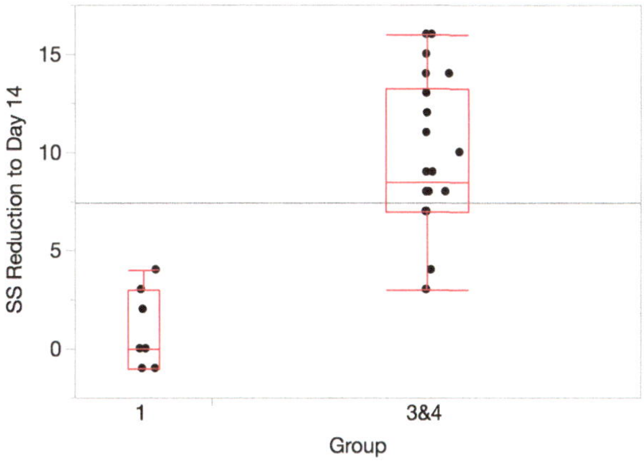

Fig. 7.2 Symptom severity reduction at day 14 in treatment arms. Two-sample t-test p-value is <0.001

or fungal pathogens. The sensitivity of C&S technique was much lower, for example, only 2/13 culture reports revealed polymicrobial or fungal association. In addition, twenty DNA NGS results detected an anaerobic flora either primarily or as a part of a polymicrobial sequence.

Of the 22 controls, 5 had positive urine cultures while 21/22 had positive DNA NGS results. Interestingly enough, the 5 subjects with positive C&S and DNA NGS all had similar organisms. However, in 3 of these subjects DNA NGS results reported 2 or more organisms in addition to the common one found on C&S method. In patients with symptoms of acute cystitis and positive DNA NGS results, the average number of organisms as a bacterial load presented in each sample was 10^6 compared to control subjects who had an average of 10^5 ($p < 0.001$) (Fig. 7.3).

7.4 Discussion

The diagnostic techniques for UTIs have been in use for over 125 years. Since Drs. Koch and Petri developed plating and culture models in the 1880s, little has changed. Considered the gold standard in the diagnosis of UTIs, there are several reasons for re-evaluation of the culture model.

One disadvantage of urine evaluated by culture techniques include contamination which occurs if the test yields more than 2 isolates in quantities greater than or equal to 10,000 CFU/mL. According to the review of current laboratory practices, contamination rate of urine cultures varies from 0.8% to 41.7% with the median rate of 15.0% [16]. DNA sequencing detected a great majority of specimens in this study, (34/44) as being polymicrobial (average 2.8) whereas only (2/13) culture specimens showed more than one organism.

Urine culture sensitivity ranges from 23% to 77% based on patients with symptoms of cystitis [17]. Studies also point out that results of urine cultures are more sensitive depending on the amount of bacteria present. Urine culture testing does not permit the reliable detection of $<10^5$ cfu/mL [18]. In turn this may miss those

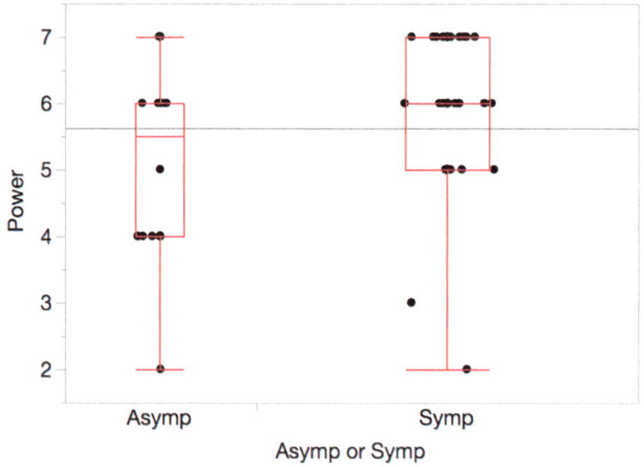

Fig. 7.3 One-way symptomatic versus asymptomatic comparison of power of DNA at entry. Two-sample *t*-test, *p*-value = 0.0216

patients that present with lower bacterial counts leading to the misdiagnosis of a UTI or missing the infection completely [19]. DNA next generation sequencing reports on bacterial loads as low (10^2–10^4), medium (10^5–10^7), and high quantities ($\geq 10^7$). DNA sequencing specimens were quantified as 10^2–10^7. The culture reports in our study were quantified as 10^5–10^7. We found that several urine specimens diagnosed with DNA sequencing techniques will include many aerobic and anaerobic bacteria with as little as 10^2–10^4 organisms. The DNA sequencing model may contain several organisms, all of which are quantified into the percentage of the specimen that they make up, with a minimum result being 2%.

Asymptomatic bacteriuria can occur with low counts of uropathogens or may present as so-called urethral syndrome. Other causes of asymptomatic bacteriuria include infections with organisms such as *Mycoplasma*, *Trichomonas*, *Chlamydia*, Gonococci, *Candida*, Mycobacteria, Schistosomiasis, and Tuberculosis, which are difficult to diagnosis with typical urine culture techniques and often times missed [20]. The advantages of DNA testing are the ability to assess for these and other organisms including a reference bank of over 25,000 organisms.

Precise antibiotic therapy will help to limit bacterial resistance, improve symptom scores faster, and decrease the time of treatment and ultimately cost. The term of antibiotic stewardship was introduced two decades ago to search for the best methods necessary to prevent and control the problem of antimicrobial resistance. Despite an implementation of new antibiotics in clinical practice, the problem of increased resistance reduces the chance of efficient prophylaxis and treatment. A choice of targeted antibiotic(s) with optimization of its regimen, dose, and time frame has become a main prerequisite of successful treatment. It can be achieved by better identification of true uropathogens through better understanding of the urinary tract microbiome. The clinical application of DNA next generation sequencing may allow us to improve the targeting of pathogenic bacterial strains while avoiding eradication of beneficial commensal flora.

This study reveals several new concepts in the diagnosis and treatment of UTIs. All 44 patients showed positive results in DNA sequencing tests, while only 13/44 patients had positive urine culture tests. Clinically those patients with persistent symptoms of a UTI and negative urine cultures (15/22 patients) will be treated empirically or will be asked to repeat the study. This leads to the loss of time, ultimately increasing health care costs. On a head-to-head comparison, symptom scores were statistically significantly better for those patients whose treatment was based on DNA results versus traditional culture studies. Patients treated in arm A, subset 2, (culture negative, DNA test positive) improved with respect to symptom scores when they started treatment on day 8.

The other advantage of DNA sequencing test was an additional high sensitivity to detect anaerobic bacteria in 20/44 patients. The distribution of this infection was as follows: Ten of the 20 patients had an anaerobic bacteria accounting for the primary infectious component of the urine, and another 10 were secondary, associated with aerobic or facultative anaerobic bacteria. Basically, anaerobic UTIs were often overseen as a causative factor for a number of reasons. These include the difficulty to ascertain these organisms because of the inconsistent use of adequate methods to isolate and identify them. It is more costly and time consuming to diagnose them with traditional methods. As well it is not performed on a routine basis as initial reports suggesting anaerobic bacteria were a rare cause of UTIs and they are a normal part of the genitourinary flora [21, 22]. After introduction of novel genomic techniques, a detection rate of anaerobic bacteria was increased especially with the use of 16S ribosomal RNA sequencing in both symptomatic and asymptomatic patients [23–25]. This has led to the suggestion of a microbiota, that are pathogens in a particular environment in case of an acute cystitis when urine is either normal or potentially pathological [26, 27].

In this study patients treated with antibiotics clinically improved whether they had primary anaerobic, aerobic, or a combination of bacteria. We know that urethritis or urethral syndrome may mimic symptoms of a UTI. DNA testing therefore may help when diagnosing and treating symptoms of a UTI and urine cultures are negative.

Why however do some patients present with symptoms with only 10^2–10^4 organisms while some who have 10^7 organisms have no symptoms whatsoever? Is there a threshold which when passed causes symptoms of a UTI? Are there underlying abnormalities that create the milieu for symptoms of a UTI? Participants who were asymptomatic had an average of $10^{5.09}$ organisms whereas symptomatic patients averaged $10^{5.88}$ bacteria, a statistically significant finding as noted previously. Asymptomatic bacteriuria is common but varies widely in the general population based on age, sex, and the presence of genitourinary abnormalities. Its prevalence can range from 1–5% in healthy premenopausal women up to 27% in women with diabetes based on traditional culture studies [28].

The cost of a new diagnostic test is extremely important in establishing an effective tool in treating UTIs to define the cost/benefit ratio. The price of comparative testing between DNA next generation sequencing and urine cultures in this study was 40% that of urine cultures. The cost of the DNA NGS including PCR and 16sRNA testing was in total US $199. The cost of an aerobic urine culture in the Florida Hospital system is US $60. When including fungal and anaerobic cultures, the total cost is over US $500.

A variety of clinical scenarios may challenge physicians with an opportunity to utilize DNA sequencing in both research and practical settings in the future. In fact, the patients with simple uncomplicated UTIs are normally treated empirically. But many patients who have persistent symptoms of cystitis despite treatment and have negative urine cultures can benefit from DNA sequencing testing. In cases with suspected "superbugs" or anaerobic bacteria, DNA sequencing may also prove more beneficial in accurate diagnosis of cystitis, urethritis, or urethral syndrome. DNA sequencing can help to evaluate for low bacterial loads or resistant infections not otherwise diagnosed with traditional methods. Finally other options for DNA sequencing that may prove beneficial in the future include semen studies and extra prostatic secretions for chronic prostatitis, renal stones to evaluate for causative factors of calculi formation, to evaluate the urinary milieu for interstitial cystitis patients, and samples from asymptomatic people to help establish a urinary microbiome.

In the body of the literature, we did not find a study that has performed a head-to-head comparison of these two diagnostic techniques. The significant limitation of the study is the small sample size with low statistical power of the results, and a larger study needs to be done with a bigger sample size to achieve more robust conclusions of this promising study. We believe that this area of aerobic and anaerobic UTIs, polymicrobial sequences, and bacterial loads common in this study calls for further investigation and research.

7.5 Conclusion

Results of the first head-to-head comparison trial revealed symptom scores which were significantly better for those patients whose treatment was based on DNA results versus traditional culture studies. The sensitivity of the DNA technique was significantly higher than standard C&S method. Thus, all 44 patients demonstrated positive results in DNA sequencing tests, while only 13/44 patients had positive urine culture tests. Furthermore, in the cohort of patients with DNA positive and negative culture tests, the treatment outcomes were improved with respect to symptom scores when they started treatment on day 8. That ultimately accelerated recovery time and possibly decreased the frequency of development of chronic cystitis afterward, optimizing the cost/efficacy ratio. The other advantage of the DNA test is an increased sensitivity in the diagnosis of anaerobic flora that was detected in 20/44 DNA results. Ultimately, in this study the DNA test allowed us to achieve better treatment outcomes in patients treated with antibiotics for primary anaerobic, aerobic, or a combination of bacteria. Therefore, DNA testing may help when diagnosing and treating symptoms of acute cystitis especially when urine cultures are negative.

References

1. Thoureen T, Scott S, Best J. Urinary tract infection. Monograpgh. AHC Media. 2015. https://www.ahcmedia.com/articles/135127-urinary-tract-infection
2. Patton JP, Nash DB, Abrutyn E. Urinary tract infection: economic considerations. Med Clin North Am. 1991;75:495–513.
3. Haley RW, Culver DH, White JW, Morgan WM, Emori TG. The nationwide nosocomial infection rate. A new need for vital statistics. Am J Epidemiol. 1985;121:159–67.
4. Schappert SM, Rechtsteiner EA. Ambulatory medical care utilization estimates for 2007. Vital Health Stat. 2011;13:1–38.
5. Badalato G, Kaufmann M. Adult urinary tract infection. American Urological Association. AUA Medical Scholl Curriculum. 2016. https://www.auanet.org/education/adult-uti.cfm.
6. Jancel T, Dudas V. Management of uncomplicated urinary tract infections. West J Med. 2002;176:51–5.
7. Nickel JC. Practical management of recurrent urinary tract infections in premenopausal women. Rev Urol. 2005;7:11–7.
8. Baron EJ, Miller JM, Weinstein MP, et al. A guide to utilization of the microbiology laboratory for diagnosis of infectious diseases: 2013 recommendations by the Infectious Diseases Society

of America (IDSA) and the American Society for Microbiology (ASM)(a). Clin Infect Dis. 2013;57:e22–e121.
9. Schmiemann G, Kniehl E, Gebhardt K, Matejczyk MM, Hummers-Pradier E. The diagnosis of urinary tract infection: a systematic review. Dtsch Arztebl Int. 2010;107:361–7.
10. Kunin CM, White LV, Hua TH. A reassessment of the importance of "low-count" bacteriuria in young women with acute urinary symptoms. Ann Intern Med. 1993;119:454–60.
11. Arav-Boger R, Leibovici L, Danon YL. Urinary tract infections with low and high colony counts in young women. Spontaneous remission and single-dose vs multiple-day treatment. Arch Intern Med. 1994;154:300–4.
12. Organization WH. WHO's report on antibiotic resistance reveals serious. Geneva: Worldwide Threat to Public Health; 2014.
13. Andriole VT. The quinolones: past, present, and future. Clin Infect Dis. 2005;41(Suppl 2):S113–9.
14. Lu PL, Liu YC, Toh HS, et al. Epidemiology and antimicrobial susceptibility profiles of gram-negative bacteria causing urinary tract infections in the Asia-Pacific region: 2009-2010 results from the Study for Monitoring Antimicrobial Resistance Trends (SMART). Int J Antimicrob Agents. 2012;40(Suppl):S37–43.
15. Clayson D, Wild D, Doll H, Keating K, Gondek K. Validation of a patient-administered questionnaire to measure the severity and bothersomeness of lower urinary tract symptoms in uncomplicated urinary tract infection (UTI): the UTI symptom assessment questionnaire. BJU Int. 2005;96:350–9.
16. Bekeris LG, Jones BA, Walsh MK, Wagar EA. Urine culture contamination: a College of American Pathologists Q-probes study of 127 laboratories. Arch Pathol Lab Med. 2008;132:913–7.
17. Hooton TM, Roberts PL, Cox ME, Stapleton AE. Voided midstream urine culture and acute cystitis in premenopausal women. N Engl J Med. 2013;369:1883–91.
18. Gatermann S, Fünfstück R, Handrick W. Harnwegsinfektion—Mikrobiologisch-infektologische Qualitätsstandards. In: Harnwegsinfektion. Mauch M, Podbielski A, Hermann M, (editors). Urban&Fisher. Munchen, Jena. 2005:8–21.
19. Stamm WE, Counts GW, Running KR, Fihn S, Turck M, Holmes KK. Diagnosis of coliform infection in acutely dysuric women. N Engl J Med. 1982;307:463–8.
20. Franz M, Horl WH. Common errors in diagnosis and management of urinary tract infection. II: clinical management. Nephrol Dial Transplant. 1999;14:2754–62.
21. Headington JT, Beyerlein B. Anaerobic bacteria in routine urine culture. J Clin Pathol. 1966;19:573–6.
22. Wilson ML, Gaido L. Laboratory diagnosis of urinary tract infections in adult patients. Clin Infect Dis. 2004;38:1150–8.
23. Hilt EE, McKinley K, Pearce MM, et al. Urine is not sterile: use of enhanced urine culture techniques to detect resident bacterial flora in the adult female bladder. J Clin Microbiol. 2014;52:871–6.
24. Pearce MM, Hilt EE, Rosenfeld AB, et al. The female urinary microbiome: a comparison of women with and without urgency urinary incontinence. MBio. 2014;5:e01283–14.
25. Willner D, Low S, Steen JA, et al. Single clinical isolates from acute uncomplicated urinary tract infections are representative of dominant in situ populations. MBio. 2014;5:e01064–13.
26. Cho I, Blaser MJ. The human microbiome: at the interface of health and disease. Nat Rev Genet. 2012;13:260–70.
27. Ursell LK, Metcalf JL, Parfrey LW, Knight R. Defining the human microbiome. Nutr Rev. 2012;70(Suppl 1):S38–44.
28. Nicolle LE, Bradley S, Colgan R, et al. Infectious Diseases Society of America guidelines for the diagnosis and treatment of asymptomatic bacteriuria in adults. Clin Infect Dis. 2005;40:643–54.

Recurrent Urinary Tract Infection in Young Woman

8

Liliana Mereu and Saverio Tateo

8.1 Definition

A urinary infection (UTI) occurs when uropathogenic bacteria replace the normal flora of the peri-urethral area and ascend to cause cystitis. Infrequently, this infection goes up to the kidney to cause pyelonephritis [1].

A UTI is recurrent when it follows the complete clinical resolution of a previous UTI [2]. Recurrent urinary infection (RUTI) can be defined as 3 episodes of UTI with urine culture positive in the previous 12 months or 2 episodes within the 6 months [3].

Uncomplicated UTI occurs in a healthy person in the absence of structural or functional abnormalities of the urinary tract [4]. All other UTIs are considered complicated UTIs. Repeated pyelonephritis should be considered as complicated UTI [5].

8.2 Etiology

UTI is caused by improved adherence, infection, and colonization of uropathogens. The usual bacteria include *Escherichia coli*, *Enterococcus faecalis*, *Staphylococcus saprophyticus*, *Klebsiella pneumoniae*, and *Proteus mirabilis*. Citrobacter and enterococci are less likely causes of UTI in women [1].

The classic theory for the development of UTI is that the uropathogen is part of the endogenous rectal flora, and it colonizes the vagina and the urethra. In

L. Mereu (✉)
Unit of Obstetrics and Gynecology, Policlinico G. Rodolico - San Marco, CHIRMED Department, University of Catania, Catania, Italy
e-mail: Liliana.mereu@unict.it

S. Tateo
Service de Ginécologie, Obstétrique, Centre Hospitalier de Troyes, Troyes, France

T. E. Bjerklund Johansen, T. Cai (eds.), *Guide to Antibiotics in Urology*,
https://doi.org/10.1007/978-3-319-92366-6_8

susceptible women, gastrointestinal tract and vagina may represent a reservoir for uropathogenic bacteria [6].

In general the pathogenesis of RUTI can be related to bacterial re-infection or persistence. In bacterial persistence, the same pathogen may be cultured in the urine 2 weeks after sensitivity-adjusted therapy. Bacterial re-infection is a recurrence with a different organism or with the same organism in more than 2 weeks after treatment [7].

An alternative hypothesis is the survival of bacteria in the bladder through the progression of transient intracellular bacterial communities (IBC) into persistent quiescent intracellular reservoirs (QIR) [8–12].

Urinary colonization rates are higher among women: first, the vagina and the anus are close to the urethral opening, and women have more peri-urethral tissue where bacteria grow; second, the bacteria are more likely to ascend to the female bladder than the male bladder because of the shorter urethral length. Clinical studies demonstrate that vaginal microbiota may influence the susceptibility to RUTI. It has been suggested that the urinary tract is routinely exposed to vaginal bacteria as *Gardnerella vaginalis*, a dominant member of the vaginal microbiota in some women [13].

Risk factors for recurrent UTI in young women are female sex, prior *E. coli* UTI, sexual intercourse, diaphragm/spermicide/cervical cap use, oral contraceptive, vaginal infection, trauma/manipulation, diabetes, obesity, genetic factors anatomic abnormality as shorter anal-urethral distance <4,5 cm, B and AB blood groups, and cell-mediated immunity [14–19].

8.3 Epidemiology

RUTI in woman is a common presentation to urologists, gynecologists, and family doctors. Survey data suggest that 1 in 3 women will have had a diagnosed and treated UTI by age 24 and more than 50% will be affected in their lifetime; 20–30% of women will have recurrence [20]. In a 6-month study of college-aged women, 27% of these UTIs were found to recur once and 3% a second time [21].

The economic implications of UTI are quite high, predominantly related to the high incidence of UTI. The direct costs include outpatient doctor visits, antimicrobial prescription hospital expenses, as well as non-medical cost associated with sick days and morbidity.

8.4 Diagnosis

Common symptoms of a UTI are dysuria, urinary frequency, urgency, supra-pubic pain, and possible hematuria. Systemic symptoms are usually absent. The urine may have a bad smell and appear cloudy [22]. Irritative voiding symptoms are present in 25–30% of women with RUTIs. The probability of finding a positive urinary culture in the presence of the above symptoms and the absence of vaginal discharge is around 81% [23].

Differential diagnoses include vaginitis, urethritis, interstitial cystitis, and pelvic inflammatory disease. Many organisms such as *Chlamydia*, *Neisseria gonorrhoeae*, *Candida*, bacterial vaginosis, and Herpes simplex may be involved and mimic cystitis [24].

Clinical symptoms of a RUTI have to be distinguishing from irritative voiding symptoms without infection. Women with RUTIs were more likely to have symptoms after intercourse, a previous history of pyelonephritis, absence of nicturia, and experience prompt resolution of symptoms after antibiotic therapy than those women without infection. Women with RUTIs were more unlikely to report nicturia and have symptoms between episodes of UTI than women with irritative voiding symptoms. The presence of dysuria, urinary frequency, and urgency suggests a non-infectious cause as seen in interstitial cystitis, urethral syndrome, or detrusor muscle over-activity [25].

A woman with RUTIs should undergo an initial clinical evaluation including a history taking and a physical and pelvic examination to evaluate urogenital anatomy, to detect pelvic organ prolapse, atrophy of the vagina or vaginosis. Specific aspects as to be taken into consideration for complete evaluation: positive family history of diabetes mellitus (DM), obesity, and women with suspected urine retention should be evaluated for post-void residual urine volume.

Diagnosis of RUTI depends on the characteristic of clinical features, presence of three positive urinary cultures within the previous 12 months, and the presence of neutrophilis in the urine (pyuria). Urinalysis, urine culture, and sensitivity testing are the standard diagnostic investigations to detect the causative organism and to determine specific antimicrobial therapy.

The standard definition of UTI on culture is >100,000 colony-forming units (cfu)/mL. In acute cystitis, even 1000 cfu/mL and in acute pyelonephritis 10,000 cfu/mL may be sufficient for diagnosis in a symptomatic patient [26]. Culture has a sensitivity of 80% and a specificity of 90% [6].

When working up RUTI, culture and sensitivity analysis should be performed also when symptomatic, to confirm a UTI and in 2 weeks from sensitivity-adjusted treatment to guide further treatment and exclude persistence.

The use of urine dipstick analysis to evaluate the presence of nitrates can be helpful with a sensitivity of 19–48% and a specificity of 92–100%. A negative result does not rule out infection in a symptomatic patient [27]. The presence of leukocyte esterase (pyuria) produced by neutrophilis may be associated with UTI but also other not uropathogens organism can cause pyuria; the sensitivity and specificity of this test, in women with UTI, is 72–97% and 41–86%, respectively [6].

8.5 Management

8.5.1 Counselling

Women with RUTIs should be educated about re-infection and relapse. Patients should be advised and encouraged to drink plenty of fluids (2–3 L per day) and to urinate frequently to help flush bacteria from the bladder.

Preventive measures related to sexual intercourse as clean the genital areas before and after sex and to wipe from front to back may reduce the recurrence rate. In general, avoiding multiple sexual partners will reduce the risk of both UTIs and sexually transmitted infections.

Women should be encouraged to avoid spermicidal contraceptives, diaphragms that may irritate the vagina and urethra and facilitate the colonization of bacteria within the urinary tract.

Skin allergens introduced to the genital area, such as bath liquids, vaginal creams and lotions, sprays, or soaps are better avoided as they could alter vaginal flora [16, 28, 29].

8.5.2 Therapy

Antimicrobial therapy is the core treatment for UTIs. In order to ensure compliance and be patient-friendly, the drug should be given for a short period of time to prevent

Table 8.1 Antibiotic management of RUTIs

Antibiotic	Dosage	Effectiveness	Resistance rate
First-line agent			
Fosfomicin (monuril)	3 g onc dic	91	Up to 0.6
Nitrofurantoin	100 mg twice a day for 5 days	93	Up to 1.6
Trimethoprim/ sulfamethoxazole	160/800 twice a day per day for 3 days	93	Up to 24.2
Second-line agent			
Fluoroquinolones	Ciprofloxacin 250 twice a day for 3 days Levofloxacin 250–500 mg per day for 3 days	90	Up to 17 Up to 6
Third-line agent			
Beta-lactams	Amoxicillin/clavulanate 500/125 twice a day for 3 days Cefaclor: 250 mg three times per day for 5 days Cefdinir: 300 mg twice a day for 3 days Cefpodoxime: 100 mg twice a day for 3 days Cephalexin: 500 mg twice a day for 7 days	89	Varies by medication

resistance. The eradication can be achieved within hours if the antibiotics are maintained at sufficient urine levels. Antibiotics should be chosen according to the sensibility of the infecting bacteria and the concentrations of uropathogens in the urine [30].

Oral antibiotic therapy resolves 94% of uncomplicated UTIs, although recurrence is not uncommon.

As shown in Table 8.1 for first-line therapy in case of uncomplicated UTIs may be chosen: a 3-day regimen of trimethoprim sulfamethoxazole (TMP-SMX) or a 5-day course of nitrofurantoin. A 3- to 7-day regimen of beta-lactams may be indicated if first-line therapies cannot be used. Although a 3-day course of fluoroquinolones can be quite effective, it is not recommended as first-line therapy because of the emerging resistance, potential side effects, and high cost. Fluoroquinolones may be considered in women with low tolerance or an allergic reaction to first-line antibiotics. Fosfomycin trometamol has been shown to be a safe and effective alternative for the treatment of UTIs, also in pregnant, elderly, and pediatric patients, but it seems to be less effective. Because of its poor efficacy, amoxicillin and ampicillin should not be used for the empirical treatment of UTIs [31].

Persistent bacteriuria after resolution of clinical symptoms should be considered asymptomatic bacteriuria and should not be further treated in non-pregnant women. Treatment of asymptomatic bacteriuria may increase the risk of UTI recurrence by altering normal flora [32]. Hence, a follow-up urinalysis and urine culture is not indicated in women with uncomplicated UTIs, but should be performed in those women who are suffering from RUTIs or a complicated UTI.

A Cochrane review has shown that antibiotics in comparison to placebo are more effective in preventing recurrences in pre- and postmenopausal women with RUTIs [31].

A variety of antibiotics are used for the prevention and management of RUTIs:

Ampicillin, amoxicillin, and sulfonamides are not the drugs of choice for empirical treatment because of the widespread of resistance in 15–20% of *E. coli* [2, 33, 34].

Nitrofurantoin or amoxicillin/clavulanic acid remain effective in terms of sensitivity, but nitrofurantoin needs to be avoided in patients with complicated UTI, as pyelonephritis because of its poor serum and tissue levels.

The rate of *E. coli* resistance to fluoroquinolones, even in uncomplicated UTIs, varies between countries with rates reported as 0.5–7.6% in Europe [35], 15% in Korea, [36] and up to 35% in some parts of India [37].

Penicillins and cephalosporins are considered safe during pregnancy, while trimethoprim, sulfonamides, and fluoroquinolones should be avoided.

Fluoroquinolones and TMP-SMX prevent RUTI by inhibiting the recovery rate of uropathogens from the fecal reservoir while nitrofurantoin has a role in the treatment of RUTI by sterilizing the urine and reduce bacterial attachment [38, 39].

Various prophylaxis regimens such as patient self-treatment, post-coital prophylaxis, and continuous prophylaxis are important strategies in preventing RUTIs.

Patient self-treatment is recommended in cases of ≤2 episodes of UTIs annually, whereas continuous antimicrobial prophylaxis, or post-coital prophylaxis, is

Table 8.2 Recommended prophylactic regimens for RUTIs

Medication	Continuous dosage	Post-coital dosage	Acute self-treatment
Commonly used first-line agents			
Nitrofurantoin	50–100 mg per day	50–100 mg	
Trimethoprim/ sulfamethoxazole	40/200 mg per day 40/200 mg × 3 weekly	40/200 mg 80/400 mg	160/800 mg × 2/day per 3 days
Occasionally used first-line agents			
Cefaclor	250 mg daily	–	
Cephalexin	125–250 daily	125–250 mg	
Trimethoprim	100 mg daily	–	
Agents not commonly used for prophylaxis			
Ciprofloxacin	125 mg per day	125 mg	250 mg × 2/day per 3 days
Fosfomicin	3 gr every 10 days	–	
Ofloxacin	–	100 mg	
Norfloxacina	200 mg daily	200 mg	
Cinoxacin	250–500 daily	250 mg	200 mg × 2/day per 3 days

generally considered in ≥3 episodes of UTIs per year [40]. Table 8.2 shows possible regiments for RUTI prophylaxis.

- Patient self-treatment decreases overall antibiotic consumption and may be utilized in women who are not suitable for long-term daily prophylaxis. Self-therapy should be proposed to women who are motivated and have good compliance. Patient has to be informed to consult a physician in case of pregnancy, symptoms change, increase recurrence of episodes, or no change in symptoms within 48 h of treatment.
- Post-coital prophylaxis could be a strategy in case of cystitis related to sexual intercourse. Post-coital treatment consists in taking a course of antibiotics within 2 h of intercourse decreasing cost and side effects.
- Continuous daily or thrice weekly prophylaxis for 6 months or more is another alternative for prophylaxis.

Prophylaxis should be started after eradication of infection. Optimal prophylactic antibiotic is unknown, for the right choice allergies, prior susceptibility, local resistance patterns, cost, and side effects have to be considered. Side effects could be vaginal and oral candidiasis, gastrointestinal symptoms, skin rash, and severe nausea. There is no evidence to guide treatment after 6–12 months, although low dose trimethoprim/sulfamethoxazole has been tried for up to 5 years [41]. Those patients who wish to continue antibiotic prophylaxis for longer periods should be advised that there is no long-term safety data, a small chance of severe side effects, and resistant developing infections [42, 43]. When prophylaxis is discontinued, more than 50% of women will have another infection within 3 months [44].

Urine IBCs and filaments may be prognostic indicators of specific clinical outcomes; women with these findings may benefit from different management or prophylaxis strategies such as longer treatment or use of antibiotics with intracellular penetration. The recognition of uropathogenic *E. coli* as a potential intracellular pathogen challenges our current treatment regimens for UTI and stimulates the development of new antimicrobials or treatment regimens/strategies.

8.5.3 Alternative Strategies

Various alternative strategies have been studied for the prevention of RUTIs.

Although smaller studies have shown that **cranberry** juice or tablets can prevent RUTIs in premenopausal women, an updated Cochrane review showed that evidence for its benefit in preventing UTIs is small [45]. Recent trials demonstrated that cranberry has a protective effect regarding catheter associated urinary tract infection in the postoperative period [46, 47].

Recent studies indicate that the rate of cystitis among women treated with **acupuncture** was one-third the rate of that among untreated women and half the rate among women treated by false acupuncture. Therefore, acupuncture may prevent RUTIs in healthy adult women [48].

Reid et al. showed in vitro that **lactobacillus** can prevent uropathogen infections [49]. Other trials have showed that specifically *L. rhamnosus* gr-1 and *L. fermentum* rc-14 can colonize the vagina preventing UTIs. Nevertheless, more clinical studies are needed to clarify the role of lactobacillus in RUTI prevention [50, 51].

Methenamine hippurate (MH) is used for prophylaxis and treatment of RUTIs. Methenamine is hydrolyzed by acid urine to ammonia and formaldehyde that acts as a bactericide. MH are well tolerated and have mild adverse effects, such as gastrointestinal upsets, rashes, anorexia, and stomatitis. Patients should be informed about adequate hydration, side effects, and the need to avoid milk products and antacids to maintain the urine acidic. A recent Cochrane review on the use of MH concluded that short-term use is effective in preventing RUTIs [52].

Vitamin C can acidify urine and has been related with decreased risk of UTI. It also works synergistically with MH, providing an acidic environment. There is data to suggest that vitamin C can also have a bacteriostatic effect within urine, mediated by reduction of urinary nitrites to reactive nitrogen oxides [53].

D-mannose is a natural sugar which may have clinical benefit. Mannose receptors are part of the mucopolysaccharide layer on uroepithelial cells in the urinary tract. The mechanism of action is to prevent adhesion and invasion of urothelial cells by *E. coli* binding its mannose receptor. A randomized placebo-controlled non-blinded clinical trial has shown that a daily dose of 2 g d-mannose was superior to placebo and as effective as 50 mg nitrofurantoin in preventing UTI [54].

Vaccines are being explored as a prevention strategy. At present there are no widely available vaccines due to limited clinical success. Several vaccines, made from combinations of heat killed uropathogenic strains, have had partial success or are under development, delivered through injection, vaginal suppositories of intra-nasal sprays [55, 56]. OM-89 [Uro-Vaxom(R)] vaccinations have been demonstrated to be better than placebo with minimal side effects. The European Association of Urology guidelines have recommended immuno-prophylaxis in female patients with RUTIs [57].

Intravesical instillation of hyaluronic acid and chondroitin sulfate has been used in case of interstitial cystitis, overactive bladder syndrome, radiation cystitis, and prevention of RUTI. Treatment involved hyaluronic acid 1.6% and chondroitin sulfate 2% with one instillation per week for the first month, every 2 weeks instillations for the second month, and finally monthly instillations until remission of symptoms. Various studies demonstrated significantly reduced rates of recurrence and increased symptomatic relief, quality of life, and bladder capacity compared to standard therapy only [58]. Further research is required, and due to significant cost, it is limited at this stage to multi-resistant, difficult to eradicate UTIs.

8.5.4 Pregnancy and Recurrent UTI

Pregnant women with bacteriuria have a higher risk of preterm delivery and low birth weight infant [59]. The recommendation is to follow up the women with culture 1 week after the end of the therapy and monthly until the completion of the pregnancy [32].

Indications for prophylaxis are women with a pre-pregnancy history of RUTI, persistent symptomatic or asymptomatic bacteriuria after two antibiotic treatment, and after one UTI in women with risk factors for urinary complications (diabetes or sickle cell trait). The agents that may be used during pregnancy are nitrofurantoin (50 mg) or cephalexin (250 mg) [60, 61].

References

1. Echolls RM, Tosiello RL, Haverstock DC, et al. Demographic, clinical, and treatment parameters influencing the outcome of acute cystitis. Clin Infect Dis. 1999;29:113–9.
2. Hooton TM, Stamm WE. Diagnosis and treatment of uncomplicated urinary tract infection. Infect Dis Clin N Am. 1997;11:551–81.
3. Epp A, Larochelle A, Lovatsis D, et al. Recurrent urinary tract infection. J Obstet Gynaecol Can. 2010;32:1082–101.
4. Dason S, Dason JT, Kapoor A. Guidelines for the diagnosis and management of recurrent urinary tract infection in women. Can Urol Assoc J. 2011;5:316–22.
5. Campbell MF, Wein AJ, Kavoussi LR. Campbell-Walsh urology. 9th ed. Philadelphia, PA: W.B. Saunders; 2007.
6. Epp A, Alrcohelle A. 250-urinary tract infection. J Obstet Gynaecol Can. 2017;39(10):e422–31. https://doi.org/10.1016/j.jogc.2017.08.017.
7. Hotoon TM. Recurrent urinary tract infection in women. Int J Antimicrob Agents. 2001;17:259–68.
8. Rosen DA, Hooton TM, Stamm WE, Humphrey PA, Hultgren SJ. Detection of intracellular bacterial communitiesin human urinary tract infection. PLoS Med. 2007;4(12):e329. www.plosmedicine.org. December 1949

9. Russo TA, Stapleton A, Wenderoth S, Hooton TM, Stamm WE. Chromosomal restriction fragment length polymorphism analysis of Escherichia Coli strains causing recurrent urinary tract infection in young women. J Infect Dis. 1995;172:440–5.
10. Ejrnaes K, Sandvang D, Lundgreen B, Ferry S, Holm S, Monsen T, et al. Pulsed-field gel electrophoresis typing of Escherichia coli strains from samples collected before and after pivmecillinam or placebo treatment of uncomplicated community-acquired urinary tract infection in women. J Clin Microbiol. 2006;44:1776–81.
11. Vosti KL. A prospective longitudinal study of the behavior of serologically classified isolates of Escherichia coli in women with recurrent urinary tract infection. J Infect. 2007;55:8–18.
12. Beerepoot MA, den Heijer CD, Penders I, Prins IM, Stobberingh EE, Geerlings SE. Predictive value of Escherichia coli susceptibility in strains causing asymptomatic bacteriuria for women with recurrent symptomatic urinary tract infections receiving prophylaxis. Clin Microbiol Infect. 2012;18:E84–90.
13. Gilbert NM, O'Brien VP, Lewis AL. Transient microbiota exposures activate dormant Escherichia coli infection in the bladder and drive severe outcomes of recurrent disease. PLoS Pathog. 2017;13(3):e1006238. https://doi.org/10.1371/journal.ppat.1006238.
14. Scholes D, Hooton TM, Roberts PL, Stapleton AE, Gupta K, Stamm WE. Risk factors for recurrent urinary tract infection in young women. J Infect Dis. 2000;182:1177–82.
15. Foxman B, Barlow R, D'Arcy H, et al. Urinary tract infection: self-reported incidence and associated costs. Ann Epidemiol. 2000;10:509–15.
16. Hooton TM, Scholes D, Hughes JP, Winter C, Roberts PL, Stapleton AE, et al. A prospective study of risk factors for symptomatic urinary tract infection in young women. N Engl J Med. 1996;335:468–74.
17. Sheinfeld J, Schaeffer AJ, Cordon Cardo C, Rogatko A, Fair WR. Association of the Lewis blood group phenotype with recurrent urinary tract infections in women. N Engl J Med. 1989;320:773–7.
18. Df K, Blackwell CC, Brettle RP, Weir DM, Winstanley FP, Elton RA. ABO blood group secretor state and susceptibility to recurrent urinary tract infection in women. Br Med J. 1982;285:7–9.
19. Smithson A, Sarrias MR, Barcelo J, Suarez B, Horcajada JP, Soto SM, et al. Expression of interleukin 8 receptors (CXCR1 and CXCR2) in premenopausal women with recurrent urinary tract infections. Clin Diagn Lab Immunol. 2005;12:1358–63.
20. Foxman B. Epidemiology of urinary tact infections: incidence, morbiditi and economic cost. Am J Med. 2002;113:5S–13S.
21. Foxman B. Recurring urinary tract infection: incidence and risk factors. Am J Public Health. 1990;80:331–3.
22. Franco VMA. Recurrent urinary tract infections. Best Pract Res Clin Obstet Gynecol. 2005;19:861–73.
23. Stamm WE, Wagner KF, Amstel R. Causes of acute urethral syndrome in women. N Engl J Med. 1980;303:409–15.
24. Bent S, Nallamothu BK, Simel DL, et al. Does this women have an acute urinary tract infection? JAMA. 2002;287:2701–10.
25. Mohsin R, Siddiqui KM. Recurrent urinary tractinfections in females. J Pak Med Assoc. 2010;60:55–9.
26. Giesen LG, Cousins G, Dimitrov BD, et al. Predicting acute uncomplicated urinary tract infection in women: a systematic review of the diagnostic accuracy of symptoms and signs. BMC Fam Pract. 2010;11:78.
27. Simmerville JA, Mactyed WC, Pahira JJ. Urinalysis a comprehensive revie. Am Fam Physician. 2005;71:1153–62.
28. Jacobson SH. A five-year prospective follow-up of women with non-obstructive pyelonephritic renal scarring. Scand J Urol Nephrol. 1991;25:51–3.
29. Rocco F, Franchini V. Antimicrobial therapy for treatment of UTI in the elderly. Eur Urol. 1991;19:7–15.
30. Arnold JJ, Hehn LE, Klein DA. Common questions about recurrent urinary tract infection in women. Am Fam Physician. 2016;93:560–9.

31. Albert X, Huertas I, Pereiro I, Sanfelix J, Gosalbes V, Perrotta C. Antibiotics for preventing recurrent urinary tract infection in non-pregnant women. Cochrane Database Syst Rev. 2004;2004:CD001209.
32. Cai T, Mazzoli S, Mondaini N, Meaci F, Nesi G, d'elia C, Malossini G, Boddi V, Bartoletti R. The role of asymptomatic bacteriuria in young women with recurrent urinary tract infections: to treat or not to treat? Clin Infect Dis. 2012;55:771–7.
33. Drekonja DM, Johnson JR. Urinary tract infections. Prim Care. 2008;35:345–67.
34. Gupta K, Scholes D, Stamm WE. Increasing prevalence of antimicrobial resistance among uropathogens causing acute uncomplicated cystitis. JAMA J Am Med Assoc. 1999;281:736–8.
35. Kahlmeter G, Poulsen HO. Antimicrobial susceptibility of Escherichia coli from community-acquired urinary tract infections in Europe: the ECO*SENS study revisited. Int J Antimicrob Agents. 2012;39:45–51.
36. Shin J, Kim J, Wie SH, Cho YK, Lim SK, Shin SY, et al. Fluoroquinolone resistance in uncomplicated acute pyelonephritis: epidemiology and clinical impact. Microb Drug Resist. 2012;18:169–75.
37. Rizvi M, Khan F, Shukla I, Malik A, Shaheen. Rising prevalence of antimicrobial resistance in urinary tract infections during pregnancy: necessity for exploring newer treatment options. J Lab Physicians. 2011;3:98–103.
38. Stamm WE, Gounts GW, Wagner K, Martine D, Gregory D, McKevitt M, et al. Antimicrobical prophylaxis of recurrent urinary tract infections:a double-blind, placebo-controlled trial. Ann Inter Med. 1980;92:770–5.
39. Nicolle LE, Harding GK, Thomson M, et al. Efficacy of five years of continuous, low-dose trimethoprimsulfamethoxazole prophylaxis for urinary tract infection. J Infect Dis. 1988;157:1239–42.
40. Stapleton A, Stamm WE. Prevention or urinary tract infections. Best Pract And research. Clin Obstet Gynecol. 2005;19:861–73.
41. Nicolle LE. Prophylaxis: recurrent urinary tract infection in women. Infection. 1992;20:S203–5.
42. Cetti RJ, Venn S, Woodhouse CR. The risks of long-term nitrofurantoin prophylaxis in patients with recurrent urinary tract infection: a recent medico-legal case. BJU Int. 2009;103:567–9.
43. Hooton TM. Recurrent urinary tract infection in women. UpToDate 2011. http://www.uptodate.com/contents/recurrent-urinary-tract-infection-in-women. Accessed 21 Sept 2011.
44. Gupta K, Hooton TM, Roberts PL, Stamm WE. Patient-initiated treatment of uncomplicated recurrent urinary tract infections in young women. Ann Intern Med. 2001;135:9–16.
45. Jepson RG, Craig JC. Cranberries for preventing urinary tract infections. Cochrane Database Syst Rev. 2008:CD001321.
46. Alreak T, Soedal LIF, Faghereim SU, Digranes A, Baerheim A. Acupunture treatment in the prevention of uncomplicated recurrent lower urinary tract infection in adult women. Am J Public Health. 2002;92:1609–11.
47. Thomas D, Rutman M, Cooper K, Abrams A, Finkelstein J, Chughtai B. Does cranberry have a role in catheter-associated urinary tract infections? Can Urol Assoc J. 2017;11:E421–4. https://doi.org/10.5489/cuaj.4472.
48. Foxman B, Cronenwett AEW, Spino C, Berger MB, Morgan DM. Cranberry juice capsules and urinary tract infection post surgery: results of a randomized trial. Am J Obstet Gynecol. 2015;213(2):194.e1–8. https://doi.org/10.1016/j.ajog.2015.04.003.
49. Reid G, Bruce AW. Probiotics to prevent urinary tract infections: the rationale and evidence. World J Urol. 2006;24:28–32.
50. Uehara S, Monden K, Nomoto K, Deno Y, Kariyama R, Kumon H. A pilot study evaluating the safety and effectiveness of lactobacillus vaginal suppositories in patients with recurrent urinary tract infection. Int J Antimicrob Agents. 2006;28:S30–4.
51. Falagas ME, Betsi GI, Tokas T, Athanasius S. Probiotics for prevention of recurrent urinary tract infections in women. Drugs. 2006;66:1253–61.
52. Lee BS, Bhuta T, Simpson JM, Craig JC. Methenamine hippurate for preventiv urinary tract infections. Chocrane database. Sys Rev. 2012;10:CD003265.

53. Carlsson S, Govoni M, Wiklund NP, et al. In vitro evaluation of a new treatment for urinary tract infections caused by nitrate-reducing bacteria. Antimicrob Agents Chemother. 2003;47:3713–8.
54. Kraicec Bm Papes D, Altarac S. D –mannose powder for prophylaxis of recurrent urinary tract infections in women: randomized cliniucal trial. World J Urol. 2014;32:79.
55. Uehling DT, Hopkins WJ, Elkahwaji JE, et al. Phase 2 clinical trial of a vaginal mucosal vaccine for urinary tract infections. J Urol. 2003;170:867.
56. Hopkins WJ, Elkahwaji J, Baierle LM, et al. Vaginal mucosal vaccine for recurrent urinary tract infections in women: results of a phase 2 clinical trial. J Urol. 2007;177:1349.
57. Naber KG, Cho YH, Matsumoto T, et al. Immunoactive prophylaxis of recurrent urinary tract infections: a meta analysis. Int J Antimicrob Agents. 2009;33:111–9.
58. Ciani O, Arendsen E, Romancik M, et al. Intravesical administration of combined hyaluronic acid (HA) and chondroitin sulfate (CS) for the treatment of female recurrent urinary tract infections: a European multicentre nested case-control study. BMJ Open. 2016;6:e009669.
59. Romero R, Oyarzun E, Mazor M, et al. Meta-analysis of the relationship between asymptomatic bacteriuria and preterm delivery/low birth wwight. Obstet Gynecol. 1989;73:576–82.
60. Pfau A, Sacls TG. Effective prophylaxis for recurrent urinary tract infections during pregnancy. Clin Infect Dis. 1992;12:810–4.
61. Ovalle A, Levancini M. Urinary tract infections in regnancy. Curr Opin Urol. 2001;11:55–9.

Pyelonephritis: In- and Outpatients

9

Gernot Bonkat and Georg Müller

9.1 Introduction

Acute pyelonephritis is defined as an inflammation of the kidney caused by a bacterial infection of the renal parenchyma and/or pelvis. Acute pyelonephritis is considered as complicated when additional factors could promote such infection or make their treatment more difficult. Those factors include age above 65 years, diabetes, presence of urinary tract abnormalities or obstruction, pregnancy, transplantation, immunosuppression, multiresistant bacteria, hospital-acquired infection, symptoms for seven or more days, presence of an indwelling urethral catheter, stent, and nephrostomy tube or urinary diversion. In addition, in male patients, pyelonephritis is always considered as complicated. Finally, pyelonephritis and especially obstructive pyelonephritis has a strong potential to cause sepsis and ultimately death if untreated, and thus although it is quite common, pyelonephritis must be considered as a serious urological situation [1, 2].

Overall pyelonephritis also occurs mostly in women. Men, children, and pregnant women represent only a small percentage of all cases. Acute pyelonephritis has an estimated incidence of 10.5 million–25.9 million cases globally. Data for the USA account for a range comprised between 459,000 and 1,138,000 cases. As mentioned above, pyelonephritis might become a severe or lethal situation if it evolves toward a sepsis. Indeed, several studies estimated that the hospitalization rate ranges from 9 to 12 per 10,000 for women and from 1 to 3 per 10,000 for males [3]. However, in men mortality is higher in (1.6% of hospitalized cases) compared to

G. Bonkat (✉)
alta uro AG, Merian Iselin Klinik, Department of Biomedical Engineering, University Basel, Basel, Switzerland
e-mail: bonkat@alta-uro.com

G. Müller
alta uro AG, Merian Iselin Klinik, Basel, Switzerland
e-mail: mueller@alta-uro.com

T. E. Bjerklund Johansen, T. Cai (eds.), *Guide to Antibiotics in Urology*,
https://doi.org/10.1007/978-3-319-92366-6_9

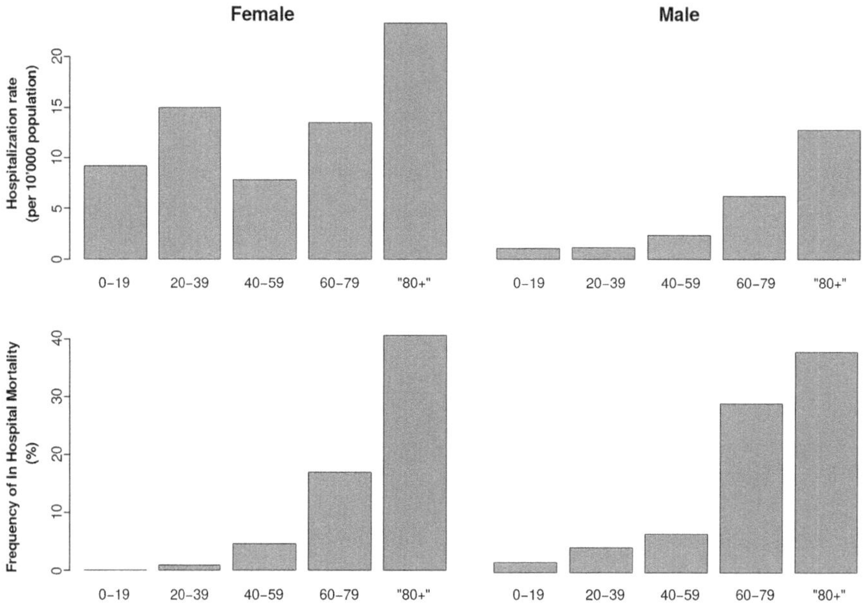

Fig. 9.1 Barplots showing the hospitalization rate and the in-hospital death rate for male and female with pyelonephritis. (Data from [4])

women (0.7% of hospitalized cases). All in all this results in cost of ca 2.14 billion USD for the USA only, thus emphasizing even more the public health and economic importance of the disease [3, 4]. However, one must keep in mind that such data are general and age is a crucial factor (see Fig. 9.1).

9.2 Diagnosis

Most publications commonly agree that flank pain, fever, and costovertebral angle tenderness with or without lower urinary tract symptoms (e.g., dysuria, urgency, and frequency) are the classic presenting features of pyelonephritis. In addition, gastrointestinal symptoms such as nausea, vomiting, diarrhea, or abdominal pain can also contribute to the diagnostic [3, 5, 6].

The diagnostic may be more difficult in immune-suppressed or immune-compromised patients as fever will not be marked. Similarly, in elderly patient with fever is not always marked as well. To make diagnostic even more difficult in elderly, several of these symptoms might be chronic or unrelated. Indeed, urinary tract symptoms such as incontinence, frequency, or urgency may be chronic. In addition, bacteriuria is commonly observed at older ages especially in elderly patients who are catheterized. In such patients care must be taken to exclude other possible diagnostic and make appropriate verifications when appropriate.

In addition to the physical examination of the patient, imaging and laboratory tests are very helpful in diagnosing pyelonephritis. Imaging will allow to identify structural abnormalities, such as obstruction from a stone or an abscess. In addition, in diabetic patients emphysematous pyelonephritis (necrotizing infection of the kidney with gas formation that occurs in renal parenchyma, collecting system or perinephric tissue) is common. It has been speculated that hyperglycemia might be responsible for gas through anaerobic gas production by microbes. As a consequence, imaging should be considered in diabetic patients with uncontrolled or poorly controlled glycemia [5, 7]. It was also shown that growth rate in urine and artificial urine was much higher when glucose was added [8] again supporting the use of imaging in diabetic patients.

In terms of laboratory assays, at early stage, when there is a suspicion of pyelonephritis, a rapid dipstick might already prove quite helpful. Dipstick studies have reported quite a wide range of sensitivity and specificity, and one must remain careful about negative results. Still considering the usually high CFU count and WBC count, it could be useful in the context of pyelonephritis; however, this would need to be thoroughly investigated. Considering further laboratory investigations, it is commonly admitted that a CFU count of 10′000 cfu/mL with a WBC count of 10/mm^3 (=10′000/mL or 1/HPF) is indicative of pyelonephritis when combined to the symptoms mentioned in the physical examination. Flow cytometry can deliver such result quite rapidly; however, bacterial culture is needed to isolate the causative pathogen and perform drug susceptibility testing (EAU guidelines). Finally, a blood culture is needed when bacteremia and sepsis are suspected. It must be noted that the CFU count threshold might be lowered (to 1000 CFU/mL) in cases where obstructive pyelonephritis is suspected, or if the patient had received previous antimicrobial therapy, or if extreme urine acidification is observed [9]. Finally, if fastidious microorganisms are suspected (ureaplasma, mycoplasma, mycobacterium), such threshold should be lowered as well, and incubation time before reading culture results should be increased.

9.3 Microbiology of Pyelonephritis

The microbiology of pyelonephritis is essentially dominated by *Escherichia coli* that represent up to 81% of isolates in female outpatients. Figure 9.2 is demonstrating the difference in uropathogen spectrum between male and females. Other enterobacteriaceae are also commonly isolated especially from the genus *Klebsiella* that can represent up to 7.3% of isolate in male inpatients [10]. Noteworthy, although *E. coli* isolates still represent a majority of isolates in male patients, other pathogens are more common, and their presence should be considered before initiating empirical antimicrobial therapy. In *E. coli* it was shown that isolate from pyelonephritis exhibited more frequently the presence of specific virulence compared to "unrelated" fecal isolates. Among those virulence factors, the presence of specific adhesins (P-, S-, and type-1 fimbriae), toxins (uropathogenic-specific protein, hemolysin, and cytotoxic necrotizing factor 1), capsule, and siderophores were found [11–14].

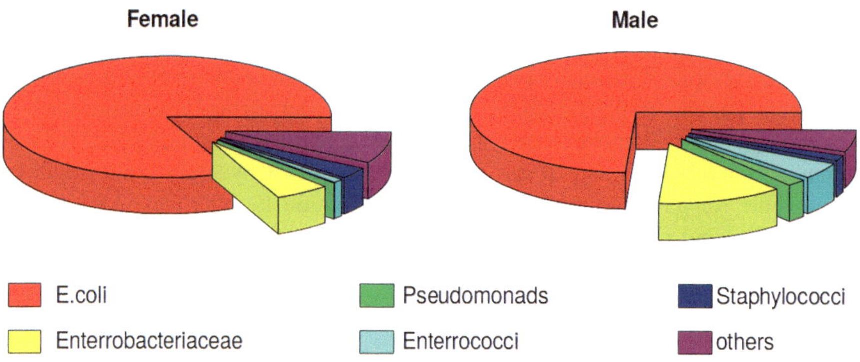

Fig. 9.2 Pie chart showing the difference in uropathogen spectrum between male and female. Although *E. coli* largely dominate the spectrum, it is less frequent in males where other Enterobacteriaceae are encountered more often [10]

In contrast, pathogenesis of other uropathogens has been much less studied. Other species such as *Proteus* spp., *K. pneumoniae*, and *S. saprophyticus* adhere to uroepithelial cells through different adhesive mechanisms. For *K. pneumoniae*, it was shown that the adhesin fimH and capsular polysaccharides played an important role in adhesion to epithelial cell from the urinary tract [15, 16]. *Proteus* spp., *K. pneumoniae*, and *S. saprophyticus* each produce urease promoting the release of ammonia and CO_2 and thus increasing urinary pH. That process can eventually worsen the situation by promoting the precipitation of minerals (such as struvite) that could ultimately form kidney stones. Finally, with respect to the pathogenesis of other uropathogens, it has been noted in [15] that "patients with diabetes are more likely to have infections involving *Klebsiella* spp., whereas patients with urinary catheters are more frequently diagnosed with *Pseudomonas* infection."

Fungal uropathogenic isolates especially yeast such as *Candida* species are rarely isolated [17, 18]. Mostly isolates are linked to nosocomial infections. However, such isolate should be considered with care as non-albicans *Candida* species such as *C. glabrata*, *C. tropicalis*, and *C. parapsilosis* and *C. krusei* can have higher (intrinsic) resistance to antifungal than *C. albicans* [19]. Increase glucose levels in blood and urine in diabetic patients might favor such yeast and lead to emphysematous pyelonephritis. Indeed, higher glucose concentration in urine has been shown to lead to an increased growth rate of *Candida albicans* (REF Lukas paper 1). Overall, the pathogen spectrum has been shown to shift drastically between acute uncomplicated pyelonephritis compared to complicated pyelonephritis. Indeed, in the later, *E. coli* is much less present, and yeast, enterococci, pseudomonads, and other enterobacteriaceae are isolated much more often [20] (Fig. 9.3). This certainly advocates for a very careful selection of antimicrobials when complicated pyelonephritis is suspected (or diagnosed).

Still, a compilation of case reports and clinical data on emerging pathogens is missing. Similarly, the role of the urinary tract microbiome in promoting or protecting from UTI and eventually from pyelonephritis has been subject to very few studies yet.

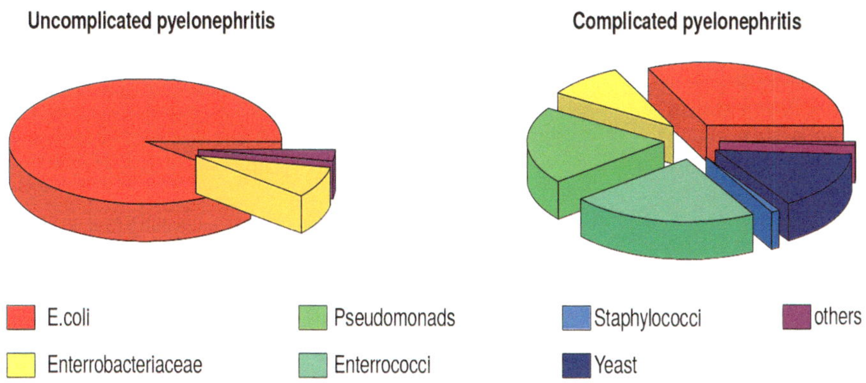

Fig. 9.3 Pie chart showing the difference in uropathogens spectrum isolated between uncomplicated acute pyelonephritis and complicated pyelonephritis. Although *E. coli* largely dominate the spectrum of uncomplicated pyelonephritis, it is less frequent in complicated cases [20]

9.4 Treatment

If the patient's conditions are sufficiently good, that is, fever and leukocytosis are mild, home treatment can be safely considered. It is possible that prior to home treatment a parenteral treatment is given in hospital and continued at home with a similar oral treatment. However, hospitalization is necessary if the patient shows/indicates additional risk factors involving a complicated pyelonephritis or presents clinical signs of sepsis [5]. Among the additional risk factors to be considered, the presence of comorbid conditions (e.g., renal dysfunction, urologic disorders, diabetes mellitus, advanced liver or cardiac disease), male sex, metabolic derangement (e.g., acidosis renal dysfunction), pregnancy, abdominal pain, or vomit or inability to take liquids by mouth are the one commonly encountered in the literature [6]. Very few variations in the uropathogens spectrum isolated from pyelonephritis patients over previous years have been observed. On the contrary, significant changes in the resistance patterns to antimicrobials have been noted [15]. Therefore, it is of much importance to have an up-to-date local drug susceptibility pattern. Table 9.1 summarizes the antimicrobial treatment option for the inpatient and outpatient.

9.4.1 Outpatient Treatment

Currently, EAU and ISDA guidelines recommend fluoroquinolones and cephalosporins for oral empirical therapy of uncomplicated pyelonephritis (see Table 9.1). Oral cephalosporins achieve significantly lower concentrations than intravenous cephalosporins. However, fluoroquinolones resistance being common, the local susceptibility toward this antimicrobial should be below 10% to use it safely. If high resistance to fluoroquinolones exists in the institution, other acceptable choices

Table 9.1 Regimens for empirical parenteral antimicrobial therapy in uncomplicated pyelonephritis

Antimicrobial	Inpatient (parenteral)	Outpatient (oral)
First-line treatment		
Ciprofloxacin	400 mg twice daily	500 mg twice daily (7 days)
Ciprofloxacin extended-release		1000 mg once daily (7 days)
Levofloxacin	750 mg once daily	750 mg once daily (5 days)
Trimethoprim/ sulfamethoxazole		160 mg/800 mg twice daily (14 days)
Cefpodoxime	2000 mg thrice daily	200 mg twice daily (10 days)[a]
Ceftibuten	1000–2000 mg thrice daily	400 mg once daily (10 days)[a]
Second-line treatment		
Cefepime	1000–2000 mg twice daily	
Piperacillin/tazobactam	2500–4500 mg twice daily	
Ceftolozane/tazobactam	1500 mg thrice daily	
Ceftazidime/avibactam	2500 mg thrice daily	
Gentamicin	5 mg/kg once daily	
Amikacin	15 mg/kg once daily	
Alternative options (third line)		
Imipenem/cilastatin	500 mg thrice daily	
Meropenem	1000 mg thrice daily	
Ceftolozane/tazobactam	1500 mg twice daily	
Ceftazidime/avibactam	2500 mg twice daily	
Cefiderocol	2000 mg twice daily	
Meropenem-vaborbactam	2000 mg twice daily	
Plazomicin	15 mg/kg o.d	

[a] In case of such treatment, an initial intravenous dose of a long-acting parenteral antimicrobial (e.g., ceftriaxone) should be administered

include trimethoprim-sulfamethoxazole (160/800 mg) or an oral beta-lactam (assuming that the uropathogen has been proved susceptible). Alternatively, such alternative can also be considered if there are known allergic reactions to fluoroquinolones. Other antimicrobials that do not reach a sufficient renal tissue levels such as nitrofurantoin, fosfomycin, and pivmecillinam are not recommended and should be avoided [1, 21].

9.4.2 Inpatient Treatment

Patients with uncomplicated pyelonephritis requiring hospitalization should be treated initially with an intravenous antimicrobial regimen such as a fluoroquinolone, an aminoglycoside (with or without ampicillin), an extended-spectrum cephalosporin, an extended-spectrum penicillin, or a carbapenem (see Table 9.1). The antimicrobial used must be chosen based on local resistance patterns and optimized as soon as drug susceptibility testing results become available. The EAU guidelines also recommend that in case of suspicion of a sepsis empiric antimicrobial treatment should be also consider extended-spectrum beta-lactamases (ESBL) producing microorganisms.

For inpatients initially treated with parenteral therapy who improve clinically and can tolerate oral fluids, a switch to an oral antimicrobial therapy can be considered [1, 21–23].

Studies have noted that outpatient oral therapy is successful in 90 percent of selected patients with uncomplicated acute pyelonephritis who can tolerate oral intake, will be compliant with the treatment regimen, will return for early follow-up, and have adequate social support [24, 25]. However, these studies are older, and new data should be gathered keeping in mind the ongoing increase of antimicrobial resistance. In all cases, the response to treatment should be monitored regularly. It is expected that appropriate empiric (or if available early drug susceptibility results guided) antimicrobial therapy will produce visible improvements within 48–72 h. If no improvement is observed as expected (i.e., no progressive reduction in, or resolution of, the systemic signs and symptoms that indicated the pyelonephritis during the diagnostic), a complication of acute pyelonephritis should be considered. Alternatively, another diagnostic should be considered as well, and appropriate additional testing should be conducted immediately.

References

1. Bonkat G, Pickard R, Bartoletti R, Cai T, Bruyére F, Geerlings SE, et al. EAU Guidelines on Urological Infections 2018. European Association of Urology Guidelines 2018 Edition. presented at the EAU Annual Congress Copenhagen 2018. Arnhem: European Association of Urology Guidelines Office; 2018.
2. Johnson JR, Russo TA. Acute pyelonephritis in adults. N Engl J Med. 2018;378(1):48–59.
3. Brown P, Ki M, Foxman B. Acute pyelonephritis among adults: cost of illness and considerations for the economic evaluation of therapy. PharmacoEconomics. 2005;23(11):1123–42.
4. Foxman B, Klemstine KL, Brown PD. Acute pyelonephritis in US hospitals in 1997: hospitalization and in-hospital mortality. Ann Epidemiol. 2003;13(2):144–50.
5. Rollino C, Sandrone M, Peruzzi L, De Marchi A, Beltrame G, Ferro M, et al. Direct bacterial infection of the renal parenchyma: pyelonephritis in native kidneys, Bacterial Infections and the Kidney. Cham: Springer; 2017. p. 161–93.
6. Colgan R, Williams M, Johnson JR. Diagnosis and treatment of acute pyelonephritis in women. Am Fam Physician. 2011;84(5):519.
7. Huang A, Palmer LS, Hom D, Anderson AE, Kushner L, Franco I. Ibuprofen combined with antibiotics suppresses renal scarring due to ascending pyelonephritis in rats. J Urol. 1999;162(4):1396–8.
8. Wernli L, Bonkat G, Gasser TC, Bachmann A, Braissant O. Use of isothermal microcalorimetry to quantify the influence of glucose and antifungals on the growth of Candida albicans in urine. J Appl Microbiol. 2013;115(5):1186–93.
9. Platt R. Quantitative definition of bacteriuria. Am J Med. 1983;75(1B):44–52.
10. Czaja CA, Scholes D, Hooton TM, Stamm WE. Population-based epidemiologic analysis of acute pyelonephritis. Clin Infect Dis. 2007;45(3):273–80.
11. Johnson JR. Virulence factors in Escherichia coli urinary tract infection. Clin Microbiol Rev. 1991;4(1):80–128.

12. Marrs CF, Zhang L, Tallman P, Manning SD, Somsel P, Raz P, et al. Variations in 10 putative uropathogen virulence genes among urinary, faecal and peri-urethral Escherichia coli. J Med Microbiol. 2002;51(2):138–42.
13. Pham T, Kaul A, Hart A, Goluszko P, Moulds J, Nowicki S, et al. dra-related X adhesins of gestational pyelonephritis-associated Escherichia coli recognize SCR-3 and SCR-4 domains of recombinant decay-accelerating factor. Infect Immun. 1995;63(5):1663–8.
14. Bauer RJ, Zhang L, Foxman B, Siitonen A, Jantunen ME, Saxen H, et al. Molecular epidemiology of 3 putative virulence genes for Escherichia coli urinary tract infection–usp, iha, and iroN E. coli. J Infect Dis. 2002;185(10):1521–4.
15. Ronald A. The etiology of urinary tract infection: traditional and emerging pathogens. Am J Med. 2002;113(Suppl 1A):14S–9S.
16. Schembri MA, Blom J, Krogfelt KA, Klemm P. Capsule and fimbria interaction in Klebsiella pneumoniae. Infect Immun. 2005;73(8):4626–33.
17. Krishnasamy PV, Liby C 3rd. Emphysematous pyelonephritis caused by Candida tropicalis. Am J Med. 2010;123(4):e7–8.
18. Fox L, Nelson AC, Ghanem G. Candida krusei emphysematous pyelonephritis possibly due to Dapagliflozin therapy. Infect Dis Clin Pract. 2018;26:363.
19. Pappas PG, Kauffman CA, Andes DR, Clancy CJ, Marr KA, Ostrosky-Zeichner L, et al. Clinical practice guideline for the management of candidiasis: 2016 update by the Infectious Diseases Society of America. Clin Infect Dis. 2016;62(4):e1–50.
20. Ramakrishnan K, Scheid DC. Diagnosis and management of acute pyelonephritis in adults. Am Fam Physician. 2005;71(5):933–42.
21. Gupta K, Hooton TM, Naber KG, Wullt B, Colgan R, Miller LG, et al. International clinical practice guidelines for the treatment of acute uncomplicated cystitis and pyelonephritis in women: a 2010 update by the Infectious Diseases Society of America and the European Society for Microbiology and Infectious Diseases. Clin Infect Dis. 2011;52(5):e103–e20.
22. Hooton TM. Uncomplicated urinary tract infection. N Engl J Med. 2012;366(11):1028–37.
23. Mombelli G, Pezzoli R, Pinoja-Lutz G, Monotti R, Marone C, Franciolli M. Oral vs intravenous ciprofloxacin in the initial empirical management of severe pyelonephritis or complicated urinary tract infections: a prospective randomized clinical trial. Arch Intern Med. 1999;159(1):53–8.
24. Safrin S, Siegel D, Black D. Pyelonephritis in adult women: inpatient versus outpatient therapy. Am J Med. 1988;85(6):793–8.
25. Bach D, van den Berg-Segers A, Hubner A, van Breukelen G, Cesana M, Pletan Y. Rufloxacin once daily versus ciprofloxacin twice daily in the treatment of patients with acute uncomplicated pyelonephritis. J Urol. 1995;154(1):19–24.

Part III

Treatment of Urinary Tract Infections with Risk Factors and Urosepsis

Management of Catheter-Associated Urinary Tract Infections

10

András Magyar, Péter Tenke, and Béla Köves

10.1 General

In this chapter we aim to discuss the main aspects in terms of diagnostics, treatment, and prevention of catheter-associated urinary tract infections (CA-UTIs).

Urinary tract infections (UTIs) are considered complicated in the presence of risk factors such as diabetes mellitus, immunosuppression, and functional or anatomical abnormalities including the presence of urinary foreign bodies. Presence of these complicating factors makes the UTIs more difficult to treat than the uncomplicated infections [1–3]. Complicated UTIs that develop in patients with indwelling catheters, or who have been catheterized within the past 48 h, are considered CA-UTIs. Female sex, microbial colonization of the drainage bag, catheter insertion outside the operating room, catheter care violations, serious illness, older age, diabetes mellitus, and elevated serum creatinine levels at the time of catheterization increase the risk of development of CA-UTIs [4–10].

Despite the increased risk for infection, bladder catheterization, with appropriate indication, plays an important role in management of patients with urinary retention, especially after spinal cord injury as a result of trauma. The renal-related mortality in these patients has been reduced from 95% to 3% since the last century. However, as a result of widespread, often unnecessary use of urinary catheters, CA-UTIs have become the most common health care–associated infections worldwide. General hospitals play a huge role in the spread of CA-UTIs, where 15–25% of patients undergo urinary catheterization for an average duration of 2–4 days [4, 11–13]. The duration of the catheterization is a major risk factor for infection, as the risk of bacteriuria increases by 3–8% each day after a urinary catheter is placed, and by the first month bacteriuria develops universally [4, 14–17]. CA-UTIs develop in one-quarter of hospitalized patients with catheter-associated bacteriuria, while

A. Magyar (✉) · P. Tenke · B. Köves
Department of Urology, Jahn Ferenc South Pest Teaching Hospital, Budapest, Hungary
e-mail: urologia@jahndelpest.hu

T. E. Bjerklund Johansen, T. Cai (eds.), *Guide to Antibiotics in Urology*,
https://doi.org/10.1007/978-3-319-92366-6_10

bacteremia appears in 1–4% of the cases [15, 18–22], which is a significant risk for the patients, since the mortality rate of hospital-acquired bacteremia is around 10% [21]. Moreover, twenty percent of hospital-acquired bacteremias arise from the urinary tract, and the majority of these infections is catheter-associated, especially in chronically catheterized patients, who undergo endoscopic surgery, such as transurethral resection of the prostate [23, 24]. The risk of infectious complications is increased by 10 times [25], while the death rate following TURP and similar operations is approximately doubled in this patient group. The fact that CA-UTIs are often caused by multidrug-resistant bacteria might also play a major role in the increased risk. Besides the increased mortality rate, long-term catheterization is associated with an increased rate of upper urinary tract inflammation, frequent febrile episodes, catheter obstruction, renal and bladder stone formation, infection with urease-producing uropathogens, local genitourinary infections, fistula formation, incontinence, and bladder cancer [12, 26, 27].

The literature on CA-UTIs is problematic, because authors often confuse terminology on catheter-associated bacteriuria (asymptomatic colonization) and CA-UTIs (symptomatic infection), even though there is a key difference between these conditions, especially from the therapeutic point of view [28]. Asymptomatic bacteriuria is a benign condition, which should not be treated, unless the patient is pregnant or undergoes certain urologic procedures.

10.2 Pathogenesis

10.2.1 The Source of Infection

At the time of catheter insertion, there is an increased risk that the patient's fecal or skin flora is inoculated into the bladder from the personnel's hand or from the environment [29]. This is especially common in patients who have inadequate cleansing of the perineum and distal urethra.

The most common mechanism of bacterial colonization is transurethral ascent. Bacteria can migrate on both surfaces of the catheters: along the extraluminal surface between the urethra and the catheter surface, or by reflux from the contaminated bags along the lumen of the catheter. Two-thirds of the uropathogens which cause catheter-associated bacteriuria are acquired extraluminally, and one-third intraluminally [30]. Some data suggest that colonization via the urethral route occurs more often in women [9, 31]. However, the intraluminal ascent of bacteria is faster (32–48 h) than the extraluminal (72–168 h) [32]. As a result, bacteria found in the drainage bag soon appear in the bladder [4, 15, 33].

The main risk factor of development of CA-UTIs is the duration of catheterization. In open-drainage catheter systems, the bacteriuria develops within 4 days, while in closed catheter systems the rate of bacteriuria increases by 3–8% per day [5, 34]. Later, the formation of bacterial biofilm between the catheter and the urethra provides a favorable environment for continuous bacterial invasion and proliferation via the extraluminal route.

10.2.2 The Pathomechanism of Colonization

After a catheter is placed, it continuously provides a route for the bacteria into the urinary tract and serves as a surface that promotes microbial adhesion to the bladder. Moreover, catheterization bypasses and reduces the effectiveness of the host-defense mechanisms, and provides easier access for the pathogens to the bladder, since uroepithelial cells from catheterized patients are more receptive to binding of bacteria, uroepithelial mucosa is disrupted, exposing new binding sites for bacterial adhesins [35, 36]. After the attachment to the surface of the catheter, the pathogens undergo a phenotypical change resulting in an enhanced production of exopolysaccharides, which leads to bacterial biofilm formation. Furthermore, within 1–3 days after adhesion to the catheter surface, the biofilms can also migrate to the bladder wall. Inside the biofilm, the pathogen microcolonies are protected from the host defense system and the mechanical flush of the urine flow. The biofilm also inhibits the diffusion of antibiotics to the multimicrobial colonies [6, 35]. Repeated unsuccessful antibiotic treatments lead to the selection of multidrug-resistant bacteria. From the therapeutic point of view, it is also notable that urine cultures obtained through a catheter with a biofilm do not always reflect the bacterial population growing within the bladder [37–39]. The planktonic free-floating bacteria can be detected by conventional urine culturing; however, sessile pathogens within the biofilm cannot be detected by routine methods [40–45]. One-quarter of bacteria cultured from urine collected through the catheter are not present in urine simultaneously obtained by suprapubic bladder puncture [37].

10.3 Considerations Regarding the Spectrum and Antibiotic Resistance of Bacteria in Catheterized Patients

10.3.1 Bacterial Spectrum

CA-UTIs are caused by a different spectrum of uropathogens than uncomplicated UTIs. While in patients without catheters, uropathogens are more likely to be of enteric origin (*Escherichia coli*, *Enterobacteriaceae*), in presence of urinary catheters there is an increased chance of infections caused by non-enteric bacteria, such as *Pseudomonas aeruginosa* due to biofilm formation. *E. coli* remains the most common uropathogen in both catheterized and non-catheterized patients, but Gram-positive bacteria such as *Enterococcus species* are among the leading causes of UTI in the presence of catheters. Candiduria can be isolated in 3–32% of patients, catheterized for short periods of time, which is usually asymptomatic and often does not require any treatment [20, 46].

Time is a major factor in the bacterial colonization. It has been shown that concentrations of bacteria increase with the duration of the catheterization and then decrease significantly when a new catheter is inserted [39]. In short-term catheterization (<30 days), the bacteriuria is mostly caused by single organisms and is usually asymptomatic. Moreover, the colonization is often caused by less virulent bacteria, and the bacterial spectrum mostly depends on the locally prevailing flora of the community or hospital. In long-term catheterization (30 days or longer), however, the bacteriuria is polymicrobial in up to 95% of the cases, the biofilm formation occurs universally, and the bacteria are more likely to be resistant to antibiotics. *E. coli* is the most common bacteria, but other organisms such as *Providencia stuartii* [17], *Acinetobacter*, *Enterococcus*, and *Candida* spp. may also frequently be found. There is a higher rate of urease-producing bacteria with stronger biofilm forming activity, such as *Proteus mirabilis*, *Pseudomonas aeruginosa*, *Klebsiella pneumoniae*, or *Morganella morganii*. Crystalline biofilm formation, struvite stone formation, and catheter encrustation are often caused by urease-producing organisms. The bacterial spectrum of the catheters can be different to the free-floating bacteria in the urine, as some bacteria colonize only the catheter and dwell within the biofilm. In the case of chronic catheterization, cultures obtained before catheter replacement showed a 110-fold higher rate of *P. mirabilis*, *P. stuartii*, *M. morganii*, *P. aeruginosa*, and *Enterococci* compared to cultures obtained from freshly replaced catheters [39].

10.3.2 Bacterial Resistance to Antibiotics

CA-UTIs are often caused by highly antimicrobial resistant bacteria, such as ESBL-positive or multidrug-resistant pathogens. The biofilm formation during long-term catheterization might serve as one of the main reasons of the high bacterial resistance rates. Patients with indwelling catheters often receive antimicrobials, which cannot reach the bacteria protected by the bacterial biofilm. The lower antibiotic exposure and the repeated antibiotic treatments facilitate the development of bacterial resistance versus antibiotics. The spread of bacterial resistance is more rapid as the rate of genetic material exchange is increased among the bacteria within the biofilms [35].

Bacteria in biofilms, especially those that can hydrolyze urea in the urine to free ammonia, cause alkaline urine and often form encrustations of the catheters, as the increased urine pH facilitates hydroxyapatite or struvite stone formation. The encrustations will soon result in catheter obstruction, which may increase the risk for epididymitis, prostatitis, and scrotal abscess [6, 47].

10.4 Diagnosis and Treatment of CA-UTIs

Diagnosis of CA-UTI in catheterized patients (urethral, suprapubic, or intermittent) is based on positive urine culture accompanied by symptoms suggesting UTI, with no other identified source of infection. Development of UTI in patients who have been catheterized within the previous 48 h is also considered as CA-UTI.

Diagnosis of CA-UTI may be difficult, since the symptoms of complicated UTIs (e.g., dysuria, urgency, frequency, flank pain, costovertebral angle tenderness, suprapubic pain, and fever) may be atypical in the presence of urinary catheters.

Furthermore, a very heterogeneous group of patients may be affected. Patients with neurogenic disorders, septic patients catheterized to relieve urinary tract obstruction, and catheterized for surgical procedures often develop CA-UTI. Clinical presentations may vary from simple post-operative CA-UTI, which can disappear after removal of the catheters, to severe pyelonephritis or sepsis, or Fournier gangrene, requiring intensive care and surgical intervention. In addition, concomitant complicating factors, such as diabetes mellitus, may worsen the outcome.

10.4.1 Standard Diagnostic Evaluation

Symptoms referable to the urinary tract, fever, or leukocytosis, odorous or cloudy urine have little predictive value for the diagnosis of CA-UTI. In CA-UTIs the classic symptoms of UTI, such as dysuria, frequent and urgent urination, mostly appear only after the catheter has been removed. Diagnosis is especially difficult in patients with neurogenic bladders, due to absence of sensation in the pelvis. In chronically catheterized patients, febrile episodes are only found in less than 10% of the cases. Thorough inspection and evaluation of the symptoms is necessary to exclude sources of infection other than the urinary tract. In the case of septic patients, blood culturing is recommended. It is also notable that if bladder catheterization lasts longer than 10 years, the patient should be screened for bladder cancer, due to its increased risk.

10.4.1.1 Clinical Symptoms that Might be Associated with CA-UTI

- New onset or worsening of fever.
- Rigors.
- Altered mental status.
- Malaise, or lethargy with no other identified cause.
- Flank pain.
- Costovertebral angle tenderness.
- Acute hematuria.
- Pelvic discomfort.
- Dysuria, urgent or frequent urination and suprapubic pain or tenderness (in those whose catheters have been removed in the past 48 h).
- Autonomic dysreflexia, sense of unease, increased spasticity may indicate CA-UTI in patients with spinal cord injury.

10.4.1.2 Pyuria

The presence, absence, or degree of pyuria cannot be used to distinguish catheter-associated bacteriuria from CA-UTI. The sensitivity of pyuria for catheter-associated bacteriuria is low, around 47%, the specificity is 90%, and the positive predictive value is 32% [48]. In long-term catheterization, levels of pyuria do not change substantially during symptomatic episodes [49].

In catheterized patients, dipstick testing for nitrites and leukocyte esterase cannot be used as a diagnostic tool either [50].

10.4.1.3 Microbiology

There are some basic rules concerning the collection of the urine from catheterized patients, depending on the duration of catheterization. In patients with short-term catheterization, urine specimens can be collected through the catheter port using aseptic technique [46]. In the case of long-term catheterization, the urine specimen for culturing should be obtained from the freshly changed catheter. Before the initiation of antibiotic treatment, the catheter should be replaced, if the duration of the catheterization was at least 2 weeks long at the onset of the symptomatic infection [37–39, 51]. Culture specimens should not be collected from drainage bags.

There is no standardized threshold for the bacterial count to be considered positive. However, if UTI symptoms are present at $\geq 10^3$ cfu/mL bacteria in a single catheter urine or in a midstream voided urine (if the catheter has been removed in the past 48 h), uninfected and infected bladder urine can be differentiated with 97% sensitivity and 97% specificity [52]. It is important to emphasize that in catheterized patients, pyuria or the presence or absence of odorous or cloudy urine is not diagnostic for CA-UTI, and in asymptomatic catheterized patients there is no need for routine urine culturing either [28, 53].

10.4.2 Asymptomatic Bacteriuria in Catheterized Patients

Catheters placed in the urinary tract inevitably lead to bacteriuria, and bacterial colonization of permanent urethral catheters and stents cannot be prevented with antibiotic prophylaxis. Bladder catheterization also increases the risk of symptomatic UTI [54]. If there are no symptoms of CA-UTI, the bacteriuria is considered asymptomatic. Catheter-associated asymptomatic bacteriuria is defined by 10^5 cfu/mL of a bacterial species in a single urine specimen obtained from a catheterized patient with no symptoms for UTI.

There is no benefit from screening or treating asymptomatic bacteriuria with antibiotics, except during pregnancy or in certain cases of antibiotic prophylaxis for surgical procedures (traumatic urinary tract interventions such as transurethral resection of the prostate), as it will only lead to development of drug-resistant organisms [47]. Screening and treatment of asymptomatic bacteriuria may also be advised on placement or exchanges of nephrostomy tubes and indwelling urethral stents, but is not recommended on uncomplicated placement and exchanges of indwelling catheters [55, 56].

In catheterized patients, pyuria or the presence or absence of odorous or cloudy urine is not diagnostic for CA-UTI and in itself should not be treated with antibiotics [28, 53]. Instead of antimicrobial therapy, alternate interventions, such as improved continence management or hydration, should be instituted [57, 58].

Depending on the patient's condition, it is important to minimalize the number of days wearing an indwelling urethral catheter as much as possible. After the catheter has been successfully removed, bacteriuria will spontaneously disappear in one-third to one-half of the cases [59, 60].

10.4.3 Symptomatic CA-UTIs

CA-UTIs are caused by a wider spectrum of pathogens than uncomplicated UTIs, and an increased rate of antibiotic-resistant bacteria can be expected. For this reason, before the initiation of antibiotic treatment in CA-UTIs, urine culturing should be performed to confirm that an empirical regimen provides appropriate coverage, as well as because it later gives the opportunity to modify the treatment based on the antimicrobial susceptibility data [61]. Collection of the urine specimens for culturing should be obtained from a freshly placed catheter [28]. A prospective, randomized, controlled trial revealed that in long-term catheterization, the replacement of the catheter at the onset of CA-UTI results in faster recovery and a lower rate of CA-UTI recurrence within 28 days after treatment [51]. If the catheterization can be discontinued, the catheter must be removed and midstream urine should be sent for culturing.

It is difficult to estimate the optimal treatment duration, since there is a big variety of clinical manifestations of CA-UTIs, such as cystitis, prostatitis, pyelonephritis, abscess formation, and bacteremia. Antibiotic resistance of the causative pathogen, co-morbid conditions, and patient response should also be taken into account.

Treatment duration should be limited to reduce selection pressure for drug-resistant flora in long-term catheterized patients, especially with mild infections. In patients with fast and complete response to antibiotic therapy, treatment should last 7 days in general. If the patient is a younger woman and the symptoms are limited to the lower urinary tract, the catheter should be removed and then followed by a 3 days long antibiotic treatment. In otherwise healthy patients a 5 days long treatment for CA-UTI with levofloxacin is a valid option. The therapy should be prolonged up to 2 weeks when the resolution of the symptoms shows delayed tendency [28]. The optimal treatment duration for patients with spinal cord injury is between 3 and 14 days.

In many cases, the catheter cannot be removed. If CA-UTI develops in these patients, replacement of the catheter is required, in order to fasten up the resolution of symptoms and to decrease the bacterial burden. Prior to antibiotic treatment, if the catheter can be removed, a midstream urine specimen collection is preferred [28]. The empirical treatment is usually initiated with broad-spectrum antibiotics based on local susceptibility patterns, depending on the patient's health status. After receiving culture results, antibiotic treatment should be adjusted to the antibiotic susceptibility pattern of the causative pathogen, preferably by switching to narrower spectrum antibiotics. In septic patients, blood samples must also be taken for culturing. If the patient does not have a prompt clinical response within 72 h of the treatment, re-evaluation of the symptoms and further diagnostics may be necessary. Urine culture or urinalysis for follow-up of resolved CA-UTIs is not required. Funguria is often present in catheterized patients; however, its relevance is still not completely known; thus, it is hard to predict when funguria should be treated.

10.5 Non-antibiotic Treatments and Strategies, Alternatives, and Prevention

10.5.1 Clear Indications, Limitation of Catheter Use

Prevention of CA-UTI should receive high priority in infection prevention programs. The most important aspect is to limit the use of urinary catheterization. Catheterization should be restricted to clear indications. Acceptable indications for urinary catheter use are (1) significant acute or chronic urinary retention, where surgical correction is not an option and the medical therapy was not effective, (2) if accurate monitoring is necessary and other options are not available for critically ill patients, (3) for fluid challenge in acute renal failure, and (4) before prolonged surgeries and for special indications in certain operations.

The duration of catheterization should always be minimized, and unnecessary catheterization should be avoided. As a general rule, catheters should be removed as early as possible. After non-urological operations, removal of the catheter on the same day is the optimal solution. It is recommended to use portable bladder scan devices to determine any residual urine in postoperative patients, as opposed to applying instant catheterization for this purpose. Nurse-based or electronic physician reminder systems and automatic stop-orders could limit inappropriate urinary catheterization. Urinary incontinence should not be managed with urinary catheterization, except in selected cases on the request of a well-informed patient.

10.5.2 Strict Protocol, Institutional Strategies, and Education

To reduce the contamination rate at institutions, written catheter care protocols are necessary; staff education and assessment of the adherence to the infection control guidelines is essential. Adherence to protocols for catheter care was associated with a lower incidence of CA-UTI [62, 63]. During the care of catheterized patients, the staff should observe the following rules. The indwelling catheters should be introduced under antiseptic conditions, and the risk of urethral trauma should be minimized through the use of adequate lubricant and the smallest possible catheter. The catheterized urinary tract should always be treated as an open wound, and the staff must be aware of the constant risk of cross-infection between catheterized patients [64–66]. Strict application of aseptic techniques, use of closed catheter systems, sterile equipment, such as sterile disposable gloves, and frequent hand disinfection are mandatory. While using closed catheter drainage, breaks in the integrity of the system should be kept to a minimum. Opening the drainage system should be limited to drainage bag exchanges, bladder wash-out, or urine sampling if necessary. Preconnected systems can also be useful. The drainage bag and connecting tube should be kept below the level of the bladder. The timing of catheter changes depends on the patient, the catheter type, and manufacturer. In some patients ("blockers"), catheter blockage occurs more often, and their catheter must be changed more frequently [67, 68]. The catheterized patients should also receive sufficient fluids orally.

10.5.3 Alternatives to Urethral Catheters

Prevention of CA-UTIs may be accomplished by alternatives to indwelling catheterization. If long-term urine deviation is unavoidable, placement of an epicystostomy or intermittent catheterization is the preferred option over chronic urethral catheterization. Suprapubic catheterization is often indicated in patients undergoing urological procedures, significant retention during prostatitis, urethral trauma, and also provides better patient comfort. Intermittent catheterization is a popular option in the management of neuropathic bladder, but requires cooperative and skilled patients. However, the majority of patients managed with intermittent catheterization also become bacteriuric [69]: bacteriuria is acquired at the rate of 1–3% per catheterization, and is universal by the end of the third week [70–73]. It has been shown that suprapubic catheters are superior to indwelling urethral catheters in terms of bacteriuria and the lack of risk for urethral strictures [74]. Urethral stents and condom catheters are also alternatives to indwelling urinary catheters. Condom catheters can be useful in male patients without outlet obstruction. Their application is a valid option for male patients who require short-term catheterization and have minimal postvoid residual volume.

The material of the catheter is also important. Silicone catheters may have advantages over latex catheters as they are associated with less cytotoxicity, inflammation, urethritis, stricture formation, penile discomfort, and obstruction from encrustations, but do not seem to reduce the development of bacteriuria [75].

10.5.4 Other, less Common Methods

The urine of catheterized patients cannot be permanently sterilized with antibiotics, and chronic antibiotic suppressive therapy is not effective [47]. The data are insufficient concerning the use of methenamine salts for prophylaxis being effective; however, some observations suggest that their application may be considered in patients who wear catheters for less than 1 week following gynecologic surgery [28]. The benefit of cranberry products for reducing CA-UTIs has not been proven; therefore, they should not be used routinely in CA-UTI. Routine metal cleansing with povidone-iodine solution, as well as the use of silver sulfadiazine, polyantibiotic cream, green soap, and water have no advantage. Catheter irrigation with antimicrobials or saline and addition of antimicrobials or antiseptics to the drainage bag is not recommended either.

10.6 Research on CA-UTIs

10.6.1 Catheter-Associated Asymptomatic Bacteriuria and CA-UTI

CA-UTIs require further research using standardized methodologies. Researchers often assess the effectiveness of novel interventions and tools by their ability to reduce catheter-associated asymptomatic bacteriuria, but fail to explore the effect they have on CA-UTIs. However, most of the patients with catheter-associated asymptomatic bacteriuria do not develop CA-UTI, although it is presumed that the presence of bacteriuria might be relevant in the development of symptomatic infections, but the connection between the two conditions is uncertain. Since CA-UTIs often show atypical symptoms, better diagnostic tools are needed to distinguish CA-UTIs from bacteriuria.

10.6.2 New Catheter Types and Materials

One hundred years ago, Foley introduced the self-retaining urethral catheter. As it was initially used with open drainage, bacteriuria developed within 4 days [76]. With the introduction of closed-catheter systems, development of bacteriuria became slower, but was still universal in 30 days [12, 32, 77]. Recently, a lot of new catheter types have been introduced with the aim to reduce bacteriuria and the number of CA-UTI episodes, such as catheters coated with different chemical materials. Antibiotic-impregnated catheters could decrease the frequency of bacteriuria in short term, did not prevent development of symptomatic CA-UTI. Silver alloyed catheters showed benefits also only at short-term [78]. Phosphorylcholine and heparin coating could also inhibit encrustation and biofilm formation in short-term [79–81]. However, these modifications might have benefits in short-term catheterization at intensive care units [82]. Unfortunately, their effect on morbidity is not assured, and none of them showed advantage in long-term. For this reason, research on new types of catheters that can reduce bacteriuria, the rate of symptomatic UTIs, and the biofilm formation on catheter surface is necessary. New antimicrobial agents, effective against bacteria dwelling in the biofilm on catheter surface, should be developed. Biomaterials and mechanical catheter surface modifications to prevent adherence of bacterial cells are still under development; however, reduction of catheter encrustation especially caused by *P. mirabilis* biofilms represents a major scientific challenge [83, 84]. Upcoming research on mechanical modification of catheter surface shows promising results, due to their ability to inhibit bacterial biofilm adhesion, but they require further research, whether they can reduce the number of CA-UTI episodes in long-term [85]. Inoculation of organisms of low virulence into the bladder to create a protective flora is a promising and exciting novel field of research [86, 87].

10.7 Conclusions

Urinary catheterization is the most important predisposing factor for nosocomial UTI, as indwelling catheters provide surface for bacterial colonization, decrease the effectiveness of host-defense mechanisms, and provide a transient presence of uropathogens in the bladder. The colonized catheter surface enhances the attachment of bacterial adhesins with the host cell binding receptors, damages the uroepithelial mucosa, exposing new binding sites for the bacteria, and reduces the virulence requirements of any bacterial strain to induce infection. Once a catheter is inserted in the urinary tract, the bacteria develop a polymetric matrix on the catheter surface. As a consequence, an own bacterial community develops encapsulated and protected by the bacterial biofilm, increasing the risk of UTI. During long-term catheterization, the microcolonies within the biofilms become polymicrobial. The biofilms inherently protect uropathogens from antimicrobials and the host immune response promoting the selection of antibiotic-resistant bacteria, which makes treatment of CA-UTIs even more difficult. Furthermore, the symptoms of UTI are often nonspecific in catheterized patients and pyuria or bacteriuria alone are not diagnostic for catheter-associated bacteriuria or CA-UTI either.

However, only patients with CA-UTI should receive antibiotic treatment. In chronically catheterized patients, the catheter should be removed or replaced prior antibiotic treatment.

To reduce the rate of nosocomial CA-UTIs prevention is especially important. Since the avoidance of unnecessary catheterization is considered to be the most effective way to reduce incidence of CA-UTIs, these strategies should be prioritized at all health care facilities. Adherence to hygienic protocols for catheter care is associated with a lower incidence of CA-UTIs. As indwelling urethral catheters are prone to cause symptomatic infection, alternatives should always be considered in appropriate patients. Silicone catheters are more biocompatible, cause less tissue necrosis, and obstruct less often; therefore, they are preferred for long-term usage. Previous research on chemical modification of the catheter surface such as development of antibiotic impregnated, silver alloyed, or heparinized catheters showed good results in short-term; however, in long term they did not reduce the risk of CA-UTIs. Research on mechanical modification of catheter surface shows promising results in terms of reduction of bacterial biofilm formation.

Acknowledgments The book chapter was written based on the latest existing international guidelines on catheter-associated urinary tract infections:

- European and Asian guidelines on management and prevention of catheter-associated urinary tract infections. International journal of antimicrobial agents, 2008 [47].
- European Association of Urology Guidelines on Urological infections, 2017 [88].

– Diagnosis, prevention, and treatment of catheter-associated urinary tract infection in adults: 2009 International Clinical Practice Guidelines from the Infectious Diseases Society of America [28].

References

1. Reyner K, Heffner AC, Karvetski CH. Urinary obstruction is an important complicating factor in patients with septic shock due to urinary infection. Am J Emerg Med. 2016;34(4):694–6.
2. Heyns CF. Urinary tract infection associated with conditions causing urinary tract obstruction and stasis, excluding urolithiasis and neuropathic bladder. World J Urol. 2012;30(1):77–83.
3. Spoorenberg V, Hulscher ME, Geskus RB, de Reijke TM, Opmeer BC, Prins JM, et al. Better antibiotic use in complicated urinary tract infections; multicentre cluster randomised trial of 2 improvement strategies. Ned Tijdschr Geneeskd. 2016;160:D460.
4. Garibaldi RA, Burke JP, Dickman ML, Smith CB. Factors predisposing to bacteriuria during indwelling urethral catheterization. N Engl J Med. 1974;291(5):215–9.
5. Maki DG, Tambyah PA. Engineering out the risk for infection with urinary catheters. Emerg Infect Dis. 2001;7(2):342–7.
6. Saint S, Chenoweth CE. Biofilms and catheter-associated urinary tract infections. Infect Dis Clin N Am. 2003;17(2):411–32.
7. Platt R, Polk BF, Murdock B, Rosner B. Risk factors for nosocomial urinary tract infection. Am J Epidemiol. 1986;124(6):977–85.
8. Huth TS, Burke JP, Larsen RA, Classen DC, Stevens LE. Randomized trial of meatal care with silver sulfadiazine cream for the prevention of catheter-associated bacteriuria. J Infect Dis. 1992;165(1):14–8.
9. Garibaldi RA, Burke JP, Britt MR, Miller MA, Smith CB. Meatal colonization and catheter-associated bacteriuria. N Engl J Med. 1980;303(6):316–8.
10. Loeb M, Hunt D, O'Halloran K, Carusone SC, Dafoe N, Walter SD. Stop orders to reduce inappropriate urinary catheterization in hospitalized patients: a randomized controlled trial. J Gen Intern Med. 2008;23(6):816–20.
11. Haley RW, Hooton TM, Culver DH, Stanley RC, Emori TG, Hardison CD, et al. Nosocomial infections in U.S. hospitals, 1975-1976: estimated frequency by selected characteristics of patients. Am J Med. 1981;70(4):947–59.
12. Warren JW. Catheter-associated urinary tract infections. Infect Dis Clin N Am. 1997;11(3):609–22.
13. Jamil F. Towards a catheter free status in neurogenic bladder dysfunction: a review of bladder management options in spinal cord injury (SCI). Spinal Cord. 2001;39(7):355–61.
14. Classen DC, Larsen RA, Burke JP, Stevens LE. Prevention of catheter-associated bacteriuria: clinical trial of methods to block three known pathways of infection. Am J Infect Control. 1991;19(3):136–42.
15. Hartstein AI, Garber SB, Ward TT, Jones SR, Morthland VH. Nosocomial urinary tract infection: a prospective evaluation of 108 catheterized patients. Infect Control. 1981;2(5):380–6.
16. Kunin CM, McCormack RC. Prevention of catheter-induced urinary-tract infections by sterile closed drainage. N Engl J Med. 1966;274(21):1155–61.
17. Warren JW, Damron D, Tenney JH, Hoopes JM, Deforge B, Muncie HL Jr. Fever, bacteremia, and death as complications of bacteriuria in women with long-term urethral catheters. J Infect Dis. 1987;155(6):1151–8.
18. Saint S. Clinical and economic consequences of nosocomial catheter-related bacteriuria. Am J Infect Control. 2000;28(1):68–75.

19. Garibaldi RA, Mooney BR, Epstein BJ, Britt MR. An evaluation of daily bacteriologic monitoring to identify preventable episodes of catheter-associated urinary tract infection. Infect Control. 1982;3(6):466–70.
20. Tambyah PA, Maki DG. Catheter-associated urinary tract infection is rarely symptomatic: a prospective study of 1,497 catheterized patients. Arch Intern Med. 2000;160(5):678–82.
21. Bryan CS, Reynolds KL. Hospital-acquired bacteremic urinary tract infection: epidemiology and outcome. J Urol. 1984;132(3):494–8.
22. Edgeworth JD, Treacher DF, Eykyn SJ. A 25-year study of nosocomial bacteremia in an adult intensive care unit. Crit Care Med. 1999;27(8):1421–8.
23. Ibrahim AI. Hospital acquired pre-prostatectomy bacteriuria: risk factors and implications. East Afr Med J. 1996;73(2):107–10.
24. Gould CV, Umscheid CA, Agarwal RK, Kuntz G, Pegues DA, Healthcare Infection Control Practices Advisory C. Guideline for prevention of catheter-associated urinary tract infections 2009. Infect Control Hosp Epidemiol. 2010;31(4):319–26.
25. Grabe MHS. Bacteriuria, a risk factor in men with bladder outlet obstruction. In: Kass EM, Svanborg E, editors. Host parasite interaction in urinary tract infection. University of Chicago press; 1986. p. 303–6.
26. Rudman D, Hontanosas A, Cohen Z, Mattson DE. Clinical correlates of bacteremia in a veterans administration extended care facility. J Am Geriatr Soc. 1988;36(8):726–32.
27. Kunin CM, Douthitt S, Dancing J, Anderson J, Moeschberger M. The association between the use of urinary catheters and morbidity and mortality among elderly patients in nursing homes. Am J Epidemiol. 1992;135(3):291–301.
28. Hooton TM, Bradley SF, Cardenas DD, Colgan R, Geerlings SE, Rice JC, et al. Diagnosis, prevention, and treatment of catheter-associated urinary tract infection in adults: 2009 International Clinical Practice Guidelines from the Infectious Diseases Society of America. Clin Infect Dis. 2010;50(5):625–63.
29. Cohen A. A microbiological comparison of a povidone-iodine lubricating gel and a control as catheter lubricants. J Hosp Infect. 1985;6(Suppl A):155–61.
30. Tambyah PA, Halvorson KT, Maki DG. A prospective study of pathogenesis of catheter-associated urinary tract infections. Mayo Clin Proc. 1999;74(2):131–6.
31. Daifuku R, Stamm WE. Association of rectal and urethral colonization with urinary tract infection in patients with indwelling catheters. JAMA. 1984;252(15):2028–30.
32. Warren JW, Tenney JH, Hoopes JM, Muncie HL, Anthony WC. A prospective microbiologic study of bacteriuria in patients with chronic indwelling urethral catheters. J Infect Dis. 1982;146(6):719–23.
33. Nickel JC, Grant SK, Costerton JW. Catheter-associated bacteriuria. An experimental study. Urology. 1985;26(4):369–75.
34. Saint S, Lipsky BA. Preventing catheter related bacteriuria: should we? Can we? How? Arch Intern Med. 1999;159(8):800–8.
35. Jacobsen SM, Stickler DJ, Mobley HL, Shirtliff ME. Complicated catheter-associated urinary tract infections due to Escherichia coli and Proteus mirabilis. Clin Microbiol Rev. 2008;21(1):26–59.
36. Daifuku R, Stamm WE. Bacterial adherence to bladder uroepithelial cells in catheter-associated urinary tract infection. N Engl J Med. 1986;314(19):1208–13.
37. Bergqvist D, Bronnestam R, Hedelin H, Stahl A. The relevance of urinary sampling methods in patients with indwelling Foley catheters. Br J Urol. 1980;52(2):92–5.
38. Grahn D, Norman DC, White ML, Cantrell M, Yoshikawa TT. Validity of urinary catheter specimen for diagnosis of urinary tract infection in the elderly. Arch Intern Med. 1985;145(10):1858–60.
39. Tenney JH, Warren JW. Bacteriuria in women with long-term catheters: paired comparison of indwelling and replacement catheters. J Infect Dis. 1988;157(1):199–202.
40. Biering-Sorensen F. Urinary tract infection in individuals with spinal cord lesion. Curr Opin Urol. 2002;12(1):45–9.

41. Choong S, Whitfield H. Biofilms and their role in infections in urology. BJU Int. 2000;86(8):935–41.
42. Costerton JW. Introduction to biofilm. Int J Antimicrob Agents. 1999;11(3–4):217–21; discussion 37–9
43. Donlan RM. Biofilm formation: a clinically relevant microbiological process. Clin Infect Dis. 2001;33(8):1387–92.
44. Kumon H. Management of biofilm infections in the urinary tract. World J Surg. 2000;24(10):1193–6.
45. Reid G. Biofilms in infectious disease and on medical devices. Int J Antimicrob Agents. 1999;11(3–4):223–6; discussion 37–9
46. Nicolle LE. Catheter associated urinary tract infections. Antimicrob Resist Infect Control. 2014;3:23.
47. Tenke P, Kovacs B, Bjerklund Johansen TE, Matsumoto T, Tambyah PA, Naber KG. European and Asian guidelines on management and prevention of catheter-associated urinary tract infections. Int J Antimicrob Agents. 2008;31(Suppl 1):S68–78.
48. Tambyah PA, Maki DG. The relationship between pyuria and infection in patients with indwelling urinary catheters: a prospective study of 761 patients. Arch Intern Med. 2000;160(5):673–7.
49. Steward DK, Wood GL, Cohen RL, Smith JW, Mackowiak PA. Failure of the urinalysis and quantitative urine culture in diagnosing symptomatic urinary tract infections in patients with long-term urinary catheters. Am J Infect Control. 1985;13(4):154–60.
50. Schwartz DS, Barone JE. Correlation of urinalysis and dipstick results with catheter-associated urinary tract infections in surgical ICU patients. Intensive Care Med. 2006;32(11):1797–801.
51. Raz R, Schiller D, Nicolle LE. Chronic indwelling catheter replacement before antimicrobial therapy for symptomatic urinary tract infection. J Urol. 2000;164(4):1254–8.
52. Lipsky BA, Ireton RC, Fihn SD, Hackett R, Berger RE. Diagnosis of bacteriuria in men: specimen collection and culture interpretation. J Infect Dis. 1987;155(5):847–54.
53. Geerlings SE, van den Broek PJ, van Haarst EP, Vleming LJ, van Haaren KM, Janknegt R, et al. Optimisation of the antibiotic policy in The Netherlands. X. The SWAB guideline for antimicrobial treatment of complicated urinary tract infections. Ned Tijdschr Geneeskd. 2006;150(43):2370–6.
54. DeGroot-Kosolcharoen J, Guse R, Jones JM. Evaluation of a urinary catheter with a preconnected closed drainage bag. Infect Control Hosp Epidemiol. 1988;9(2):72–6.
55. Cooper FP, Alexander CE, Sinha S, Omar MI. Policies for replacing long-term indwelling urinary catheters in adults. Cochrane Database Syst Rev. 2016;7:CD011115.
56. Dasgupta R, Grabe M. Preoperative antibiotics before endourologic surgery: current recommendations. J Endourol. 2009;23(10):1567–70.
57. Nicolle LE. Consequences of asymptomatic bacteriuria in the elderly. Int J Antimicrob Agents. 1994;4(2):107–11.
58. Nicolle LE, Long-Term-Care-Committee S. Urinary tract infections in long-term-care facilities. Infect Control Hosp Epidemiol. 2001;22(3):167–75.
59. Schaberg DR, Weinstein RA, Stamm WE. Epidemics of nosocomial urinary tract infection caused by multiply resistant gram-negative bacilli: epidemiology and control. J Infect Dis. 1976;133(3):363–6.
60. West DA, Cummings JM, Longo WE, Virgo KS, Johnson FE, Parra RO. Role of chronic catheterization in the development of bladder cancer in patients with spinal cord injury. Urology. 1999;53(2):292–7.
61. Nicolle LE. A practical guide to antimicrobial management of complicated urinary tract infection. Drugs Aging. 2001;18(4):243–54.
62. Bonza ESJR, Munoz P, Voss A, Kluytmans J. Co-operative Group of the European Study Group on Nosocomial Infections. A European perspective on nosocomial urinary tract infections II. Report on incidence, clinical characteristics and outcome (ESGNI- 004 study). European study group on nosocomial infection. Clin Microbiol Infect. 2001;2001(7):532–42.

63. Johansen TEB, Cel M, Naber K, Stratchounski L, Svendsen MV, Tenke P, PEP and PEAP Study Investigators. European Society of Infections in Urology. Prevalence of hospital-acquired urinary tract infections in urology departments. Eur Urol. 2007;51:1100–11. [discussion 1112]
64. Zimakoff JD, Pontoppidan B, Larsen SO, Poulsen KB, Stickler DJ. The management of urinary catheters: compliance of practice in Danish hospitals, nursing homes and home care to national guidelines. Scand J Urol Nephrol. 1995;29(3):299–309.
65. Ehrenkranz NJ, Alfonso BC. Failure of bland soap handwash to prevent hand transfer of patient bacteria to urethral catheters. Infect Control Hosp Epidemiol. 1991;12(11):654–62.
66. Casewell M, Phillips I. Hands as route of transmission for Klebsiella species. Br Med J. 1977;2(6098):1315–7.
67. Platt R, Polk BF, Murdock B, Rosner B. Mortality associated with nosocomial urinary-tract infection. N Engl J Med. 1982;307(11):637–42.
68. Choong S, Wood S, Fry C, Whitfield H. Catheter associated urinary tract infection and encrustation. Int J Antimicrob Agents. 2001;17(4):305–10.
69. Terpenning MS, Allada R, Kauffman CA. Intermittent urethral catheterization in the elderly. J Am Geriatr Soc. 1989;37(5):411–6.
70. Bakke A. Clean intermittent catheterization--physical and psychological complications. Scand J Urol Nephrol Suppl. 1993;150:1–69.
71. Diokno AC, Sonda LP, Hollander JB, Lapides J. Fate of patients started on clean intermittent self-catheterization therapy 10 years ago. J Urol. 1983;129(6):1120–2.
72. Pearman JW. Urological follow-up of 99 spinal cord injured patients initially managed by intermittent catheterisation. Br J Urol. 1976;48(5):297–310.
73. Wyndaele JJ, Maes D. Clean intermittent self-catheterization: a 12-year followup. J Urol. 1990;143(5):906–8.
74. McPhail MJ, Abu-Hilal M, Johnson CD. A meta-analysis comparing suprapubic and transurethral catheterization for bladder drainage after abdominal surgery. Br J Surg. 2006;93(9):1038–44.
75. Crnich CJ, Drinka PJ. Does the composition of urinary catheters influence clinical outcomes and the results of research studies? Infect Control Hosp Epidemiol. 2007;28(1):102–3.
76. Kass EH. Asymptomatic infections of the urinary tract. Trans Assoc Am Phys. 1956;69:56–64.
77. Haley RW, Culver DH, White JW, Morgan WM, Emori TG. The nationwide nosocomial infection rate. A new need for vital statistics. Am J Epidemiol. 1985;121(2):159–67.
78. Brosnahan J, Jull A, Tracy C. Types of urethral catheters for management of short-term voiding problems in hospitalised adults. Cochrane Database Syst Rev. 2004;(1):CD004013.
79. Riedl CR, Witkowski M, Plas E, Pflueger H. Heparin coating reduces encrustation of ureteral stents: a preliminary report. Int J Antimicrob Agents. 2002;19(6):507–10.
80. Ruggieri MR, Hanno PM, Levin RM. Reduction of bacterial adherence to catheter surface with heparin. J Urol. 1987;138(2):423–6.
81. Tenke P, Riedl CR, Jones GL, Williams GJ, Stickler D, Nagy E. Bacterial biofilm formation on urologic devices and heparin coating as preventive strategy. Int J Antimicrob Agents. 2004;23(Suppl 1):S67–74.
82. Johnson JR, Kuskowski MA, Wilt TJ. Systematic review: antimicrobial urinary catheters to prevent catheter-associated urinary tract infection in hospitalized patients. Ann Intern Med. 2006;144(2):116–26.
83. Morris NS, Stickler DJ. Encrustation of indwelling urethral catheters by Proteus mirabilis biofilms growing in human urine. J Hosp Infect. 1998;39(3):227–34.
84. Morris NS, Stickler DJ, Winters C. Which indwelling urethral catheters resist encrustation by Proteus mirabilis biofilms? Br J Urol. 1997;80(1):58–63.
85. Reddy ST, Chung KK, McDaniel CJ, Darouiche RO, Landman J, Brennan AB. Micropatterned surfaces for reducing the risk of catheter-associated urinary tract infection: an in vitro study on the effect of sharklet micropatterned surfaces to inhibit bacterial colonization and migration of uropathogenic Escherichia coli. J Endourol. 2011;25(9):1547–52.
86. Darouiche RO, Hull RA. Bacterial interference for prevention of urinary tract infection. Clin Infect Dis. 2012;55(10):1400–7.

87. Koves B, Salvador E, Gronberg-Hernandez J, Zdziarski J, Wullt B, Svanborg C, et al. Rare emergence of symptoms during long-term asymptomatic Escherichia coli 83972 carriage without an altered virulence factor repertoire. J Urol. 2014;191(2):519–28.
88. Bonkat G PR, Bartoletti R, Bruyère F, Geerlings SE, Wagenlehner FM, et al. Urological infections. In: EAU guidelines London: European Association of Urology p 857–920. 2017.

Urinary Tract Infections in Kidney Transplant Patients

11

José Medina-Polo, Laila Schneidewind, Fabian P. Stangl, and Truls E. Bjerklund Johansen

11.1 Introduction

Urinary tract infections (UTIs) are more common in patients with end-stage renal disease and in those with kidney transplantation than in patients without specific risk factors. Moreover, there is a higher incidence of resistance among causative microorganisms. Infectious complications in kidney transplant recipients are associated with increased morbidity and mortality [1, 2]. Half of all kidney transplant patients are estimated to develop urinary tract infections within 3 years of transplantation [3]. The highest UTI incidence is during the first 6 months after the transplantation. Infections may be related to surgical injury, urethral catheterization, double-J stent insertion, and the most intensive immunosuppressant regimens, which significantly deplete T cell antibodies [4, 5]. Recurrent UTI is also frequent in kidney transplant recipients, with a reported incidence of 2.9–27% [4]. Recurrent UTIs

J. Medina-Polo (✉)
Department of Urology, Health Research Institute i+12, Hospital Universitario 12 de Octubre imas12, Madrid, Spain
e-mail: jose.medina@salud.madrid.org

L. Schneidewind
Department of Hematology/Oncology, University Greifswald Medical Center, Greifswald, Germany
e-mail: laila.schneidewind@med.uni-rostock.de

F. P. Stangl
Department of Urology, University Hospital of Bern, Bern, Switzerland
e-mail: fabian.stangl@stud.pmu.ac.at

T. E. B. Johansen
Institute of Clinical Medicine, University of Oslo, Oslo, Norway

Chair Research Group on Inflammation and Infection in Urology and Urology Department, Clinic for Surgery, Inflammation and Transplantation, Oslo University Hospital, Oslo, Norway
e-mail: tebj@uio.no

T. E. Bjerklund Johansen, T. Cai (eds.), *Guide to Antibiotics in Urology*,
https://doi.org/10.1007/978-3-319-92366-6_11

require multiple courses of antibiotic therapy, which can result in bacterial resistance. Immunosuppression is a risk factor for infections and antibiotic treatment may affect the levels of immunosuppressive treatment [6]. Therefore, urologists have an important role in diagnosing, preventing, and managing urinary infections in patients on the waiting list for kidney transplantation and those with transplanted grafts.

The aim of the present chapter is to review the following aspects of urinary tract infections related to kidney transplantations:

Before transplantation

- Recommendations about urological workup in candidates for kidney transplantation, focusing on urological infections.

After transplantation

- Prevention of urinary tract infections in kidney transplant recipients.
- Recommendations about diagnosing and treating asymptomatic bacteriuria in kidney transplant recipients.
- Analysis of differential characteristics of urinary tract infections in kidney transplant recipients.
- Treatment of urinary tract infections in kidney transplant recipients.

11.1.1 Urological Workup in Candidates for Kidney Transplantation with a Focus on Urological Infections

Patients with chronic kidney disease have a higher risk of urinary tract infections (UTIs) than the healthy population. Risk factors include structural and functional disorders of the urinary tract, loss of antibacterial properties of the urine, mild immunosuppression due to uremia with inhibition of protective mucosa production in the urothelium [7]. Moreover, chronic kidney disease associated with stone formation and autosomal dominant polycystic kidney disease (ADPKD) entails a higher risk for UTIs. Risk factors for UTIs after kidney transplantation are age, female sex, longer pretransplantation dialysis time, and urinary tract obstruction [1].

Patients with end-stage renal disease requires careful diagnostic workup before kidney transplantation. Several reviews have stated that the complementary tests needed depend on the characteristics of the recipient [8, 9]. In particular, patients with recurrent urinary tract infections require further studies, including measurement of urinary flow rate and evaluation of postvoid-residual urine. According to previous data, urodynamics or voiding cystourethrogram may be indicated in select cases. Urodynamic examinations are mandatory in case of bladder dysfunction as the incidence of neurogenic bladder is higher among patients with recurrent UTIs, and UTIs are frequent both before and after kidney transplantation. Moreover, UTIs may deleteriously affect graft function [10]. There might be an etiological interrelationship between neurogenic bladder and end-stage renal disease as both conditions may be due to diabetes mellitus. A key point in the diagnostic workup is to define if the patient has a normal bladder from a functional point of view. Normal bladder function consists of urine storage at low pressure, absence of leakage, and complete empty by spontaneous voiding. In contrast, an abnormal urinary bladder stores urine at high pressure, leaks, or does not empty entirely by natural voiding [6, 10]. Kidney transplantation may, however, be performed in patients with a neurogenic bladder after a proper diagnostic workup. Voiding cystourethrogram and urodynamics are recommended in case of voiding dysfunction, bladder augmentation or substitution, recurrent urinary tract infections, pyelonephritis, or vesicoureteral reflux. Urine or bladder wash cytology is indicated in the case of prior cyclophosphamide therapy or significant irritative voiding symptoms in order to rule out bladder cancer [10].

11.2 Diagnosis and Treatment of Asymptomatic Bacteriuria in Kidney Transplant Recipients

Asymptomatic bacteriuria has a high prevalence after a kidney transplantation. It is estimated to occur in up to 50% of recipients, but it only needs treatment in specific situations. Asymptomatic bacteriuria in patients with a kidney transplant is defined by the presence of >10^5 bacterial colony-forming units per milliliter (CFU/mL) on urine culture with no local or systemic symptoms of UTI [11]. International guidelines such as the European Association of Urology (EAU) and the Infectious Diseases Society of America (IDSA) guidelines state that asymptomatic bacteriuria should not be treated in kidney transplant patients after the short-term posttransplant period [12–14]. Other indications for evaluating and treatment of asymptomatic bacteriuria are recipients with a risk for developing pyelonephritis such as indwelling devices, neurogenic bladder, or combined transplants [5, 15]. Worth of notice, hospitalization for urinary tract infections occurred more frequently in patients that had been treated for asymptomatic bacteriuria. Moreover, it is reported an incidence due to resistant microorganisms up to 36%. Therefore, treatment of asymptomatic bacteriuria has been proposed in selected cases only, in order to avoid pyelonephritis and the possible effect of the infections on graft function [3, 16]. Two episodes of isolation of asymptomatic bacteriuria, glomerulonephritis, recurrent UTI, and relapsing UTI have been demonstrated as pyelonephritis risk factors [17].

The current practice of management of asymptomatic bacteriuria was evaluated in a survey by Coussement et al. with more than 200 participants. They found that 72% of the responders routinely test urine to screen for bacteriuria, and 43% treat asymptomatic bacteriuria with antibiotics within the first 6 months after kidney transplantation [18]. A similar survey about the current practice among urologists carried out by the EAU Section of Infections in Urology (ESIU) reported that 29.5% of the responders screen routinely for asymptomatic bacteriuria after kidney transplantation and 27.3% and 27.3% during the first 2 and 6 months after kidney transplant, respectively. In addition, 20.4% treat asymptomatic bacteriuria with antibiotics in the first 2 months after kidney transplant, 29.5% in the first 6 months, and 38.6% if a urological procedure or biopsy is expected.

However, a literature review demonstrated that treating asymptomatic bacteriuria might be associated with a higher incidence of hospitalization due to UTIs and a higher risk of developing antibiotic-resistant bacteria [19]. Furthermore, several randomized controlled trials have demonstrated that treating asymptomatic bacteriuria 2 and 6 months after kidney transplantation is not associated with a higher risk of acute pyelonephritis, hospital admission, or graft loss [18, 20, 21]. Therefore, the review by Coussement et al. concluded that treating asymptomatic bacteriuria is not indicated beyond 2 months after kidney transplantation as it can be associated with a higher incidence of hospitalizations. Furthermore, there is no difference in the incidence of urinary tract infections between patients who received treatment for asymptomatic bacteriuria and those without antibiotic treatment. Fosfomycin has been proposed as adequate treatment of asymptomatic bacteriuria for the cases when it is indicated [22].

11.3 Differential Characteristics of Urinary Tract Infections in Patients with a Kidney Transplant

The prevalence of UTI among kidney transplant recipients ranges from 7% to 80%, with the highest incidence in the first year after the transplantation. Risk factors for UTIs in kidney transplant recipients include female sex, old age, recurrent UTIs before transplant, vesicoureteral reflux, autosomal dominant polycystic kidney disease (ADPKD), delayed graft function, and a long time with urethral catheter or ureteral stents [11]. In addition, kidney cysts in patients with ASPKD may serve as reservoirs for bacteria and predispose for the development of UTIs. Furthermore, repeated isolation of asymptomatic bacteriuria and recurrent urinary tract infections are associated with a higher incidence of pyelonephritis and multidrug-resistant microorganisms [1]. Graft rejection episodes are also risk factors for acute pyelonephritis [7].

Escherichia coli is the most commonly isolated microorganism in patients with UTIs and kidney transplants. However, other gram-negative uropathogens are frequently isolated, and *Enterococcus* species represent up to 25–30% of the microorganisms isolated [5]. Moreover, other pathogens such as *Corynebacterium urealyticum* and viruses may also be responsible for UTIs. As trimethoprim-sulfamethoxazole is used as antibiotic prophylaxis to avoid pneumocystis carinii, there is high resistance to these antibiotics. Fluoroquinolones are also reported to have a high resistance rate, up to 50% [11].

As for UTIs in patients with no risk factors, the pathogenesis of UTI in recipients with kidney transplantation is usually related to bacteria getting to the bladder ascending from the perineal area through the urethra. In addition, patients with a kidney transplant may be predisposed to a higher risk of pyelonephritis as the ureter is usually anastomosed to the bladder without an antireflux mechanism. These patients also have a higher risk of neurogenic bladder [10, 11]. In patients with pyelonephritis, preceding episodes of uncomplicated UTIs are reported [6]. For a comprehensive description of risk factors for UTIs, we recommend using the ORENUC system. The acronym represents the following: O for patients with no known risk factors, R for recurrent UTIs without other risk factors, E for extra-urogenital risk factors, N for nephropathic disease, U for urological risk factors, and C for urinary catheter or stents [7, 12].

Risk factors for UTIs in kidney transplant recipients	
Pretransplant factors	Female gender Diabetes mellitus Urinary tract abnormalities or neurogenic bladder Glomerulonephritis Long pretransplantation dialysis time
Pretransplant factors	Ureteral stents and urethral catheters Bladder instrumentation Deceased-donor grafts Double kidney transplant Old age
Posttransplant factors	Immunosuppression Acute rejection Reduced graft function Urinary tract obstruction

Type of infections [12]:

- Simple cystitis—the presence of $>10^5$ CFU/mL on urine culture with local urinary symptoms such as dysuria, urinary frequency, urinary urgency, hematuria, and suprapubic pain but no systemic symptoms, such as fever or allograft pain, and no indwelling devices (e.g., ureteral stent, nephrostomy tube, or chronic urinary catheter).
- Complicated UTI the presence of $>10^5$ CFU/mL on urine culture with fever, allograft pain, chills, malaise, or bacteremia with identical concomitant organism in urine and blood cultures.
- Recurrent UTI: three or more episodes of symptomatic UTI over 12 months or two episodes in 6 months.

The diagnostic workup starts with an assessment of symptoms. Questionnaires are useful since the diagnosis and treatment is often based on symptoms only [23, 24]. For cases with no typical symptoms, or recurrent UTI, it is recommended to perform a urine dipstick analysis, urine microscopy, and urine culture [12]. Blood cultures should be obtained in case of complicated UTIs, fever, systemic symptoms, or pyelonephritis [11, 12]. It should be noted that urine cultures may be negative in patients with infections due to yeast, acid-fast bacilli, and *C. urealyticum* [11]. *C. urealyticum* should be suspected in cases with chronic UTI symptoms and negative conventional urine cultures, alkaline urine (pH >7), pyuria or microscopic hematuria with no other explanation, presence of struvite crystals, obstructive uropathy, and encrusting cystitis or pyelitis [11].

UTIs in kidney transplant recipients may also be caused by a virus such as herpes virus (HSV), cytomegalovirus (CMV), Epstein-Barr virus (EBV) and BK polyomavirus (BKPyV), and even influenza or parainfluenza viruses. Although CMV infections have the highest incidence, prophylaxis programs effectively minimize it. CMV infections may lead to graft rejection. Polyomaviruses may cause hemorrhagic cystitis and stenosis of the ureter [1, 5].

Ultrasound, including post-void residual urine, is recommended in patients with a history of urolithiasis, neurogenic bladder, recurrent UTIs, and UTIs that do not respond adequately to antibiotics. Computed tomography may be indicated in selected cases, where ultrasound findings are not conclusive. Urodynamics studies are indicated for bladder dysfunction and acontractility and to assess bladder capacity, compliance, or bladder outflow obstruction. Cystoscopy is used to rule out urethral or bladder abnormalities such as stenosis or bladder tumors [11].

11.4 Treatment of Urinary Tract Infections in Kidney Transplant Patients

Empirical antibiotics should be prescribed for all kidney transplant recipients with symptomatic UTIs based on local susceptibility data and previous cultures of the patient's urine. A urinalysis and urine culture are recommended before starting antibiotic therapy. Antibiotic treatment should be reviewed when urine culture results and an antibiogram are available [11]. A short duration of treatment or a single dose of antibiotic is not recommended. A treatment duration of 5–7 days is usually prescribed, and a longer duration in the early transplantation period can be required [4, 11]. According to clinical practice guidelines, fluoroquinolones should not be used as empirical treatment [12].

Fosfomycin and trimethoprim-sulfamethoxazole (TMP-SMX) are considered first-line therapy in the case of noncomplicated cystitis in non-transplant patients. However, it should be noted that TMP-SMX is frequently used as prophylaxis during the peri-transplant period, and microorganisms may have developed resistance to TMP-SMX. The basis for using fosfomycin relies on its good oral bioavailability, low resistance rates in the population, and low risk of adverse events. Moreover, fosfomycin usually shows good activity in vitro against multidrug-resistant microorganisms [22]. Amoxicillin-clavulanate and cephalosporins are also alternatives for managing UTIs in kidney transplant recipients. The glomerular filtration rate must be assessed for patients with kidney transplants, as a dose adjustment may be required [12]. Aminoglycosides should be used with caution as they have a nephrotoxic potential. The combination of loop diuretics such as furosemide and cephalosporin is nephrotoxic. Nitrofurantoin is contraindicated in patients with an estimated glomerular filtration rate of less than 30 mL/min/1.73 m^2, as the drug accumulation leads to increased side effects and reduced urinary tract recovery, which may entail treatment failure [12].

For patients with systemic symptoms, fever, and/or pyelonephritis, intravenous treatment is recommended with antibiotics, such as piperacillin-tazobactam, meropenem, vancomycin, and cefepime. Although the antibiotic treatment should be maintained for at least 2 weeks, treatment can be switched to oral administration after defervescence and the symptoms improvement [11].

11.5 Prevention of Urinary Tract Infections in Kidney Transplant Recipients

The evidence about preventing urinary tract infections in patients with kidney transplantation is limited. Most of the reviews about the prevention of recurrent UTIs do not include kidney transplantation recipient [25]. According to EAU guidelines on urological infections, alternatives such as local or oral probiotics containing strains for vaginal flora regeneration, cranberry products, D-mannose, and endovesical installations with hyaluronic acid and chondroitin sulfate have a weak recommendation level [12]. Pagonas et al. studied the effect of cranberry juice and L-methionine in 82 kidney transplant recipients with recurrent urinary tract infections and reported that cranberry juice might reduce the number of urinary tract infection episodes by 63.9% and L-methionine reduced the annual number of UTIs by 48.7%. The best outcomes were reported for cranberry juice 50 mL daily and L-methionine 500 mg combined. However, the study has several limitations as only 82 patients were included, no more than 40 per group [26].

In ordinary patients, prophylactic strategies with strong recommendation for prevention of recurrent urinary infections include vaginal estrogen replacement in postmenopausal women and immunoactive prophylaxis [12]. Regarding immunoactive prophylaxis, many studies are based on the formula OM-89, containing 18 serotypes of *Escherichia coli* lysed bacteria. It consists of one tablet daily for 3 months, and a booster course can be added every 10 days for 6–9 months. The proposed mechanism of action is the stimulation of dendritic cells, neutrophils, and phagocytosis by macrophages [25]. There are other alternatives, such as the sublingual formula MV140 or an intramuscular/vaginal tablet. Published studies focusing on kidney transplantation recipients are scarce [27]. Zgoura et al. included 28 patients, 14 with three subcutaneous injections of inactivated bacteria and 14 controls. The study reported a reduced incidence of urinary tract infections with higher isolation of non-*E. coli* bacteria in the control group [28]. A study on sublingual vaccination with the formula MV-140 for 6 months in 43 kidney transplant recipients reported a reduction in the incidence of urinary tract infections from 4.2 to 2.7 episodes per year. From the total of patients, 46.5% had fewer infections, and only 16.3% were free of urinary tract infections after 1 year. Another important point is that 39.5% of patients included in the study had urinary tract structural or functional abnormalities [29]. Antibiotic prophylaxis is recommended in case of failure with nonantibiotic measures. Several drugs have been evaluated, such as nitrofurantoin or fosfomycin 3 g once weekly for longer than 6 months [4].

Urinary catheters are one of the main risk factors for infections in the early postoperative period. Both urethral catheters and ureteral stents are used. It is recommended that urethral catheters are removed in the first week after the kidney transplant, unless any other patient characteristics require prolonged bladder drainage. The routine use of ureteral stents may prevent urological complications such as urinary fistula. However, it should be removed as soon as possible. Siskind et al. removed the urethral catheter on postoperative day one after kidney transplant from living donors without a higher rate of urine leakage. Moreover, ureteral stents were not used routinely in this group of patients [30].

It is worrisome that a recent survey among urologists reported a long period of catheterization before catheter removal: less than 1 week by 38.6% of respondents, 1–2 weeks by 34.1%, and 2–3 weeks by 25% before the urethral catheter was removed. On the other hand, the ureteral double J stent was removed between 1 and 2 weeks by 14.3%, 2–3 weeks by 28.6%, and 3–4 weeks by 57.1% (Fig. 11.1) [1].

Finally, it should be mentioned that antimicrobial prophylaxis following kidney transplantation needs to be optimized in terms of antibiotic selection and duration. Although antimicrobial prophylaxis reduces bacteriuria and the incidence of early urinary infections after kidney transplantation, a longer prophylaxis duration has not proved beneficial [31].

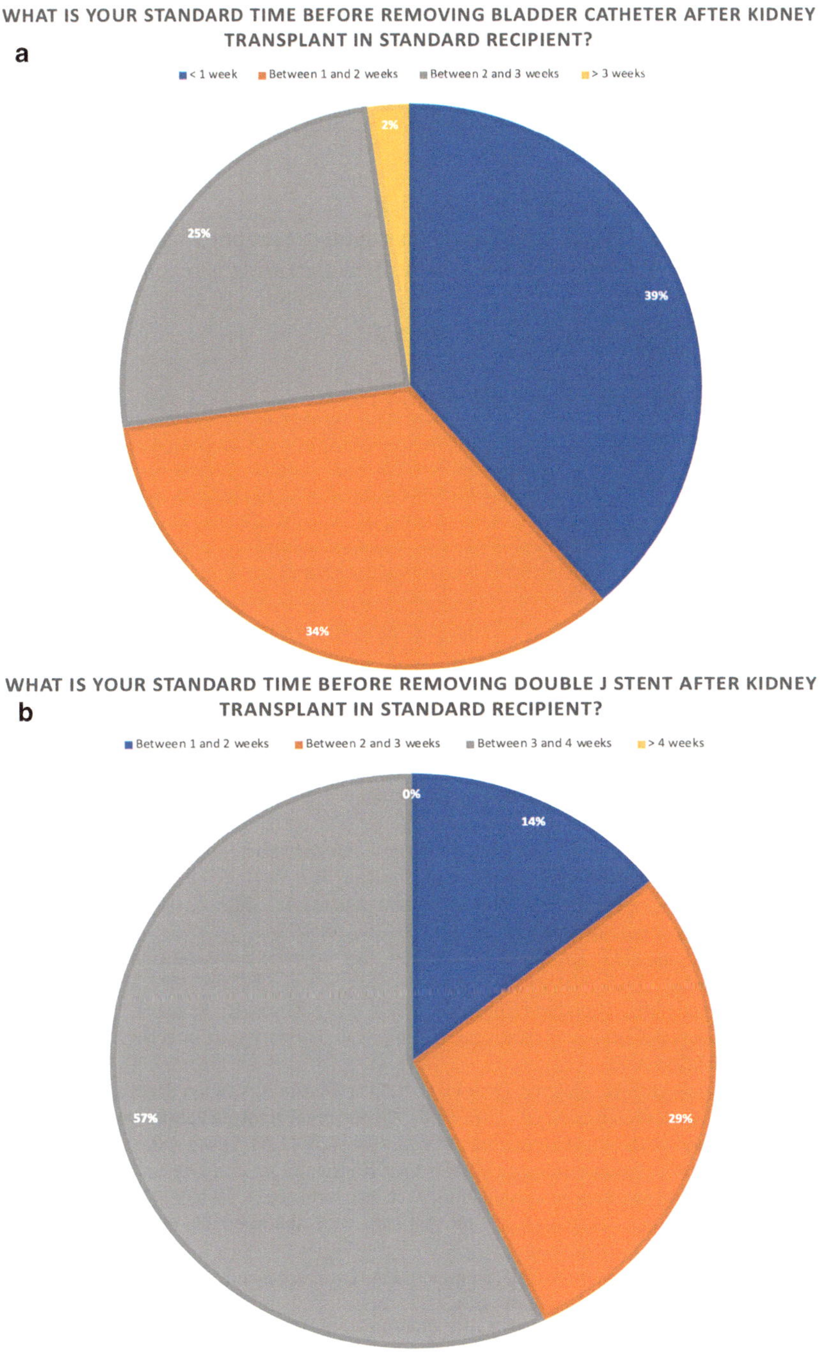

Fig. 11.1 Results of the survey carried out by ESIU among urologists involved in kidney transplantation to evaluate the current practice about the time before removing bladder catheter (**a**) and double J stent (**b**) after kidney transplant

11.6 Conclusions

The main conclusions regarding the management of urinary tract infections in immunocompromised patients with chronic kidney disease and kidney transplant may be summarized as follows:

- Treat any infection before transplantation.
- Perioperative antibiotic prophylaxis on a short-prescription basis is required.
- Perioperative low-dose trimethoprim-sulfamethoxazole is recommended as prophylactic regimen.
- Urinary catheters require prompt removal.

Statements Relating to Our Ethics and Integrity Policies

Funding Statement: None.

Conflict of Interest Disclosure: None.

References

1. Tandogdu Z, Cai T, Koves B, Wagenlehner F, Bjerklund-Johansen TE. Urinary tract infections in immunocompromised patients with diabetes, chronic kidney disease, and kidney transplant. Eur Urol Focus. 2016;2:394–9.
2. Naqvi SB, Collins AJ. Infectious complications in chronic kidney disease. Adv Chronic Kidney Dis. 2006;13:199–204.
3. Kidney Disease: Improving Global Outcomes (KDIGO) Transplant Work Group. KDIGO clinical practice guideline for the care of kidney transplant recipients. Am J Transplant. 2009;9(Suppl 3):S1–S155.
4. Chacón-Mora N, Pachón Díaz J, Cordero Matía E. Urinary tract infection in kidney transplant recipients. Enfermedades Infecc Microbiol Clínica. 2017;35(4):255–9.
5. Gan VHL, Shoskes DA. UTI in renal transplant patients. In GMS; 2018 [cited 2023 Feb 21]. https://books.publisso.de/publisso_gold/book/52/chapter/12
6. Lorenz EC, Cosio FG. The impact of urinary tract infections in renal transplant recipients. Kidney Int. 2010;78(8):719–21.
7. Wagenlehner FME, Bjerklund Johansen TE, Cai T, Koves B, Kranz J, Pilatz A, et al. Epidemiology, definition and treatment of complicated urinary tract infections. Nat Rev Urol. 2020;17(10):586–600.
8. Cabello Benavente R, Quicios Dorado C, López Martin L, Simón Rodríguez C, Charry Gónima P, González Enguita C. The candidate for renal transplantation work up: medical, urological and oncological evaluation. Arch Esp Urol. 2011;64(5):441–60.
9. Parra López ML, Lozano-Blasco JM, Martínez-Rodríguez J, León-Dueñas E, Medina-López RA. Renal transplant recipient evaluation. Arch Esp Urol. 2021;74(10):941–52.
10. Barry JM. Kidney transplantation into patients with abnormal bladders. Transplantation. 2004;77(7):1120–3.
11. Santos CAQ, Brennan DC, Vella J, Blumberg EA, Lam AQ, Bond S. Urinary tract infection in kidney transplant recipients. UpToDate 2023
12. Bonkat G, Bartoletti R, Bruyère F, Cai T, Geerlings SE, Köves B, Schubert S, Wagenlehner F, Devlies W, Horváth J, Mantica G, Mezei T, Pilatz A, Pradere B, Veeratterapillay R, Smith EJ, Blok B, Castro-Diaz D, Del Popolo G, Groen J, Hamid R, Karsenty G, Kessler TM, Pannek J, Ecclestone H, Musco S, Padilla-Fernández B, Sartori A, Schouten N, Smith EJ. EAU Guidelines on Urological Infections. 2022. ISBN 978-94-92671-16-5.

13. Nicolle LE, Bradley S, Colgan R, Rice JC, Schaeffer A, Hooton TM, et al. Infectious Diseases Society of America guidelines for the diagnosis and treatment of asymptomatic bacteriuria in adults. Clin Infect Dis. 2005;40(5):643–54.
14. Nicolle LE. Asymptomatic bacteriuria. Curr Opin Infect Dis. 2014;27(1):90–6.
15. Coussement J, Scemla A, Abramowicz D, Nagler EV, Webster AC. Antibiotics for asymptomatic bacteriuria in kidney transplant recipients. Cochrane Database Syst Rev. 2018;2(2):CD011357.
16. Snydman DR. Posttransplant microbiological surveillance. Clin Infect Dis. 2001;33(Suppl 1):S22–5.
17. Fiorante S, López-Medrano F, Lizasoain M, Lalueza A, Juan RS, Andrés A, et al. Systematic screening and treatment of asymptomatic bacteriuria in renal transplant recipients. Kidney Int. 2010;78(8):774–81.
18. Coussement J, Kamar N, Matignon M, Weekers L, Scemla A, Giral M, et al. Antibiotics versus no therapy in kidney transplant recipients with asymptomatic bacteriuria (BiRT): a pragmatic, multicentre, randomized, controlled trial. Clin Microbiol Infect. 2021;27(3):398–405.
19. Green H, Rahamimov R, Goldberg E, Leibovici L, Gafter U, Bishara J, et al. Consequences of treated versus untreated asymptomatic bacteriuria in the first year following kidney transplantation: retrospective observational study. Eur J Clin Microbiol Infect Dis. 2013;32(1):127–31.
20. Origüen J, López-Medrano F, Fernández-Ruiz M, Polanco N, Gutiérrez E, González E, et al. Should asymptomatic bacteriuria be systematically treated in kidney transplant recipients? Results from a randomized controlled trial. Am J Transplant. 2016;16(10):2943–53.
21. Sabé N, Oriol I, Melilli E, Manonelles A, Bestard O, Polo C, et al. Antibiotic treatment versus no treatment for asymptomatic bacteriuria in kidney transplant recipients: a multicenter randomized trial. Open Forum Infect Dis. 2019;6(6):243.
22. Ruiz-Ruigómez M, Fernández-Ruiz M, Silva JT, Vidal E, Origüen J, Calvo-Cano A, et al. Efficacy and safety of oral fosfomycin for asymptomatic bacteriuria in kidney transplant recipients: results from a Spanish multicenter cohort. Antimicrob Agents Chemother. 2023;95(5):e02267-20. https://doi.org/10.1128/AAC.02267-20.
23. Alidjanov JF, Abdufattaev UA, Makhsudov SA, Pilatz A, Akilov FA, Naber KG, et al. The acute cystitis symptom score for patient-reported outcome assessment. Urol Int. 2016;97(4):402–9.
24. Alidjanov JF, Naber KG, Pilatz A, Radzhabov A, Zamuddinov M, Magyar A, et al. Additional assessment of acute cystitis symptom score questionnaire for patient-reported outcome measure in female patients with acute uncomplicated cystitis: part II. World J Urol. 2020;38(8):1977–88.
25. Prattley S, Geraghty R, Moore M, Somani BK. Role of vaccines for recurrent urinary tract infections: a systematic review. Eur Urol Focus. 2020;6(3):593–604.
26. Pagonas N, Hörstrup J, Schmidt D, Benz P, Schindler R, Reinke P, et al. Prophylaxis of recurrent urinary tract infection after renal transplantation by cranberry juice and L-methionine. Transplant Proc. 2012;44(10):3017–21.
27. Lorenzo-Gómez MF, Foley S, Nickel JC, García-Cenador MB, Padilla-Fernández BY, González-Casado I, et al. Sublingual MV140 for prevention of recurrent urinary tract infections. NEJM Evid. 2022;1(4):EVIDoa2100018. https://doi.org/10.1056/EVIDoa2100018.
28. Zgoura P, Waldecker C, Bauer F, Seibert FS, Rohn B, Schenker P, et al. Vaccination against urinary tract infection after renal transplantation. Transplant Proc. 2020;52(10):3192–6.
29. Shabaka A, de la Manzanara VL, Zapata N, Santiago JL, Pérez-Flores I, de los Ángeles Moreno de la Higuera M, et al. Clinical and immunological response to sublingual vaccination for the prevention of recurrent urinary tract infections in kidney transplant patients: results after 1 year of follow-up. Transplantation. 2018;102(Supplement 7):S320.
30. Siskind E, Sameyah E, Goncharuk E, Olsen EM, Feldman J, Giovinazzo K, et al. Removal of Foley catheters in live donor kidney transplant recipients on postoperative day 1 does not increase the incidence of urine leaks. Int J Angiol. 2013;22(1):45–8.
31. Strohaeker J, Aschke V, Koenigsrainer A, Nadalin S, Bachmann R. Urinary tract infections in kidney transplant recipients—is there a need for antibiotic stewardship? J Clin Med. 2021;11(1):226.

Management of the Urosepsis Syndrome 12

Florian M. E. Wagenlehner

12.1 Introduction

Sepsis is the most severe form of nosocomial and community-acquired infections and can be caused in principle by any pathogen. Even with adequate antibiotic therapy and modern intensive care, mortality is still around 25% [1]. Most sepsis cases are caused by bacterial infections of the respiratory tract, followed by intra-abdominal infections, vascular catheter-associated infections, skin and soft tissue infections, as well as infections of the genitourinary tract [2]. In a prospective cohort study, out of 112 patients with sepsis, 36 (32%) had urosepsis [3]. Although organ failure in urosepsis occurred earlier than in other sepsis foci, patients with urosepsis had a lower 28-day mortality rate (6 vs. 37%). In multivariate analysis, sepsis focus (urosepsis, odds ratio (OR) = 0.019) and sequential organ failure assessment (SOFA) score (OR = 1.9) were significantly associated with survival [3].

12.2 Bacterial Spectrum

The most common pathogens cultured in urosepsis are *Escherichia coli* and other enterobacteria. After urological procedures or in patients with urinary catheter discharge, multidrug-resistant *Pseudomonas* spp., *Proteus* spp., *Serratia* spp., *Enterobacter* spp., *Enterococcus* spp., and staphylococci may also be taken into account [4]. A point prevalence study of urogenital infections in 70 countries (Global Prevalence Study of Infections in Urology—GPIU study) showed that antimicrobial resistance differed with different severity levels of the infection. The more severe the infection, the higher was antimicrobial resistance. The highest

F. M. E. Wagenlehner (✉)
Clinic for Urology, Pediatric Urology and Andrology, Justus-Liebig-University Gießen, Gießen, Germany
e-mail: florian.wagenlehner@chiru.med.uni-giessen.de

T. E. Bjerklund Johansen, T. Cai (eds.), *Guide to Antibiotics in Urology*,
https://doi.org/10.1007/978-3-319-92366-6_12

resistance rates were seen in septic patients. Basically, resistance to commonly prescribed antibiotics was high, ranging from 8% (imipenem) to 62% (aminopenicillin/beta-lactamase inhibitors (BLI)). Forty-five percent of *Enterobacteriaceae* and 21% of *P. aeruginosa* isolates were multiresistant [5]. This study also shows that resistance data cannot be easily extrapolated from non-septic to septic urinary tract infections. Therefore, local detailed resistance statistics should be provided for patients with urosepsis, which serves as the basis for selection of empirical therapy [5].

12.3 Third Sepsis Definition

Based on fundamental scientific and clinical findings, the sepsis criteria were revised 2016 and a new definition of sepsis was created [6]. Decisive for the definition of "sepsis" is no longer the systemic inflammatory response syndrome (SIRS) but the organ damage induced by an inadequate host response (organ dysfunction) [7]. The four SIRS criteria (fever or hypothermia, tachycardia, tachypnea, leukocytosis, or leukopenia) indicate a systemic inflammatory response; however, this can still be in a physiological context. Apart from that, the SIRS criteria proved to be too little specific to diagnose sepsis. In particular, there was no significant correlation between mortality and number or the presence of positive SIRS criteria [1].

Sepsis is now defined as a life-threatening organ dysfunction caused by a dysregulated host response to infection—roughly equivalent to the "severe sepsis" of earlier definitions. Organ dysfunction can be detected by changing the Sequential Organ Failure Assessment (SOFA) score by 2 points. A "septic shock" is further used when maintaining the mean arterial pressure (>65 mmHg) is only possible with vasopressors.

As a measure of internal validation of the new definition of sepsis, a new score was also presented, which allows easy risk assessment of patients at higher risk for poor outcomes and, since laboratory values are not required, is also suitable for practical use as a bedside and pint of care test. The so-called quick (q) SOFA score, contains three quick-to-find parameters:

1. New confusion, defined as the Glasgow Coma Scale of <14
2. Tachypnea, defined as a respiratory rate of >22/min and
3. Hypotension of a systolic blood pressure <100 mmHg [8].

12.4 Diagnosis

There is no specific biomarker for sepsis or urosepsis. Nevertheless, the classic inflammatory parameters in the blood, such as procalcitonin, CRP, interleukin-6, and white blood cell count, are used, in conjunction with clinical signs and laboratory parameters indicating organ failure, e.g., lactate. The determination of lactate is also recommended in the new treatment guidelines. Lactate can be used as a parameter for correct management, as lactate clearance controlled fluid therapy has proven to be advantageous [9]. The determination of procalcitonin should be a diagnostic standard in suspected urosepsis [10]. It can also be used for treatment control, and in pyelonephritis, normalized procalcitonin levels can be used to stop antibiotic treatment. Further, diagnostic measures should include urine cultures and blood cultures prior to antibiotic treatment [11, 12].

Furthermore, early and targeted urological imaging diagnostics for the detection or localization of complicating factors, such as obstructive uropathy due to ureteral stones, for example, or abscesses or infected urinomas, can readily be diagnosed by CT scan, for example. Those complicating factors are often accessible to minimally invasive interventional techniques that must be performed immediately.

12.5 Treatment

The essential therapeutic pillars in the treatment of urosepsis patients is the rapid empiric antibiotic treatment, the early focus control and the supportive therapy consisting of volume and oxygen administration, administration of vasopressors, and organ replacement therapy, if needed [13].

12.5.1 Antibiotic Treatment

Early adequate antibiotic therapy has been shown to improve survival in patients with septic shock [14]. This is also predominantly included in the Surviving Sepsis Campaign Guidelines and the European Association of Urology guidelines [9]. The European Association of Urology guidelines recommend initial empiric antimicrobial therapy to provide broad antimicrobial coverage against all likely causative pathogens and should be adapted on the basis of culture results, once available. The dosage of the antimicrobial substances is of paramount importance in patients with sepsis syndrome and should generally be high, with the exception of patients in renal failure. Antimicrobials must be administered no later than 1 h after clinical assumption of sepsis [4, 15]. Recommended antibiotics for empiric therapy of urosepsis are as follows: cefotaxime 2 g t.i.d, ceftazidime 1–2 g t.i.d, ceftriaxone 1–2 g q.d, cefepime 1–2 g b.i.d, piperacillin/tazobactam 2.5–4.5 g t.i.d, ceftolozane/tazobactam 1.5 g t.i.d, ceftazidime/avibactam 2.5 g t.i.d, gentamicin 5 mg/kg q.d, amikacin 15 mg/kg q.d, ertapenem 1 g q.d, imipenem/cilastatin 0.5/0.5 g t.i.d, meropenem 1 g t.i.d, doripenem 0.5 g t.i.d [15].

The advantage of combination therapy lies above all in the broadening of the spectrum, rather than possible synergism. If the isolated pathogen is sensitive to a single substance (monotherapy), a combination therapy usually brings no further advantage but possibly additional toxicity.

A routine, initial combination therapy is recommended by the Surviving Sepsis Campaign therefore with little evidence, only in septic shock [9, 16]. Whether a substance is suitable for initial monotherapy depends on the regional resistance situation. Resistance should therefore be monitored in the own institution. In one study in urosepsis, resistance rates were significantly higher than in other clinical diagnosis of healthcare-associated UTI [5]. It is therefore not appropriate to use the pathogen spectrum and resistance rates of other UTIs as representative of urosepsis to decide on empirical treatment of urosepsis. In particular, the spread of bacteria that form "extended spectrum beta-lactamases" (ESBL) and carbapenemases has dramatically increased. According to the Surviving Sepsis Campaign, piperacillin/tazobactam and carbapenems are suitable for monotherapy in sepsis [9, 16]. In contrast, the Surviving Sepsis Campaign is critical of the use of monotherapy with unprotected cephalosporines in sepsis, given the spread of ESBL-producing organisms. Cephalosporine/beta-lactamase combinations, such as ceftolozane/tazobactam and ceftazidime/avibactam, are active against a variety of ESBLs and can be used in this indication [17, 18]. Other, non-protected cephalosporines should be combined with a fluoroquinolone or an aminoglycoside (preferred) [9, 13, 16]. If a combination therapy is given, it should be de-escalated to a monotherapy after 48–72 h.

12.5.2 Focus Control

Common risk factors for urosepsis are urinary tract dysfunctions, such as those caused by obstructions (e.g., urolithiasis, tumors, catheter obstruction, prostate enlargement, urethral stricture, or congenital anomalies). Urinary tract interventions and transrectal prostate biopsies may also lead to urosepsis [19]. Important is the recommended early interventional focus control, which should be as minimally invasive as possible. In a multicenter study, early interventional focus rehabilitation was as important as early antibiotic therapy [20] and even showed a greater influence for patient survival than the early antibiotic therapy. This is especially true for urosepsis, as up to 78% of urosepsis have obstructive uropathy, mostly due to urolithiasis (43%), urological tumors (18%), benign prostatic hypertrophy (25%), or abscessed infection [21].

12.5.3 Supportive Therapy

Supportive therapy includes fluid therapy with crystalloids, or albumin, if crystalloids are not adequately increasing blood pressure. As vasopressors, norepinephrine should be used primarily. Hydrocortisone should be given only if fluid and vasopressors do not achieve a mean arterial pressure of ≥65 mmHg. Blood products should be given to target a hemoglobin level of 7–9 g/dL. Mechanical ventilation should be applied with a tidal volume 6 mL/kg and plateau pressure ≤ 30 cm H_2O and a high positive end-expiratory pressure. Sedation should be given minimally, and neuromuscular blocking agents should be avoided. Glucose levels should be targeted at ≤180 mg/dL. Deep vein thrombosis prevention should be given with low-molecular-weight heparin subcutaneously. Stress ulcer prophylaxis should be applied in patients at risk, using proton pump inhibitors and enteral nutrition should be started early.

12.6 Conclusion

Urosepsis is a frequent diagnosis and can be managed successfully, if organized effectively. The new sepsis criteria have to be implemented into clinical practice to allow early diagnosis of the sepsis syndrome. Antibiotic treatment and focus control have to be started as early as possible. Both have shown to be able to reduce mortality. The algorithm for urosepsis includes surveillance, preventive measures, and organizational aspects to provide early and encompassing management.

References

1. Kaukonen KM, Bailey M, Pilcher D, Cooper DJ, Bellomo R. Systemic inflammatory response syndrome criteria in defining severe sepsis. N Engl J Med. 2015;372(17):1629–38.
2. Martin GS. Sepsis, severe sepsis and septic shock: changes in incidence, pathogens and outcomes. Expert Rev Anti-Infect Ther. 2012;10(6):701–6.
3. Qiang XH, Yu TO, Li YN, Zhou LX. Prognosis risk of urosepsis in critical care medicine: a prospective observational study. Biomed Res Int. 2016;2016:9028924.
4. Bodmann KF, Grabein B, e.V. EdP-E-GfC. S2k Leitline: Kalkulierte parenterale Initialtherapie bakterieller Erkrankungen be Erwachsenen-Update 2017. AWMF Leitlinie 2017; AWMF RegNo 082–006.
5. Tandogdu Z, Bartoletti R, Cai T, Cek M, Grabe M, Kulchavenya E, et al. Antimicrobial resistance in urosepsis: outcomes from the multinational, multicenter global prevalence of infections in urology (GPIU) study 2003-2013. World J Urol. 2016;34(8):1193–200.
6. Singer M, Deutschman CS, Seymour CW, Shankar-Hari M, Annane D, Bauer M, et al. The third international consensus definitions for sepsis and septic shock (sepsis-3). JAMA. 2016;315(8):801–10.
7. Weis S, Carlos AR, Moita MR, Singh S, Blankenhaus B, Cardoso S, et al. Metabolic adaptation establishes disease tolerance to sepsis. Cell. 2017;169(7):1263–75. e14
8. Seymour CW, Liu VX, Iwashyna TJ, Brunkhorst FM, Rea TD, Scherag A, et al. Assessment of clinical criteria for sepsis: for the third international consensus definitions for sepsis and septic shock (sepsis-3). JAMA. 2016;315(8):762–74.
9. Rhodes A, Evans LE, Alhazzani W, Levy MM, Antonelli M, Ferrer R, et al. Surviving sepsis campaign: international guidelines for management of sepsis and septic shock: 2016. Intensive Care Med. 2017;43(3):304–77.
10. van Nieuwkoop C, Bonten TN, van't Wout JW, Kuijper EJ, Groeneveld GH, Becker MJ, et al. Procalcitonin reflects bacteremia and bacterial load in urosepsis syndrome: a prospective observational study. Crit Care. 2010;14(6):R206.
11. Norman DC. Fever in the elderly. Clin Infect Dis. 2000;31(1):148–51.
12. High KP, Bradley SF, Gravenstein S, Mehr DR, Quagliarello VJ, Richards C, et al. Clinical practice guideline for the evaluation of fever and infection in older adult residents of long-term care facilities: 2008 update by the Infectious Diseases Society of America. J Am Geriatr Soc. 2009;57(3):375–94.
13. Pletz MW, Weis S, Forstner C, Wagenlehner F. Urosepsis. Urol A. 2018;57:79.

14. Kumar A, Roberts D, Wood KE, Light B, Parrillo JE, Sharma S, et al. Duration of hypotension before initiation of effective antimicrobial therapy is the critical determinant of survival in human septic shock. Crit Care Med. 2006;34(6):1589–96.
15. Bonkat G, Bartoletti R, Bruyere F, Cai T, Geerlings SE, Köves B, Schubert S, Wagenlehner F, Mezei T, Pilatz A, Pradere B. Veeratterapillay R. EAU guidelines on urological infections. EAU Guidelines 2018.
16. Rhodes A, Evans LE, Alhazzani W, Levy MM, Antonelli M, Ferrer R, et al. Surviving sepsis campaign: international guidelines for management of sepsis and septic shock: 2016. Crit Care Med. 2017;45(3):486–552.
17. Wagenlehner FM, Sobel JD, Newell P, Armstrong J, Huang X, Stone GG, et al. Ceftazidime-avibactam versus doripenem for the treatment of complicated urinary tract infections, including acute pyelonephritis: RECAPTURE, a phase 3 randomized trial program. Clin Infect Dis. 2016;63(6):754–62.
18. Wagenlehner FM, Umeh O, Steenbergen J, Yuan G, Darouiche RO. Ceftolozane-tazobactam compared with levofloxacin in the treatment of complicated urinary-tract infections, including pyelonephritis: a randomised, double-blind, phase 3 trial (ASPECT-cUTI). Lancet. 2015;385(9981):1949–56.
19. Wagenlehner FM, van Oostrum E, Tenke P, Tandogdu Z, Cek M, Grabe M, et al. Infective complications after prostate biopsy: outcome of the global prevalence study of infections in urology (GPIU) 2010 and 2011, a prospective multinational multicentre prostate biopsy study. Eur Urol. 2013;63(3):521–7.
20. Bloos F, Ruddel H, Thomas-Ruddel D, Schwarzkopf D, Pausch C, Harbarth S, et al. Effect of a multifaceted educational intervention for anti-infectious measures on sepsis mortality: a cluster randomized trial. Intensive Care Med. 2017;43(11):1602–12.
21. Hofmann W. Urosepsis and uroseptic shock. Z Urol Nephrol. 1990;83(6):317–24.

13 The Treatment of Urinary Tract Infections Caused by ESBL-Producing Gram-Negative Bacteria, Vancomycin-Resistant Enterococci (VRE), and Other Multidrug-Resistant Bacteria

Fabian P. Stangl, Jennifer Kranz, Florian M. E. Wagenlehner, Jonas Marschall, Sören Schubert, José Medina-Polo, Laila Schneidewind, and Truls E. Bjerklund Johansen

F. P. Stangl (✉)
Department of Urology, Inselspital, University Hospital Bern, Bern, Switzerland
e-mail: fabian.stangl@alumni.pmu.ac.at

J. Kranz
Department of Urology and Pediatric Urology, RWTH Aachen University, Aachen, Germany

Department of Urology and Kidney Transplantation, Martin-Luther-University, Halle, Germany
e-mail: Jennifer.Kranz@rwth-aachen.de

F. M. E. Wagenlehner
Clinic for Urology, Pediatric Urology and Andrology, Justus-Liebig-University Giessen, Giessen, Germany
e-mail: Florian.Wagenlehner@chiru.med.uni-giessen.de

J. Marschall
Division of Infectious Diseases, Washington University School of Medicine, St. Louis, MO, USA
e-mail: jmarscha@wustl.edu

S. Schubert
Department of Medical Microbiology and Hospital Hygiene, Max-Von-Pettenkofer Institute, LMU Munich, Munich, Germany
e-mail: Schubert@med.uni-muenchen.de

J. Medina-Polo
Department of Urology, Health Research Institute i+12, Hospital Universitario 12 de Octubre imas12, Madrid, Spain
e-mail: jose.medina@salud.madrid.org

T. E. Bjerklund Johansen, T. Cai (eds.), *Guide to Antibiotics in Urology*,
https://doi.org/10.1007/978-3-319-92366-6_13

Abbreviations

AmpC-E	AmpC beta-lactamase-producing *Enterobacterales*
AMS	Antimicrobial stewardship
BL-BLI	Beta-lactam-beta-lactamase inhibitor
CAUTI	Catheter-associated urinary tract infection
CDC	Centers for Disease Control and Prevention
CRAB	Carbapenem-resistant *Acinetobacter baumannii*
CRE	Carbapenem-resistant *Enterobacterales*
CRPA	Carbapenem-resistant *Pseudomonas aeruginosa*
CTX-M	Cefotaxime-Munich
cUTI	Complicated urinary tract infection
DTR-*P. aeruginosa*	Difficult-to-treat resistance *P. aeruginosa*
ESBL-E	Extended-spectrum beta-lactamase-producing *Enterobacterales*
ESIU	European Section of Infections in Urology
FDA	Food and Drug Administration
IDSA	Infectious Diseases Society of America
KPC	*Klebsiella pneumoniae* carbapenemase
MBL	Metallo-beta-lactamase
MDR	Multidrug-resistant
MIC	Minimum inhibitory concentration
MRSA	Methicillin-resistant *Staphylococcus aureus*
OPAT	Outpatient parenteral antimicrobial therapy
PBP's	Penicillin-binding proteins
SHV	Sulfhydryl variable gene
SIRS	Systemic inflammatory response syndrome
TEM	Temoniera gene
TMP-SMX	Trimethoprim-sulfamethoxazole
t-RNA	Transfer ribonucleic acid
UTI	Urinary tract infection
VRE	Vancomycin-resistant enterococci

L. Schneidewind
Department of Urology, University Medical Center Rostock, Rostock, Germany
e-mail: laila.schneidewind@uni-greifswald.de

T. E. Bjerklund Johansen
Institute of Clinical Medicine, University of Oslo, Oslo, Norway

Institute of Clinical Medicine, University of Aarhus, Aarhus, Denmark
e-mail: t.e.b.johansen@medisin.uio.no

13.1 Definition and Epidemiology

Antibiotic resistance is a significant problem worldwide, and it has been identified as one of the most pressing public health concerns of our time [1]. In the field of urology, antibiotic resistance poses a particular challenge due to the high prevalence of extended-spectrum beta-lactamase (ESBL)-producing Gram-negative bacteria, vancomycin-resistant enterococci (VRE), and other multi-drug-resistant (MDR) bacteria [2]. These bacteria are often found in patients with lower urinary tract infections and can lead to complications such as pyelonephritis and sepsis.

ESBL, VRE, and MDR bacteria are resistant to many commonly used antibiotics, making treatment of these infections challenging and often require the use of last resort antibiotics. Moreover, inappropriate use of antibiotics in urology can lead to the development, selection, and spread of these resistant bacteria, further exacerbating the problem. Therefore, it is crucial to adopt appropriate infection prevention and control measures in urology to minimize the spread of ESBL, VRE, and MDR bacteria. These measures include implementing strict antimicrobial stewardship programs (AMS), urine sampling prior to initiation of therapy, using appropriate infection control precautions in urological procedures, and educating healthcare professionals and patients about the appropriate use of antibiotics to reduce the incidence of ESBL, VRE, and MDR infections.

The incidence of UTIs caused by ESBL and multidrug-resistant bacteria has been steadily increasing over the past few decades. In a study conducted in the United States, the proportion of *E. coli* strains resistant to at least one class of antibiotics increased from 28% in 2000 to 38% in 2010 [3]. Similarly, a study conducted in the Netherlands found that the proportion of patients with UTIs caused by ESBL-producing bacteria increased from 1.6% in 2008 to 6.0% in 2014 [4]. These trends are not unique; similar increases in ESBL and multidrug resistance have been reported in many other countries as well [5].

ESBL enzymes are capable of hydrolyzing β-lactam antibiotics, including penicillins and cephalosporins. The predominant types of ESBLs are the CTX-M, TEM, and SHV enzymes, which are encoded by different genes found on plasmids or other mobile genetic elements such transposons, and integrons, which can transfer between bacteria, allowing the spread of resistance. They are detected in Gram-negative bacteria, such as *Escherichia coli* (*E. coli*) and *Klebsiella pneumoniae* (*K. pneumoniae*). The presence of ESBLs in bacteria can limit the efficacy of many antibiotics, leading to the development of MDR bacteria [6].

Vancomycin-resistant enterococci (VRE) are a group of bacteria that are resistant to the antibiotic vancomycin, which is to treat serious infections caused by otherwise resistant Gram-positive bacteria. The two most common types of VRE are *Enterococcus faecalis* and *Enterococcus faecium*. These bacteria can cause a range of infections, including urinary tract infections, bloodstream infections, and surgical site infections [7].

According to a study published in Clinical Infectious Diseases, the prevalence of VRE in the United States has increased in recent years, with a colonization prevalence rate of 0.34% among hospitalized patients in 2015, up from 0.21% in 2011. The study also found that VRE infections are associated with longer hospital stays, increased healthcare costs, and higher mortality rates [8].

VRE are considered a significant threat to public health, particularly in healthcare settings. Patients who are at increased risk of VRE infections include those who have compromised immune systems, who have undergone invasive procedures, and who have received prolonged courses of antibiotics [9].

MDR bacteria are defined as bacteria that are resistant to multiple antibiotics from different classes. MDR resistance results from a combination of mechanisms already named above, including the acquisition of plasmids carrying multiple resistance genes, the development of mutations in chromosomal genes, and the upregulation of efflux pumps, which can extrude antibiotics from the bacterial cell [10, 11].

The prevalence of MDR bacteria is also increasing worldwide, with reports indicating that up to 60% of *E. coli* isolates from UTIs are MDR in some parts of the world. According to the Centers for Disease Control and Prevention (CDC), the prevalence of MDR bacteria in UTIs has been increasing, with up to 10% of *E. coli* isolates being MDR in 2020 in the United States. Healthcare-associated infections are a major source of MDR bacteria, with reports indicating that up to 70% of healthcare-associated infections are caused by MDR bacteria [12, 13].

The evolution of MDR bacteria is also facilitated by the widespread use of antibiotics in healthcare settings, including hospitals, long-term care facilities, and outpatient clinics, where bacteria can acquire resistance mechanisms through horizontal gene transfer from other bacteria carrying resistance genes, and genetic mutations. Overuse and misuse of antibiotics, leading to the selection and spread of resistant strains of bacteria is an additional driver of resistance development. Especially prior treatment of infections with Cephalosporins or Piperacillin/Tazobactam has been identified as a major risk factor for patients having an infection with multidrug-resistant uropathogens [14].

This chapter aims to comprehensively address treatment options for UTI caused by multiresistant microorganisms and to enable healthcare professionals to initiate effective empirical antibiotic therapy.

13.2 Comprehensive List of Antibiotics for ESBL, VRE, and MDR

13.2.1 Aminoglycosides

13.2.1.1 Amikacin, Gentamicin, Tobramycin, and Plazomicin

Amikacin, gentamicin, tobramycin, and plazomicin are all aminoglycoside antibiotics that have activity against ESBL, VRE, and multidrug-resistant bacteria. They inhibit bacterial protein synthesis by binding to the bacterial ribosome and provide a broad spectrum of activity against Gram-negative bacteria, including *Pseudomonas aeruginosa*. The combination of aminoglycosides with beta-lactams and fluoroquinolones can increase the activity against the above-named organisms significantly. It enhances the activity of the beta-lactam or carbapenem by disrupting the bacterial cell membrane, allowing the other antibiotic to penetrate the cell wall more effectively and thereby unfold its synergistic properties.

However, caution should be exercised when using aminoglycosides in combination with other antibiotics because doing so can raise the risk of side effects such nephrotoxicity and ototoxicity. Renal function has to be taken into account when adjusting the dosage, and close observation is required.

13.2.2 Aminopenicillins

13.2.2.1 Ampicillin-Sulbactam

Ampicillin-sulbactam is a beta-lactamase inhibitor combination antibiotic commonly used in preoperative prophylaxis. It was a first line antibiotic to treat UTI caused by ESBL, VRE, and multidrug-resistant bacteria but ended up ineffective as a result of too liberal usage. Due to the pharmacokinetic properties of ampicillin, very high doses of the active agent are excreted renally [15]. Therefore, it remains a viable option for ESBL resistant to ampicillin. It is effective against a broad range of Gram-positive and Gram-negative bacteria. Adverse effects include diarrhea, nausea, and various hypersensitivity reactions including anaphylaxis [16].

13.2.2.2 Piperacillin-Tazobactam

Piperacillin-tazobactam is another beta-lactamase inhibitor combination antibiotic with similar properties to ampicillin-sulbactam but has a wider spectrum of action including activity against *Pseudomonas aeruginosa* [17].

13.2.3 Carbapenems

13.2.3.1 Imipenem-Cilastatin/Relebactam, Meropenem/Vaborbactam, and Ertapenem

Carbapenems are beta-lactam antibiotics, which inhibit cell wall synthesis by binding and inactivating penicillin-binding proteins (PBS's). Due to their potency, they are first-line antibiotics for the treatment of serious ESBL infections. Relebactam and vaborbactam are new-era beta-lactamase-inhibitors, which are added to extend the Gram-negative spectrum by inhibiting, e.g., serine carbapenemases, including *Klebsiella pneumoniae* carbapenemase (KPC). Cilastatin is a dehydropeptidase inhibitor to reduce rapid renal degradation of imipenem and prolong its half-life and increase blood levels of imipenem [18]. Ertapenem is known to have no activity against *P. aeruginosa* or *E. faecalis*, and *E. faecium*, *Stenotrophomonas maltophilia*, and methicillin-resistant *Staphylococcus aureus* (MRSA) are naturally carbapenem-resistant [19].

13.2.4 Cephalosporins

13.2.4.1 Cefepime, Cefiderocol, Ceftazidime-Avibactam/Aztreonam, and Ceftolozane-Tazobactam

All the abovementioned antibiotics have a similar mechanism of action. By binding to PBPs, which are involved in the final stages of bacterial cell wall synthesis, the cross-linking of peptidoglycans is inhibited, leading to bacterial death. Cefiderocol uses a different point of entry by binding to ferric iron and using the bacterial iron transport system to enter the cell. Aztreonam also inhibits bacterial cell wall synthesis by binding to PBPs and disrupts the cross-linking of peptidoglycan, but it is not affected by many of the beta-lactamases. Aztreonam therefore covers a broader spectrum. Except for Cefepime, all the mentioned cephalosporin antibiotics are considered novel antibiotics and have been US Food and Drug Administration (FDA) approved after 2014 [20, 21].

13.2.5 Fluoroquinolones

13.2.5.1 Ciprofloxacin and Levofloxacin

These fluoroquinolone antibiotics inhibits bacterial DNA synthesis by targeting bacterial DNA gyrase and topoisomerase IV, which are enzymes involved in DNA replication, transcription, and repair. Levofloxacin has a higher affinity for topoisomerase IV than ciprofloxacin, which makes it more effective against *Streptococcus pneumoniae* and some atypical bacteria such as *Mycoplasma pneumoniae* and *Chlamydophila pneumoniae*. Levofloxacin is also more effective against some Gram-negative bacteria including *P. aeruginosa* and *H. influenza*. Levofloxacin offers in vitro susceptibility to *E. faecalis*, but clinical cure rates are insignificant [22]. Fluoroquinolones have shown to be active against ESBL-producing *Enterobacterales*, but there are often multiple resistance traits. Increased resistance to fluoroquinolones restricts its first line use in UTI due to MDR [23].

13.2.6 Glycylcyclines

13.2.6.1 Tigecycline

Tigecycline is a tetracycline derivative with a similar mechanism of action. They have been developed to overcome resistance to tetracyclines and utilize slight alterations to inhibit protein synthesis. It binds to the 30S ribosomal subunit of the bacterial ribosome at a different site other than tetracyclines, preventing the binding of aminoacyl-tRNA molecules to the A site of the ribosome, obtaining its bactericidal effect [24].

13.2.7 Polymyxins

13.2.7.1 Colistin and Polymyxin B

Polymyxin antibiotics are parenterally administered reserve antibiotics and are used to treat multidrug-resistant Gram-negative bacterial infections such as *P. aeruginosa*, *Acinetobacter baumannii*, and *K. pneumoniae*. Both colistin and polymyxin B have a similar bactericidal mechanism of action, which involves binding the lipopolysaccharide layer of the outer membrane of Gram-negative bacteria, causing the membrane to become more permeable and allowing leakage of intracellular contents. Despite their effectiveness against some multidrug-resistant bacteria, colistin and polymyxin B are not without limitations. Overuse and misuse of these drugs can lead to the emergence of resistant strains of bacteria, e.g., carriers of the MCR-1 gene conferring colistin resistance, and some strains of bacteria are inherently resistant to these drugs. Both colistin and polymyxin B can cause serious side effects, including nephrotoxicity, neurotoxicity, and respiratory failure. They require careful dosing and monitoring to minimize the risk of toxicity and ensure adequate treatment [25].

13.2.8 Tetracyclines

13.2.8.1 Doxycycline, Minocycline, and Eravacycline

These tetracycline antibiotics inhibits bacterial protein synthesis by binding to the 30S ribosomal subunit, preventing the binding of aminoacyl-tRNA to the ribosome and thereby inhibiting the addition of amino acids to the growing peptide chain. They have a broad-spectrum of activity against both Gram-positive and Gram-negative bacteria such as carbapenem-resistant *Enterobacterales*, VRE, and. *A. baumannii*. Minocycline is an old, orally available tetracycline, whereas Eravacycline was approved in 2018 by the FDA for complicated intra-abdominal infections in adults [26].

13.2.9 Miscellaneous

13.2.9.1 Daptomycin

Daptomycin is a bactericidal cyclic lipopeptide unfolding its effect by disruption of bacterial cell membrane functions. Daptomycin has a rapid onset of action and is therefore highly suitable for complicated infections due to MRSA or VRE and especially bloodstream infections. Additionally, it offers reasonable activity against catheter colonization and biofilm formation. Since daptomycin is excreted unchanged renally, high urine concentrations are reached. In cases of prolonged treatment, therapy must be closely monitored due to the increased risk of myopathy and rhabdomyolysis [27]. It is only available as an injectable compound.

13.2.9.2 Fosfomycin

Fosfomycin is an old bactericidal epoxy antibiotic and available as an oral agent Fosfomycin-Trometamol or the parenteral agent Fosfomycin-Disodium. It interferes with bacterial cell wall biosynthesis and inhibits the first cytoplasmic step of murein synthesis [28]. Fosfomycin offers a broad spectrum of antimicrobial efficacy including ESBL, MRSA, and MDR. The parenteral use of Fosfomycin for complicated infections has increased steadily over the last decade [29, 30]. The oral form is attractive as it is given as a single dose.

13.2.9.3 Linezolid

Linezolid is a synthetic oxazolidinone reserve antibiotic and inhibits the protein-biosynthesis of Gram-positive organism. The spectrum of effectivity resembles vancomycin, and it is therefore commonly used in case of resistance against vancomycin. Linezolid can be an effective option for the treatment of MRSA in hospitalized adult patients, but it is not recommended in UTI due to its weak renal excretion. Since Linezolid is available as an oral formulation, it can be used in uncomplicated UTI due to VRE, where studies showed good clinical cure rates [31].

13.2.9.4 Nitrofurantoin

Nitrofurantoin, another old antibiotic, is exerting its effect by inhibiting bacterial protein synthesis. Its usage increased rapidly over the last years since major guidelines placed it as first-line therapy for uncomplicated UTI. Toxicity like pulmonary fibrosis remains a concern, but clinical trials did not report severe side effects in short-term use [32]. Nitrofurantoin plays an in important role in the peroral treatment of UTI caused by VRE or ESBL.

13.2.9.5 Trimethoprim-Sulfamethoxazole (TMP-SMX)

TMP-SMX has been a first-line sulfonamide antibiotic for uncomplicated UTI for decades. It's good bioavailability and tolerability and broad spectrum of effectivity against Gram-positive and negative bacteria, including activity against ESBL, made it suitable to fulfill that role. High rates of resistance, against *E. coli* of over 50% in some countries, rendered it disadvantageous for empiric therapy due to a high risk of treatment failure. Nephrotoxicity remains a concern, especially in cases of prolonged therapy [33].

13.3 Management of Uncomplicated UTI

The decision to treat uncomplicated UTI (cystitis) for suspected infection with ESBL, VRE, or MDR should be carefully weighed according to severity of symptoms. It is of particular importance to refrain from treating asymptomatic bacteriuria with the named organisms, so as to lower overall resistance pressure on the causative bacteria. In case of significant discomfort and failure of nonantibiotic management, a decision to treat should always be based on the results of urine cultures and resistance patterns.

13.3.1 ESBL

The management of UTIs caused by ESBL, VRE, and multidrug-resistant bacteria is often complicated by the limited availability of effective antibiotics. In cases of uncomplicated infection, and an otherwise healthy patient, oral antibiotics such as Fosfomycin and Nitrofurantoin have been proven to be effective in UTI due to ESBL-producing bacteria [34].

Longer courses of treatment are necessary to achieve eradication of bacterial colonization. Due to the mechanism of resistance acquisition, ESBL-producing bacteria often carry co-resistance to multiple classes of antibiotics. For example, trimethoprim-sulfamethoxazole and quinolones might be effective and could be considered as potential treatment options, and ESBL-producing bacteria carry a high percentage of co-resistance to these drugs [35, 36] (see Table 13.1 for exact dosing and duration suggestions). Nitrofurantoin and Fosfomycin are first-line options for uncomplicated ESBL UTI.

Table 13.1 Antimicrobial therapy with suggested agent, dosage, and target organism. Adapted from Infectious Diseases Society of America and European Society of Clinical Microbiology and Infectious Diseases Guidelines [41, 63]

Group and agent	Standard dosage	Target organisms
Aminoglycosides		
Amikacin	15 mg/kg/dose d IV once × 1 dose, subsequent doses and dosing interval based on pharmacokinetic evaluation	ESBL-E, AmpC-E, CRE, DTR-*P. aeruginosa*
Gentamicin	5 mg/kg/dose d IV once × 1 dose, subsequent doses and dosing interval based on pharmacokinetic evaluation	ESBL-E, AmpC-E, CRE, DTR-*P. aeruginosa*
Plazomicin	15 mg/kg/dose d IV once × 1 dose, subsequent doses and dosing interval based on pharmacokinetic evaluation	ESBL-E, AmpC-E, CRE, DTR-*P. aeruginosa*
Tobramycin	5 mg/kg/dose d IV once × 1 dose, subsequent doses and dosing interval based on pharmacokinetic evaluation	ESBL-E, AmpC-E, CRE, DTR-*P. aeruginosa*
Aminopenicillins		
Ampicillin	2 g IV/PO q6h	VRE
Ampicillin-sulbactam	3–9 g IV q8h over 4 h or 27 g IV q24h as a continuous infusion	CRAB
Piperacillin-tazobactam	4.5 g IV q8 over 4 h	
Carbapenems		
Ertapenem	1 g IV q24h, infused over 30 min	ESBL-E, AmpC-E
Imipenem-cilastatin	500 mg IV q6h, infused over 30 min	ESBL-E, AmpC-E, CRE, CRAB
Imipenem-cilastatin-relebactam	1.25 g IV q6h, infused over 30 min	CRE, DTR-*P. aeruginosa*
Meropenem-vaborbactam	4 g IV q8h, infused over 3 h	CRE

(continued)

Table 13.1 (continued)

Group and agent	Standard dosage	Target organisms
Meropenem	1–2 g IV q8h, infused over 30 min	ESBL-E, AmpC-E, CRE, CRAB
Cephalosporins		
Cefepime	2 g IV q8h, infused over 3 h	AmpC-E
Cefiderocol	2 g IV q8h, infused over 3 h	CRE, DTR-*P. aeruginosa*, CRAB, *S. maltophilia*
Ceftazidime-avibactam	2.5 g IV q8h, infused over 3 h	CRE, DTR-*P. aeruginosa*
Ceftazidime-avibactam and aztreonam	Ceftazidime-avibactam: 2.5 g IV q8h, infused over 3 h *PLUS* Aztreonam: 2 g IV q8h, infused over 3 h	Metallo-β-lactamase-producing CRE, *S. maltophilia*
Ceftolozane-tazobactam	3 g IV q8h, infused over 3 h	DTR-*P. aeruginosa*
Fluoroquinolones		
Ciprofloxacin	400 mg IV q8h–q12h or 500–750 mg PO q12h	ESBL-E, AmpC-E
Levofloxacin	750 mg IV/PO q24h	ESBL-E, AmpC-E, *S. maltophilia*
Glycylcyclines		
Tigecycline	200 mg IV × first dose, then 100 mg IV q12h	CRE, CRAB, *S. maltophilia*
Polymyxins [53]		
Colistin	Refer to international consensus guidelines on polymyxins	CRE, DTR-*P. aeruginosa*, CRAB
Polymyxin B	Refer to international consensus guidelines on polymyxins	DTR-*P. aeruginosa*, CRAB
Tetracyclines		
Doxycycline	100 mg PO q12h	VRE
Eravacycline	1 mg/kg/dose IV q12h	CRE, CRAB
Minocycline	200 mg IV/PO q12h	CRAB, *S. maltophilia*
Miscellaneous		
Daptomycin	4 mg/kg IV daily	VRE
Fosfomycin	3 g PO × 1–3 doses every 48 h or 3 × 6–8 g IV up to 20 g daily	ESBL-*E. coli*, (VRE)
Linezolid	600 mg IV/PO q12h	VRE
Nitrofurantoin	100 mg PO q12h	ESBL-*E. coli*, AmpC-E, VRE
Trimethoprim-sulfamethoxazole	960 mg IV/PO q12h	ESBL-E, AmpC-E, *S. maltophilia*

13.3.2 VRE

Enterococci resistant to vancomycin often also carry resistances to other antibiotics, most often aminopenicillins. Oral therapy of VRE-associated UTI can be managed similarly to ESBL with Nitrofurantoin as drug of choice. In case of treatment failure, Linezolid may present a second-line oral therapy in case of persistent symptoms with ongoing growth of bacteria in urine cultures [37, 38]. Even though most strains carry resistance to ampicillin, it might still be worthwhile to consider this drug in uncomplicated UTI. Resistance is furthermore species-dependent caused by different PBP's. E. faecalis in contrast to E. faecium is usually sensitive to ampicillin. The renal tubular secretion and hence the urinary concentration of ampicillin exceeds the minimum inhibitory concentration (MIC) suggested by the Clinical and Laboratory Standards Institute guidelines by far. By achieving high levels of antibiotics in the urinary tract during an adequate treatment duration, we increase both exposure and time above MIC. Although this concept is regarded controversial by some investigators, studies suggest its clinical effectivity [15]. Doxycycline might have a role in treatment of VRE biofilm with low levels of overall resistance [39].

13.3.3 MDR

Treatment principles of MDR UTI are similar to the abovementioned treatment options for ESBL and VRE. A multitude of named organisms are considered MDR and identification of drug sensitivity is of utmost importance to avoid treatment failure. Again, Fosfomycin has been proven a viable option in enteral treatment [40]. The Infectious Diseases Society of America (IDSA) suggests Nitrofurantoin and Fosfomycin in standard dosing and levofloxacin or ciprofloxacin at increased dosage for uncomplicated infections as oral treatment options, in cases of proven susceptibility [41].

13.3.4 Management of Complicated UTI

Complicated UTI (cUTI) is defined as infections in patients with immunodeficiency or suppression, pregnancy, functional anatomical alterations in the urinary tract or obstruction, diabetes, catheterized patients, or in the setting of malignant diseases. All those factors increase the risk for recurrence or prolonged courses of the disease. While *E. coli* is the most common pathogen in uncomplicated UTI, other organisms, often with complex resistance patterns, are causative for infections in cUTI. To further help with risk stratification for cUTI, the European Section of Infections in Urology (ESIU) developed a classification for UTI utilizing the ORENUC- scheme (Fig. 13.1). Management of cUTI is often complex since it commonly involves patients with comorbidities. This classification helps with decision-making and tailoring of empirical antibiotic therapy. In case of severe infection, it is advisable to manage the patient interdisciplinary and consult an infectious disease specialist, pharmacologist, or clinical microbiologist. Consensus-based therapy reduces the risk for side effects and potential drug interactions as well as treatment failure. Additionally, in every case of infection removal of indwelling catheters is recommended to avoid biofilm formation. Not only do indwelling catheters or stents

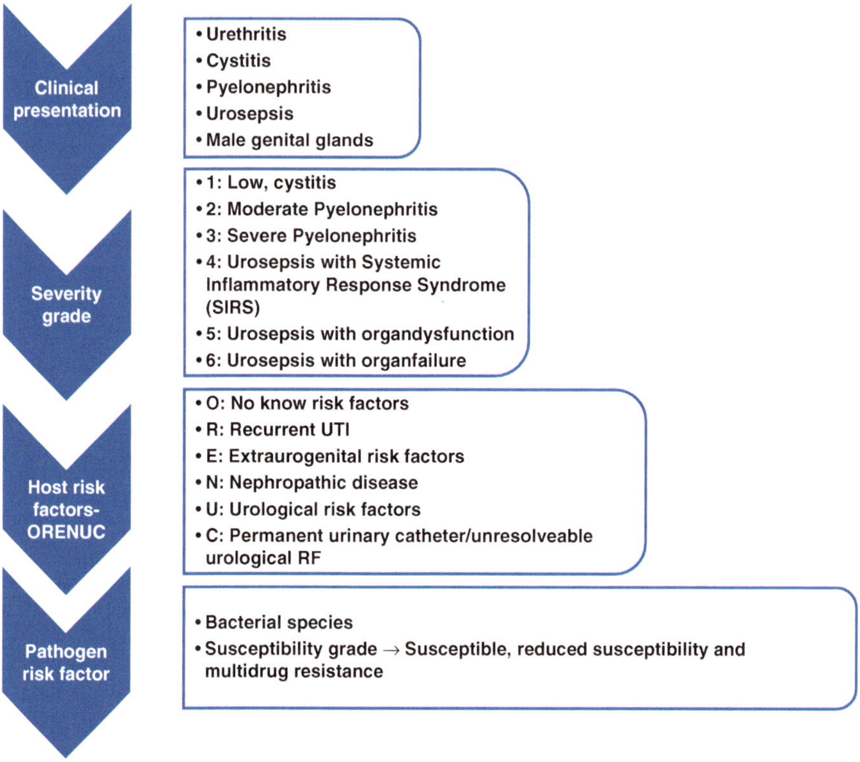

Fig. 13.1 The European Section of Infections in Urology classification of UTIs. The classification and severity assessment involves evaluation of the clinical presentation, grading the severity of the infection, and identification of host and pathogen risk factors

represent possible harbors for bacterial biofilms but also increase the risk of urolithiasis which further enables bacterial hibernation.

In case of severe infections with systemic symptoms or even signs of sepsis, decisions on empiric treatment should consider a variety of variables. Community-acquired, hospital-acquired, and catheter-associated infections all give indications on potential causative organisms and their antibiotic resistance patterns. Furthermore, patient's characteristics like allergies and kidney function play a major role in empiric treatment decision. The clinician must also consider antibiotics exposure in the recent past susceptibility data from the previous six months as well as local resistance patterns [42].

13.3.4.1 ESBL

Carbapenems are among the first choices for treatment of complicated UTI with suspected ESBL. In case of severely ill patients, carbapenems like meropenem have shown significant efficacy with low overall mortality rates [43]. Ertapenem should be used with caution because of its lack of activity against *P. aeruginosa* and *A.*

baumannii, but it may be an alternative for outpatient parenteral antimicrobial therapy (OPAT) due to its once daily administration. In case of less severely ill patients without suspected sepsis, beta-lactam-beta-lactam-inhibitors (BL-BLI) may represent a suitable treatment option if dosed correctly. Piperacillin-tazobactam provides non-inferiority compared to meropenem in case of cUTI with low severity grade [44]. Newer beta-lactam combinations such as Ceftazidime-avibactam confer high cure rates and can be considered an option but should not be first line [45]. Lastly, aminoglycosides, especially Amikacin, are a viable option for the treatment of ESBL-cUTI. This treatment must be closely monitored to avoid toxicity [46].

13.3.4.2 VRE

VRE account for a significant amount of catheter-associated UTI (CAUTI) and can form biofilms rapidly [47]. Therefore, it is of utmost importance to remove or change any indwelling catheters under suitable therapy to avoid recolonization of the urine. In case of ampicillin-susceptible VRE infection, high-dose therapy of ampicillin in combination with an aminoglycoside, e.g., gentamicin, can be used [15, 48, 49]. In case of VRE bacteremia, daptomycin and linezolid are first-line antibiotics due to low risk of treatment failure [50]. Daptomycin should be the preferred agent, given its rapid onset of effect and great activity against VRE catheter colonization and biofilm formation [39, 51].

13.3.4.3 MDR

Treatment of MDR UTI remains heavily dependent on the suspected causative organism and the resistance pattern. Severely ill patients with a history of multiresistant bacterial infections must not only be closely monitored to assess treatment success or failure, but initial empiric therapy should be broad enough to cover all potential culprits. Carbapenem-resistant *Enterobacterales* (CRE), carbapenem-resistant *A. baumannii* (CRAB), difficult-to-treat-resistant *P. aeruginosa* (DTR-P. aeruginosa), KPC, metallo-beta-lactamases (MBL), and carbapenemase-producing *P. aeruginosa* (CRPA) set tremendous hurdles in the treatment of cUTI. Polymyxin antibiotics are the first-line option for CRAB cUTI [52, 53], whereas aminoglycosides like plazomicin shows excellent activity against CRE [54]. Tigecycline is an alternative with good activity against CRE and CRAB but should be used with great caution due to its inherent resistance against *P. aeruginosa and low blood concentrations* [55]. The combination of Fosfomycin and Tigecycline or colistin remains an option for highly select cases with the most complex resistance pattern [56]. Novel BL-BLI antibiotics such as Ceftazidime-avibactam or Ceftolozane-tazobactam show potent in vitro activity against CRPA and are first-line therapeutics in these cases [57, 58]. Novel antibiotics are becoming are potential candidates for treatment of cUTI with different types of MDRO, such as Eravacycline for CRAB organisms, cefiderocol against all classes of carbapenemases including MBL and KPC, and Imipenem-relebactam and Aztreonam-avibactam for MBL. Ultimately, treatment relies heavily on the underlying resistance pattern, but reorganization and switching of therapy is common necessary [59].

13.4 Future Directions

The treatment of ESBL and multidrug-resistant UTIs continues to be a challenge for clinicians, and there is a need for new antibiotics, novel therapies, and alternative treatment approaches to combat these infections.

The development of new antibiotics, for example, murepavadin against *P. aeruginosa*, appears as a cornerstone to tackle increasing resistance. Unfortunately, incentives for pharmaceutical companies to develop new antimicrobial compounds are lacking, and the enormous cost of research and development acts as a disincentive. Governmental intervention is needed to support companies in investing in novel therapeutics. As discussed above, several novel antibiotics have been approved in recent years, including ceftazidime-avibactam, cefepime/enmetazobactam, tebipenem, meropenem-vaborbactam, plazomicin, and eravacycline [60]. Another attempt to tackle rising antibiotic resistance is the "re- or upcycling" of older, already approved therapeutics, e.g., colistin or temocillin. Often their use was dropped in the past due to an unfavorable side effects profile or the risk of significant, specific side effects. However, attributable to the lack of viable options, we must further explore these consequences.

Novel therapies, such as bacteriophages and monoclonal antibodies, are also being studied for the treatment of ESBL, VRE, and multidrug-resistant UTIs. Bacteriophages are viruses that specifically target and kill bacteria, and they have shown promise in animal studies and early clinical trials [61]. Monoclonal antibodies can target specific bacterial virulence factors, and thus enhance the effectiveness of antibiotics and reduce the risk of resistance development [62].

Finally, advances in diagnostic techniques, such as rapid molecular testing and metagenomic sequencing, may allow for more rapid identification of resistant pathogens and personalized treatment approaches according to susceptibility patterns. Rigorous AMS policies remain of utmost importance to decrease overall resistance pressure on already multidrug-resistant organisms and keep the treatment options we have in our armamentarium.

13.5 Conclusions

UTIs caused by ESBL, VRE, and multidrug-resistant bacteria represent a significant challenge for healthcare providers. As these infections continue to become more common, it is important to remain vigilant and adopt strategies to prevent their spread. By staying up to date on the latest diagnostic and treatment options, healthcare providers can offer optimal care and infection management for their patients.

Reducing unnecessary antibiotics, investing in AMS programs and interdisciplinary collaborations with infectious disease- and pharmacy specialist are measures to ensure that we will be able to treat complex UTI successfully in the future.

References

1. Murray CJ, Ikuta KS, Sharara F, Swetschinski L, Aguilar GR, Gray A, Han C, Bisignano C, Rao P, Wool E, Johnson SC. Global burden of bacterial antimicrobial resistance in 2019: a systematic analysis. Lancet. 2022;399(10325):629–55. https://doi.org/10.1016/s0140-6736(21)02724-0.
2. Picozzi S, Ricci C, Gaeta M, et al. Do we really know the prevalence of multi-drug resistant Escherichia coli in the territorial and nosocomial population? Urol Ann. 2013;5(1):25–9. https://doi.org/10.4103/0974-7796.106962.
3. Gupta K, Hooton TM, Naber KG, et al. International clinical practice guidelines for the treatment of acute uncomplicated cystitis and pyelonephritis in women: A 2010 update by the Infectious Diseases Society of America and the European Society for Microbiology and Infectious Diseases. Clin Infect Dis. 2011;52(5):e103–20. https://doi.org/10.1093/cid/ciq257.
4. van der Bij AK, Pitout JD. The role of international travel in the worldwide spread of multiresistant Enterobacteriaceae. J Antimicrob Chemother. 2012;67(9):2090–100. https://doi.org/10.1093/jac/dks214.
5. Bonomo RA, Burd EM, Conly J, et al. Carbapenemase-producing organisms: a global scourge. Clin Infect Dis. 2018;66(8):1290–7. https://doi.org/10.1093/cid/cix893.
6. Livermore DM, Canton R, Gniadkowski M, et al. CTX-M: changing the face of ESBLs in Europe. J Antimicrob Chemother. 2007;59(2):165–74. https://doi.org/10.1093/jac/dkl483.
7. Reyes K, Bardossy AC, Zervos M. Vancomycin-resistant enterococci: epidemiology, infection prevention, and control. Infect Dis Clin N Am. 2016;30(4):953–65. https://doi.org/10.1016/j.idc.2016.07.009.
8. Arias CA, Murray BE. The rise of the Enterococcus: beyond vancomycin resistance. Nat Rev Microbiol. 2012;10(4):266–78. https://doi.org/10.1038/nrmicro2761.
9. Bonten MJ, Willems R, Weinstein RA. Vancomycin-resistant enterococci: why are they here, and where do they come from? Lancet Infect Dis. 2001;1(5):314–25. https://doi.org/10.1016/s1473-3099(01)00145-1.
10. Livermore DM. Fourteen years in resistance. Int J Antimicrob Agents. 2012;39(4):283–94. https://doi.org/10.1016/j.ijantimicag.2011.12.012.
11. van Duin D, Paterson DL. Multidrug-resistant bacteria in the community: trends and lessons learned. Infect Dis Clin N Am. 2016;30(2):377–90. https://doi.org/10.1016/j.idc.2016.02.004.
12. Flores-Mireles AL, Walker JN, Caparon M, Hultgren SJ. Urinary tract infections: epidemiology, mechanisms of infection and treatment options. Nat Rev Microbiol. 2015;13(5):269–84. https://doi.org/10.1038/nrmicro3432.
13. Mazzariol A, Bazaj A, Cornaglia G. Multi-drug-resistant gram-negative bacteria causing urinary tract infections: a review. J Chemother. 2017;29(sup1):2–9. https://doi.org/10.1080/1120009x.2017.1380395.
14. Cohen-Nahum K, Saidel-Odes L, Riesenberg K, Schlaeffer F, Borer A. Urinary tract infections caused by multi-drug resistant Proteus mirabilis: risk factors and clinical outcomes. Infection. 2010;38(1):41–6. https://doi.org/10.1007/s15010-009-8460-5.
15. Shah KJ, Cherabuddi K, Shultz J, Borgert S, Ramphal R, Klinker KP. Ampicillin for the treatment of complicated urinary tract infections caused by vancomycin–resistant Enterococcus spp. (VRE): a single-center university hospital experience. Int J Antimicrob Agents. 2018;51(1):57–61. https://doi.org/10.1016/j.ijantimicag.2017.06.008.
16. Rando E, Giovannenze F, Murri R, Sacco E. A review of recent advances in the treatment of adults with complicated urinary tract infection. Expert Rev Clin Pharmacol. 2022;15(9):1053–66.
17. Ong LT. Antibiotics for complicated urinary tract infection and acute pyelonephritis: a systematic review. World J Clin Infect Dis. 2020;10:33–41.
18. Heo Y-A. Imipenem/cilastatin/relebactam: a review in gram-negative bacterial infections. Drugs. 2021;81:377–88.

19. Aurilio C, Sansone P, Barbarisi M, et al. Mechanisms of action of carbapenem resistance. Antibiotics. 2022;11(3):421.
20. Scott LJ. Ceftolozane/tazobactam: a review in complicated intra-abdominal and urinary tract infections. Drugs. 2016;76:231–42.
21. Shirley M. Ceftazidime-avibactam: a review in the treatment of serious gram-negative bacterial infections. Drugs. 2018;78:675–92.
22. Croom KF, Goa KL. Levofloxacin: a review of its use in the treatment of bacterial infections in the United States. Drugs. 2003;63:2769–802.
23. Bader MS, Loeb M, Brooks AA. An update on the management of urinary tract infections in the era of antimicrobial resistance. Postgrad Med. 2017;129(2):242–58. https://doi.org/10.1080/00325481.2017.1246055.
24. Peterson LR. A review of tigecycline—the first glycylcycline. Int J Antimicrob Agents. 2008;32(Suppl 4):S215–22. https://doi.org/10.1016/s0924-8579(09)70005-6.
25. El-Sayed Ahmed MAE, Zhong LL, Shen C, Yang Y, Doi Y, Tian GB. Colistin and its role in the Era of antibiotic resistance: an extended review (2000–2019). Emerg Microbes Infect. 2020;9(1):868–85. https://doi.org/10.1080/22221751.2020.1754133.
26. Zhanel GG, Cheung D, Adam H, et al. Review of eravacycline, a novel fluorocycline antibacterial agent. Drugs. 2016;76(5):567–88. https://doi.org/10.1007/s40265-016-0545-8.
27. Chuang YC, Lin HY, Chen PY, Lin CY, Wang JT, Chang SC. Daptomycin versus linezolid for the treatment of vancomycin-resistant enterococcal bacteraemia: implications of daptomycin dose. Clin Microbiol Infect. 2016;22(10):890.e1–7. https://doi.org/10.1016/j.cmi.2016.07.018.
28. Skarzynski T, Mistry A, Wonacott A, Hutchinson SE, Kelly VA, Duncan K. Structure of UDP-N-acetylglucosamine enolpyruvyl transferase, an enzyme essential for the synthesis of bacterial peptidoglycan, complexed with substrate UDP-N-acetylglucosamine and the drug fosfomycin. Structure. 1996;4(12):1465–74. https://doi.org/10.1016/s0969-2126(96)00153-0.
29. Castañeda-García A, Blázquez J, Rodríguez-Rojas A. Molecular mechanisms and clinical impact of acquired and intrinsic fosfomycin resistance. Antibiotics (Basel). 2013;2(2):217–36. https://doi.org/10.3390/antibiotics2020217.
30. Trinh TD, Smith JR, Rybak MJ. Parenteral Fosfomycin for the treatment of multidrug resistant bacterial infections: the rise of the epoxide. Pharmacotherapy. 2019;39(11):1077–94. https://doi.org/10.1002/phar.2326.
31. Wingler MJ, Patel NR, King ST, Wagner JL, Barber KE, Stover KR. Linezolid for the treatment of urinary tract infections caused by vancomycin-resistant enterococci. Pharmacy (Basel). 2021;9(4):175. https://doi.org/10.3390/pharmacy9040175.
32. Huttner A, Verhaegh EM, Harbarth S, Muller AE, Theuretzbacher U, Mouton JW. Nitrofurantoin revisited: a systematic review and meta-analysis of controlled trials. J Antimicrob Chemother. 2015;70(9):2456–64. https://doi.org/10.1093/jac/dkv147.
33. Raz R, Chazan B, Kennes Y, et al. Empiric use of trimethoprim-sulfamethoxazole (TMP-SMX) in the treatment of women with uncomplicated urinary tract infections, in a geographical area with a high prevalence of TMP-SMX–resistant uropathogens. Clin Infect Dis. 2002;34(9):1165–9. https://doi.org/10.1086/339812.
34. Huttner A, Kowalczyk A, Turjeman A, et al. Effect of 5-day nitrofurantoin vs single-dose fosfomycin on clinical resolution of uncomplicated lower urinary tract infection in women: a randomized clinical trial. JAMA. 2018;319(17):1781–9. https://doi.org/10.1001/jama.2018.3627.
35. Shi HJ, Wee JH, Eom JS. Challenges to early discharge of patients with upper urinary tract infections by ESBL producers: TMP/SMX as a step-down therapy for shorter hospitalization and lower costs. Infect Drug Resist. 2021;14:3589–97. https://doi.org/10.2147/idr.s321888.
36. Zykov IN, Sundsfjord A, Småbrekke L, Samuelsen Ø. The antimicrobial activity of mecillinam, nitrofurantoin, temocillin and fosfomycin and comparative analysis of resistance patterns in a nationwide collection of ESBL-producing Escherichia coli in Norway 2010-2011. Infect Dis (Lond). 2016;48(2):99–107. https://doi.org/10.3109/23744235.2015.1087648.
37. Pontefract BA, Rovelsky SA, Madaras-Kelly KJ. Linezolid to treat urinary tract infections caused by vancomycin-resistant Enterococcus. SAGE Open Med. 2020;8:2050312120970743. https://doi.org/10.1177/2050312120970743.

38. Heintz BH, Halilovic J, Christensen CL. Vancomycin-resistant enterococcal urinary tract infections. Pharmacotherapy. 2010;30(11):1136–49. https://doi.org/10.1592/phco.30.11.1136.
39. Raad II, Hanna HA, Boktour M, et al. Vancomycin-resistant Enterococcus faecium: catheter colonization, esp gene, and decreased susceptibility to antibiotics in biofilm. Antimicrob Agents Chemother. 2005;49(12):5046–50. https://doi.org/10.1128/aac.49.12.5046-5050.2005.
40. Giancola SE, Mahoney MV, Hogan MD, Raux BR, McCoy C, Hirsch EB. Assessment of Fosfomycin for complicated or multidrug-resistant urinary tract infections: patient characteristics and outcomes. Chemotherapy. 2017;62(2):100–4. https://doi.org/10.1159/000449422.
41. Tamma PD, Aitken SL, Bonomo RA, Mathers AJ, van Duin D, Clancy CJ. Infectious Diseases Society of America 2022 Guidance on the Treatment of Extended-Spectrum β-lactamase Producing Enterobacterales (ESBL-E), Carbapenem-Resistant Enterobacterales (CRE), and Pseudomonas aeruginosa with Difficult-to-Treat Resistance (DTR-P. aeruginosa). Clin Infect Dis. 2022;75(2):187–212. https://doi.org/10.1093/cid/ciac268.
42. Kadri SS, Adjemian J, Lai YL, et al. Difficult-to-treat resistance in gram-negative bacteremia at 173 US hospitals: retrospective cohort analysis of prevalence, predictors, and outcome of resistance to all first-line agents. Clin Infect Dis. 2018;67(12):1803–14. https://doi.org/10.1093/cid/ciy378.
43. Harris PNA, Tambyah PA, Lye DC, et al. Effect of piperacillin-tazobactam vs meropenem on 30-day mortality for patients with E coli or Klebsiella pneumoniae bloodstream infection and ceftriaxone resistance: a randomized clinical trial. JAMA. 2018;320(10):984–94. https://doi.org/10.1001/jama.2018.12163.
44. Guet-Revillet H, Tomini E, Emirian A, et al. Piperacillin/tazobactam as an alternative antibiotic therapy to carbapenems in the treatment of urinary tract infections due to extended-spectrum β-lactamase-producing Enterobacteriaceae: an in silico pharmacokinetic study. Int J Antimicrob Agents. 2017;49(1):62–6. https://doi.org/10.1016/j.ijantimicag.2016.09.027.
45. Sternbach N, Leibovici Weissman Y, Avni T, Yahav D. Efficacy and safety of ceftazidime/avibactam: a systematic review and meta-analysis. J Antimicrob Chemother. 2018;73(8):2021–9. https://doi.org/10.1093/jac/dky124.
46. Cho SY, Choi SM, Park SH, Lee DG, Choi JH, Yoo JH. Amikacin therapy for urinary tract infections caused by extended-spectrum β-lactamase-producing Escherichia coli. Korean J Intern Med. 2016;31(1):156–61. https://doi.org/10.3904/kjim.2016.31.1.156.
47. Sievert DM, Ricks P, Edwards JR, et al. Antimicrobial-resistant pathogens associated with healthcare-associated infections: summary of data reported to the National Healthcare Safety Network at the Centers for Disease Control and Prevention, 2009–2010. Infect Control Hosp Epidemiol. 2013;34(1):1–14. https://doi.org/10.1086/668770.
48. Arias CA, Contreras GA, Murray BE. Management of multidrug-resistant enterococcal infections. Clin Microbiol Infect. 2010;16(6):555–62. https://doi.org/10.1111/j.1469-0691.2010.03214.x.
49. Cetinkaya Y, Falk P, Mayhall CG. Vancomycin-resistant enterococci. Clin Microbiol Rev. 2000;13(4):686–707. https://doi.org/10.1128/cmr.13.4.686.
50. Balli EP, Venetis CA, Miyakis S. Systematic review and meta-analysis of linezolid versus daptomycin for treatment of vancomycin-resistant enterococcal bacteremia. Antimicrob Agents Chemother. 2014;58(2):734–9. https://doi.org/10.1128/aac.01289-13.
51. Ramaswamy DP, Amodio-Groton M, Scholand SJ. Use of daptomycin in the treatment of vancomycin-resistant enterococcal urinary tract infections: a short case series. BMC Urol. 2013;13:33. https://doi.org/10.1186/1471-2490-13-33.
52. Jiménez-Guerra G, Heras-Cañas V, Gutiérrez-Soto M, et al. Urinary tract infection by Acinetobacter baumannii and Pseudomonas aeruginosa: evolution of antimicrobial resistance and therapeutic alternatives. J Med Microbiol. 2018;67(6):790–7. https://doi.org/10.1099/jmm.0.000742.
53. Tsuji BT, Pogue JM, Zavascki AP, et al. International Consensus Guidelines for the Optimal Use of the Polymyxins: Endorsed by the American College of Clinical Pharmacy (ACCP), European Society of Clinical Microbiology and Infectious Diseases (ESCMID), Infectious Diseases Society of America (IDSA), International Society for Anti-infective Pharmacology

(ISAP), Society of Critical Care Medicine (SCCM), and Society of Infectious Diseases Pharmacists (SIDP). Pharmacotherapy. 2019;39(1):10–39. https://doi.org/10.1002/phar.2209.
54. Wagenlehner FME, Cloutier DJ, Komirenko AS, et al. Once-daily plazomicin for complicated urinary tract infections. N Engl J Med. 2019;380(8):729–40. https://doi.org/10.1056/NEJMoa1801467.
55. Pankey GA. Tigecycline. J Antimicrob Chemother. 2005;56(3):470–80. https://doi.org/10.1093/jac/dki248.
56. Bassetti M, Giacobbe DR, Giamarellou H, et al. Management of KPC-producing Klebsiella pneumoniae infections. Clin Microbiol Infect. 2018;24(2):133–44. https://doi.org/10.1016/j.cmi.2017.08.030.
57. Solomkin J, Hershberger E, Miller B, et al. Ceftolozane/tazobactam plus metronidazole for complicated intra-abdominal infections in an era of multidrug resistance: results from a randomized, double-blind, phase 3 trial (ASPECT-cIAI). Clin Infect Dis. 2015;60(10):1462–71. https://doi.org/10.1093/cid/civ097.
58. Gaibani P, Campoli C, Lewis RE, et al. In vivo evolution of resistant subpopulations of KPC-producing Klebsiella pneumoniae during ceftazidime/avibactam treatment. J Antimicrob Chemother. 2018;73(6):1525–9. https://doi.org/10.1093/jac/dky082.
59. Bassetti M, Peghin M, Vena A, Giacobbe DR. Treatment of infections due to MDR gram-negative bacteria. Front Med (Lausanne). 2019;6:74. https://doi.org/10.3389/fmed.2019.00074.
60. Wright H, Bonomo RA, Paterson DL. New agents for the treatment of infections with gram-negative bacteria: restoring the miracle or false dawn? Clin Microbiol Infect. 2017;23(10):704–12. https://doi.org/10.1016/j.cmi.2017.09.001.
61. Leitner L, Ujmajuridze A, Chanishvili N, et al. Intravesical bacteriophages for treating urinary tract infections in patients undergoing transurethral resection of the prostate: a randomised, placebo-controlled, double-blind clinical trial. (1474–4457 (Electronic)).
62. McConnell MJ. Where are we with monoclonal antibodies for multidrug-resistant infections? Drug Discov Today. 2019;24(5):1132–8. https://doi.org/10.1016/j.drudis.2019.03.002.
63. Lawandi A, Yek C, Kadri SS. IDSA guidance and ESCMID guidelines: complementary approaches toward a care standard for MDR gram-negative infections. Clin Microbiol Infect. 2022;28(4):465–9.

Antibiotic Treatment of Urogenital Tuberculosis

14

Ekaterina Kulchavenya and Truls E. Bjerklund Johansen

Abbreviations

BCG	Bacillus Calmette-Guérin
FGTB	Female genital tuberculosis
HIV	Human immunodeficiency virus
IVU	Intravenous urography
KTB	Kidney tuberculosis
MDR	Multidrug-resistant
MGTB	Male genital tuberculosis
Mtb	Mycobacterium tuberculosis
TB	Tuberculosis
UGTB	Urogenital tuberculosis
WHO	World Health Organization

E. Kulchavenya (✉)
Novosibirsk Research TB Institute, Novosibirsk, Russian Federation

Novosibirsk State Medical University, Novosibirsk, Russian Federation

T. E. Bjerklund Johansen
Urology Department, Oslo University Hospital, Oslo and Institute of Clinical Medicine, University of Oslo, Oslo, Norway

Institute of Clinical Medicine, University of Aarhus, Aarhus, Denmark
e-mail: tebj@uio.no

T. E. Bjerklund Johansen, T. Cai (eds.), *Guide to Antibiotics in Urology*,
https://doi.org/10.1007/978-3-319-92366-6_14

14.1 Introduction

Tuberculosis (TB) is a communicable disease that is a major cause of ill health. It is one of the top 10 causes of death worldwide and the leading cause of death from a single infectious agent, ranking above HIV/AIDS. This was at least the case before the COVID-19 pandemic started in March 2020. In 2019, 10 million people developed TB and 1.4 million died. The World Health Organization (WHO) emphasized that the COVID-19 pandemic threatens to reverse recent progress in reducing the global burden of TB disease. The global number of TB deaths could increase by around 0.2–0.4 million in 2020 if health services are disrupted and the number of people who are treated for TB falls by 25–50% over a period of 3 months [1].

TB is caused by the bacillus *Mycobacterium tuberculosis* (Mtb). The disease typically affects the lungs (pulmonary TB) but can also affect other sites (extrapulmonary TB). TB can affect anyone anywhere, but most people who develop the disease (about 90%) are adults. Of those who fell sick with TB in 2019, 87% were in one of 30 high TB burden countries [1].

In some regions, urogenital tuberculosis (UGTB) is the second most common—and in other regions, third most common form of TB—but a large proportion of patients is underdiagnosed and hence untreated. According to the WHO, only 38% of the estimated number of people with MDR/RR-TB were enrolled in treatment programs in 2019 [2].

UGTB includes urinary tract TB and genital TB and is associated with pulmonary or other localizations of TB in 40–65% of cases. Male genital tuberculosis (MGTB) is associated with pulmonary or renal TB in 50% of cases, but isolated forms also occur. Usually, the epididymis and prostate are involved together [3, 4]. If there is no other evidence of Mtb, UGTB may be diagnosed based on skin test, histological picture, caverns revealed by urography, and sterile pyuria.

Bacillus Calmette-Guérin (BCG), which is an attenuated *M. bovis*, is widely used for the treatment of superficial bladder cancer. In some cases, BCG treatment may be complicated by iatrogenic BCG-induced UGTB, mainly localized in the bladder or prostate, but BCG sepsis is also seen in rare cases [5–8]. Diagnosis of BCG-induced bladder TB can be made according to clinical features, such as significant dysuria and decreased bladder volume, or by histology, not by microbiology.

Before anti-TB drugs were available, UGTB was an extremely frequent disease in Russia, and every fifth patient in urology wards had kidney TB (KTB). More than one third of all pyonephrosis cases were caused by TB [9]. The anti-TB therapy for UGTB has some special features.

14.2 Materials and Methods

The present chapter is based on a narrative review of literature with keywords "urogenital tuberculosis," "prostate tuberculosis," "kidney tuberculosis," and "treatment of tuberculosis." Data were obtained from articles published in Russian and in English from journals indexed in PubMed, Google scholar, and eLibrary.

14.3 Classification

UGTB includes many forms of TB with different clinical characteristics. Each form requires tailored antibiotic therapy and management. Therefore, correct clinical classification based on diagnosis and stage is mandatory [10]. UGTB can be subclassified into kidney, urinary tract, and genital tuberculosis. Female genital tuberculosis (FGTB) is not included in this chapter.

14.3.1 Kidney Tuberculosis

There are four stages to be considered for kidney tuberculosis [11]:

Stage 1: TB of kidney parenchyma (nondestructive form, KTB-1).
Stage 2: TB papillitis (small-destructive form, KTB-2).
Stage 3: Cavernous kidney TB (destructive form, KTB-3).
Stage 4: Polycavernous kidney TB (widespread-destructive form, KTB-4).

Complications of kidney TB are chronic renal failure, fistula, and high blood pressure.

14.3.2 Urinary Tract Tuberculosis

Urinary tract TB is regarded a specific complication of KTB and is thus always secondary to KTB. Urinary tract TB first appears as an edema, and the next stages are infiltration, ulceration, and fibrosis.

TB of ureter usually develops in the lower third, but multiple lesions are possible, too. Incorrect therapy may lead to the development of ureteral stricture, which may result in loss of the kidney, even if TB is finally cured.

TB of the bladder presents with frequency, then urgency, and hematuria. BCG-induced bladder TB is a special form of iatrogenic bladder TB, which develops as a complication of BCG therapy for bladder cancer. TB of the bladder is further divided into four stages [12]:

Stage 1: Tubercle-infiltrative.
Stage 2: Erosive-ulcerous.
Stage 3: Spastic cystitis, which in fact means overactive bladder.
Stage 4: Contracted bladder up to full obliteration.

The first two stages should be treated by standard anti-TB drugs. The third stage should be treated with standard anti-TB drugs and trospium chloride, and the fourth stage needs cystectomy and urinary diversion.

TB of the urethra is nowadays not a frequent complication. It is usually diagnosed in the stage of a stricture.

14.3.3 Male Genital Tuberculosis (MGTB)

MGTB is subdivided into three categories [10]

Category 1: TB epididymitis, which may be uni- or bilateral. Bilateral TB epididymitis is always secondary to prostate TB. Isolated TB epididymitis was found in 22% as accidental surgical finding.
Category 2: TB of the testis is always secondary to infection of the epididymis. Every third patient has bilateral lesions. In 62% of patients with epididymo-orchitis, KTB is diagnosed as well. In about 12%, the disease is complicated by fistulas [10, 13].
Category 3: TB of the prostate is an underdiagnosed disease. Three quarters of men, who died from any form of TB, had prostate TB, mostly overlooked before death [14].

Prostate TB is clinically important for several reasons. It may be a sexually transmitted disease. Up to 50% of prostate TB patients have Mtb in their ejaculate if they are comorbid with hepatitis and syphilis [15], and it leads to infertility. It may cause chronic pelvic pain like any other type of prostatitis and significantly reduce the quality of life [16]. Finally, it decreases sexual function, which reduces the quality of life even more [13]. In 79% of Russian cases, prostate TB was accompanied by KTB and in 31% by TB epididymo-orchitis. Isolated prostate TB was diagnosed in only 5% [10].

TB of seminal vesicles occurs secondary to prostate TB and leads to infertility. As drainage of caseous ejaculate is difficult, TB of seminal vesicles often leads to calcifications [17]. TB of the penis is rare but can occur after sexual intercourse with infected females [18, 19] or via direct contamination through a penile wound during ritual circumcision. Penile lesions present as ulcers on the glans or penile skin. Currently, it is mainly seen as a complication of BCG therapy [20–22]. Complications of MGTB are strictures, fistula, infertility, and sexual dysfunction.

14.4 Treatment

14.4.1 Standard Antibiotic Regimens

The main principles of anti-TB chemotherapy are continuity, controllability, and follow-up of the treatment. Neglect of these principles leads to the development of drug-resistant Mtb and relapse of TB. Treatment of TB requires a combination of antimicrobials to ensure efficacy and reduce the likelihood of acquiring resistance and of treatment failure [23]. About 85% of people who develop TB disease can be successfully treated with a 6-month drug regimen. Treatment has the additional benefit of curtailing onward transmission of infection. Since 2000, TB treatment has averted more than 60 million deaths, although with access still falling short of universal health coverage, many millions have also missed out on diagnosis and care

[1]. If Mtb is susceptible, the classic oral standard quadruple regimen of isoniazid, rifampicin, pyrazinamide, and ethambutol may be effective in a rate of >90% for pulmonary TB patients [23].

Drug-resistant tuberculosis is a now a major threat to the global health security. Multidrug-resistant tuberculosis (MDR-TB) is defined as TB that is resistant, at least, to isoniazid and rifampicin. The WHO estimates that about half a million cases of multidrug or rifampicin resistant (MDR/RR-TB) are estimated to occur each year [2]. WHO-recommended treatments can only cure 50% of multidrug-resistant (MDR) tuberculosis and 30% of patients with extensively drug-resistant tuberculosis [24].

Treatment of UGTB differs from the therapy of pulmonary TB. A majority of UGTB can be managed and treated successfully with individualized therapy, which may include surgery and rehabilitation. Streptomycin and kanamycin are not recommended for UGTB because of nephrotoxicity. Among fluoroquinolones, only levofloxacin is suitable for UGTB therapy. Moxifloxacin and sparfloxacin are respiratory fluoroquinolones, so they are good for pulmonary TB but not optimal for UGTB. Para-aminosalicylic acid (PAS) is highly recommended for UGTB with involvement of pelvic organs; amoxicillin/clavulanate should be prescribed together with meropenem or imipenem, as they potentiate the anti-TB effect. Cycloserine is highly recommended, if the patient also has comorbidity with nonspecific UTI. Patients with comorbidity of HIV who are receiving anti-retrovirus therapy should be treated with rifabutin instead of rifampicin. Rifampicin and streptomycin are contraindicated for patients after organ transplantation.

All anti-TB drugs may be divided into two categories: first-line bacteriocidic drugs, for per os prescribing, injectable anti-TB drugs, and peroral second line bacteriostatic anti-TB drugs. Fluoroquinolones (ciprofloxacin (Cfx), ofloxacin (Ofx), levofloxacin (Lfx), moxifloxacin (Mfx), and gatifloxacin (Gfx)) are separated as a special class. Also, there are anti-TB drugs with unknown mechanisms of action (not recommended by WHO for ordinary use to treat MDR TB) [25]. First-line anti-TB drugs used perorally combine isoniazid (INH), rifamycin (RIF), ethambutol (EMB), and pyrazinamide (PZA). Injectable antituberculosis drugs include streptomycin (S), kanamycin (Km), amikacin (Am), capreomycin (Cm), and viomycin (Vi). The group of second-line peroral bacteriostatic anti-TB drugs combines ethionamide (Eto), protionamide (Pro), cycloserine (Cs), terizidone (Trd), *para*-aminosalicylic acid (PAS), and thioacetazone (Th). Drugs with unknown mechanisms of action are clofazimine (Cfz), amoxycillin/clavulanate (Amx/Clv), clarithromycin (Ctr), and linezolid (Lzd). In any case, no drug from any group could be used as monotherapy. Bactericidal anti-TB drugs are preferable.

Anti-TB drugs may be administered per os and parenterally; the dose is adjusted according to the weight of the patient (see Table 14.1).

Without treatment, two-thirds of affected patients will die, and the remaining one-third is likely to suffer from chronic sequelae. New oral TB drugs that are more active and less toxic are desperately needed to build new regimens that can be disseminated rapidly and successfully to the many people affected by drug-sensitive as well as drug-resistant MDR-TB in low-resource settings [23,

Table 14.1 Recommended daily dosage of anti-TB drugs for adults (mg) [26]

Drug	Patient's weight		
	33–50 kg	51–70 kg	More than 70 kg (max.)
Isoniazid	300	300–600	600
Rifampicin	450	450–600	600
Pyrazinamide	1000–1500	1500–2000	2500
Amikacin	500–750	1000	1000
Ethambutol	800–1200	1200–1600	1600–2000
Levofloxacin	500	500–750	750–1000
Prothionamide/ etionamide	500	750	750–1000
Capreomycin	500–750	750–1000	1000
PAS	3000–5000	5000–8000	8000–12,000
Cycloserine	500	500–750	750–100
Delamanid	100 mg twice daily taken with food, for 6 months		
Bedaquiline	400 mg once daily for the first 2 weeks and is then reduced to 200 mg three times weekly for the remaining 22 weeks		
Linezolid	600 mg once daily orally or intravenously		

27–31]. In particular, we need drugs that can reduce the duration treatment [24]. Current targets are less than 6 months for drug-sensitive tuberculosis and less than 12 months for drug-resistant disease. Shorter regimens will improve patient adherence, reduce cumulative drug toxicities, and reduce clinics' workloads [24].

14.4.2 New Drug Treatment Options

Below, we provide a brief characteristic of new and newly introduced old drugs for the treatment of UGTB.

1. *Nitroimidazoles*. This group consists of novel anti-TB agents and may be used both for MDR-TB and extensively drug-resistant TB (XDR-TB). XDR-TB is defined as resistance to any fluoroquinolone and to at least one of three second-line injectable drugs (capreomycin, kanamycin, and amikacin), in addition to multidrug resistance. Nitroimidazoles act through inhibition of cell wall synthesis and oxidation and include pretomanid and delamanid. Pretomanid is active against both replicating Mtb and persisters [32], but it is currently not licensed. Delamanid is, however, approved by the European Medicines Agency for the treatment of MDR-TB as part of an appropriate combination of anti-TB drugs—but only in cases where the currently approved regimen cannot be used as a result of drug resistance or intolerability.
2. *Diarylquinolines*. Bedaquiline is effective against Mtb, both during active replication and in the dormant phase, and has high activity against both MDR- and XDR-TB strains [23, 33]. It is the first new drug to be approved by the FDA for the

treatment of TB in since more than 40 years [23]. Bedaquiline should only be used as part of a regimen consisting of pyrazinamide and four second-line medications. However, such a regimen cannot be used if there is a documented resistance to fluoroquinolones in the presence of multidrug resistance [34]. The WHO does not currently recommend coadministration of bedaquiline and delamanid, because of the possible drug–drug interactions and potential cardiotoxicity [35, 36].

3. *Oxazolidinones* is a class of antibiotics that inhibits protein synthesis. Linezolid is a first-generation oxazolidinone and has excellent oral bioavailability. Initially, this class were approved for the treatment of drug-resistant Gram-positive infections. Unfortunately, their use has been complicated with severe neurological and hematological toxicity [37, 38].

Some medications are used as additional treatment such as tocopherol, Canephron, and trospium chloride for bladder TB stage 3 and Selzink for prostate TB [10]. Evaluation of the outcome of drug treatment of UGTB is difficult for several reasons. Identification of Mtb is not always possible before treatment, and healing of kidney and prostate caverns is not possible at all. A special scale has therefore been suggested for the evaluation of the outcome of drug treatment [39].

14.4.3 Surgical Treatment of UGTB

UGTB like any other UTI should be cured conservatively if diagnosed in time. However, surgery still has a role in advanced stages such as KTB stages 3–4 and bladder TB stage 4 as well as for correction of complications. The spectrum of surgical interventions for UGTB is shown in Table 14.2.

Anti-TB therapy should always be continued until the result of the histological investigation of the removed tissue is available [4, 40, 41].

Table 14.2 Surgical treatment for UGTB

Indication	Surgery
KTB-3, resistant to standard therapy (notably cavern with pyogenic layer remains, Mtb in urine, pyuria) for 2–4 months	Cavernostomy (partial nephrectomy), optimal—Laparoscopically
KTB-4	Nephrectomy, optimal—Laparoscopically
Bladder TB-4	Cystectomy (in male patients—Cystoprostatectomy) with urine diversion or bladder replacement
TB of testis with torpid course and poor effect of conservative treatment for 1–2 months	Orchidectomy
Stricture of ureter, urethra	Standard plastic operation
Fluctuation, abscess	Incision of abscess and drainage

14.5 BCG-Induced UGTB

Intravesical administration of bacillus Calmette-Guerin (BCG) is commonly used as treatment of non-muscle invasive bladder cancer and carcinoma in situ. BCG provides a significantly better prophylaxis of tumor recurrence than TUR alone, and superiority of BCG over mitomycin C for prevention of tumor recurrences has been shown as well. Instillation of BCG causes a specific inflammation of the bladder mucosa that kills cancer cells—but it should be a controlled transient and local inflammation. A loss of local control results in the spread of infection. Systemic dissemination of bacilli may lead to the development of generalized BCG-induced TB, when all organs, including meninges, are involved in TB infection. Among urogenital complications of BCG therapy, bladder TB is the most common, while TB epididymo-orchitis and TB of penis are rare.

Diagnostic criteria for BCG-induced bladder TB are dysuria and pyuria within 3 weeks after the instillation of BCG and decreasing of the bladder volume. Microbiology is not helpful. Pathohistological confirmation is crucial, but in about 50%, only fibrosis and inflammation may be found in the biopsies. Involvement of the detrusor and development of a shrunk bladder represent the clinical background for the symptoms of iatrogenic BCG-induced bladder TB.

BCG-induced bladder TB should be treated with rifampicin 0.6 and isoniazid 0.6 for 2 months. If there is also growth of a nonspecific microflora in urine, levofloxacin 0.5 daily should also be prescribed. Anti-TB therapy can be stopped after 8 weeks if patients experience symptom relief—without dysuria and urinalysis is normal. If the dynamic is good after 8 weeks but the patient has not recovered completely, anti-TB therapy should be continued for another 2 months. If results are poor after 8 weeks of treatment with rifampicin and isoniazid and bladder volume is 100 ml or less, cystectomy (in male patients—cystoprostatectomy) and urine diversion are indicated. After, anti-TB therapy with rifampicin, isoniazid, and levofloxacin should be continued for at least 2 months after surgery until full recovery with normal urinalysis and sufficient bladder volume. Algorithm of the management of BCG-induced UGTB patient [42] is shown on Fig. 14.1.

To prevent the most severe complications, BCG shouldn't be installed in case of concurrent cystitis. BCG instillation is contraindicated if a patient has dysuria and leukocyturia, and treatment with nonsteroid anti-inflammatory drugs and nitrofurantoin or fosfomycin for 3–5 days should be prescribed. BCG therapy should be paused until the symptoms of cystitis have improved. The scheduled BCG regimen shouldn't be resumed after recovering from BCG-induced TB.

Patients with BCG-induced orchiepididymitis should be treated with rifampicin 0.6 + isoniazid 0.6 + levofloxacin 0.5 daily for 2 months. In case of abscess formation, orchiectomy is indicated. Patients with symptomatic BCG-induced prostatitis should be treated with rifampicin 0.6 + isoniazid 0.6 + levofloxacin 0.5 daily for 4–6 months until symptom relief. Patients should be followed up for 2 years with control examination every 6 months. The frequency of BCG-induced granulomatous prostatitis varies from 3% to 75%. However, most patients are asymptomatic and only rarely (0.9–1.3%) have clinical complaints, findings on digital rectal

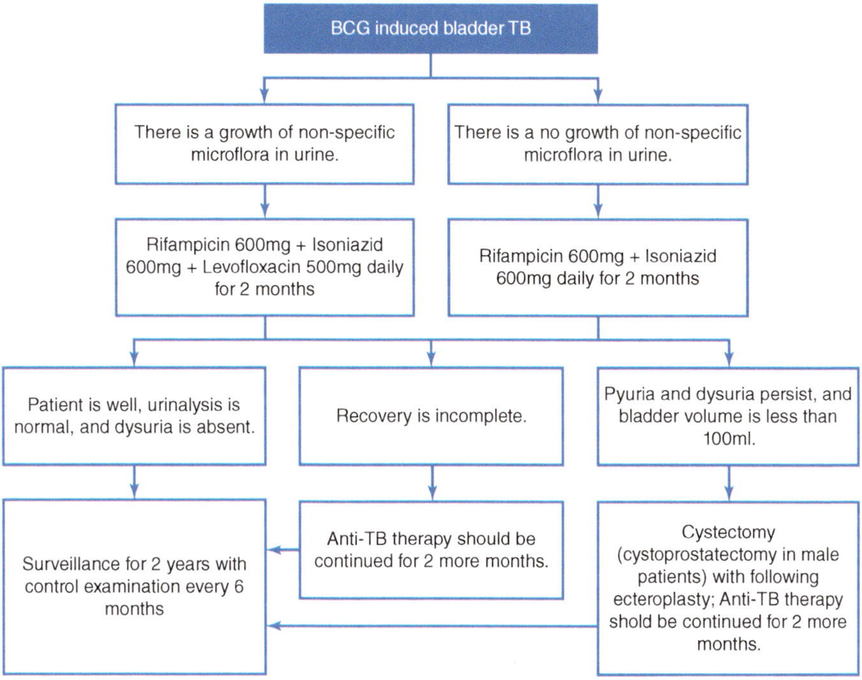

Fig. 14.1 Algorithm of the management of BCG-induced UGTB patient [42]

palpation like slight induration of the prostate, or elevated PSA level [43]. Mycobacterial prostatitis does not require anti-TB therapy, but rather, close monitoring is recommended [44, 45].

Patients with UGTB should be followed up every 6 months for 1–3 years to control if symptoms persist or recur after completion of the therapy. Control intervals will depend on the type and stage of the disease. To prevent relapse, a repeated short-course (for 2 months) therapy with isoniazid and rifampicin is recommended for patients with complicated UGTB. In MDR-UGTB, the preventive therapy is prescribed according to the sensitivity of Mtb. Specific prophylaxis against UGTB is currently not available.

14.6 Conclusions

UGTB is difficult for suspicion, diagnosis, and therapy. The index of suspicion on IGTB is low, so the correct diagnosis is delayed. It leads to the development of complications, which cannot be cured by conservative therapy and require a surgery. Even if we have a case of early diagnosed UGTB, nonoptimal therapy may result in over-fibrosis, scaring, and strictures of urinary tract, which, again, are an indication for surgery. Nevertheless, we have enough anti-TB drugs to cure UGTB.

References

1. Global tuberculosis report 2020. https://apps.who.int/iris/bitstream/handle/10665/336069/9789240013131-eng.pdf\
2. WHO consolidated guidelines on tuberculosis 2020. Module 4: treatment. https://www.who.int/publications/i/item/9789240007048
3. Kulchavenya E, Naber K, Bjerklund Johansen TE. Urogenital tuberculosis: classification, diagnosis, and treatment. Europ Urol Suppl. 2016;15(4):112–21.
4. Kulchavenya E, Kholtobin D, Shevchenko S. Challenges in urogenital tuberculosis. World J Urol. 2020;38(1):89–94. https://doi.org/10.1007/s00345-019-02767-x.
5. Bhat S, Srinivasa Y, Paul F. Asymptomatic renal BCG granulomatosis: an unusual complication of intravesical BCG therapy for carcinoma urinary bladder. Indian J Urol. 2015;31(3):259–61. https://doi.org/10.4103/0970-1591.156921.
6. Al-Qaoud T, Brimo F, Aprikian AG, Andonian S. BCG-related renal granulomas managed conservatively: a case series. Can Urol Assoc J. 2015;9(3–4):E200–3. https://doi.org/10.5489/cuaj.2664.
7. Pommier JD, Ben Lasfar N, Van Grunderbeeck N, et al. Complications following intravesical bacillus Calmette-Guerin treatment for bladder cancer: a case series of 22 patients. Infect Dis (Lond). 2015;47(10):729–35. https://doi.org/10.3109/23744235.2015.1055794. Epub 2015 Jun 16
8. Pérez-Jacoiste Asín MA, Fernández-Ruiz M, López-Medrano F, et al. Bacillus Calmette-Guérin (BCG) infection following intravesical BCG administration as adjunctive therapy for bladder cancer: incidence, risk factors, and outcome in a single-institution series and review of the literature. Medicine (Baltimore). 2014;93(17):236–54. https://doi.org/10.1097/MD.0000000000000119.
9. Marion G. Traite d'Urologie. Paris: Masson; 1940.
10. Kulchavenya E. Urogenital tuberculosis: epidemiology, diagnosis, therapy. Cham/Heidelberg/New York/Dordrecht/London: Springer; 2014. p. 137. ISBN 978-2-319-04836-9. https://doi.org/10.1007/978-3-319-04837-6.
11. Kulchavenya E. Urogenital tuberculosis: definition and classification. Ther Adv Infect Dis. 2015;2(5–6):117–22.
12. Kulchavenya E, Brizhatyuk E. Bladder tuberculosis: diagnosis and treatment. Urologiia. 2006;3:61–5. [Russian]
13. Kulchavenya E, Kim CS, Bulanova O, Zhukova I. Male genital tuberculosis: epidemiology and diagnostic. World J Urol. 2012;30(1):15–21. Epub 2011 May21. Review
14. Kamyshan IS. Guideline on urogenital tuberculosis. Kuev, 2003:363–424. [Russian].
15. Aphonin AB, Perezmanas EO, Toporkova EE, Khodakovsky EP. Tuberculous infection as sexually transmitted infection. Vestnik Poslediplomnogo Obrazovaniya. 2006;3-4:69–71. [Russian]
16. Kumar S, Kashyapi BD, Bapat SS. A rare presentation of tuberculous prostatic abscess in young patient. Int J Surg Case Rep. 2015;10:80–2. https://doi.org/10.1016/j.ijscr.2015.03.028.
17. Stasinou T, Bourdoumis A, Owegie P, Kachrilas S, Buchholz N, Masood J. Calcification of the vas deferens and seminal vesicles: a review. Can J Urol. 2015;22(1):7594–8.
18. Elkhachine Y, Sinaa M, Sakkah A, Hallab I, Ouarssani A, Jakar A, Elbenaye J. Tuberculose du gland [tuberculosis of the glans penis]. Ann Dermatol Venereol. 2020;147(10):672–5. French. https://doi.org/10.1016/j.annder.2020.06.021.
19. Banerji JS. Primary tuberculosis of the glans penis in an immunocompetent male. Lancet Infect Dis. 2020;20(4):509. https://doi.org/10.1016/S1473-3099(19)30753-4.
20. Sinha RK, Mukherjee S, Kamal MR, Karmakar D. Tuberculosis of the glans penis healing with meatal stenosis. BMJ Case Rep. 2014;2014. pii: bcr2013202155 https://doi.org/10.1136/bcr-2013-202155.
21. Linden-Castro E, Pelayo-Nieto M, Alias-Melgar A. Penile tuberculosis after intravesical bacille Calmette-Guérin immunotherapy. Urology. 2014;84(2):e3. https://doi.org/10.1016/j.urology.2014.04.037. Epub 2014 Jun 21

22. Sharma VK, Sethy PK, Dogra PN, et al. Primary tuberculosis of glans penis after intravesical Bacillus Calmette Guerin immunotherapy. Indian J Dermatol Venereol Leprol. 2011;77(1):47–50.
23. Krutikov M, Bruchfeld J, Migliori GB, et al. New and repurposed drugs. In: Migliori GB, Bothamley G, Duarte R, et al., editors. Tuberculosis (ERS monograph). Sheffield: European Respiratory Society; 2018. p. 179–204. https://doi.org/10.1183/2312508X.10021517].
24. Wallis RS, Maeurer M, Mwaba P, Chakaya J, Rustomjee R, Migliori GB, Marais B, Schito M, Churchyard G, Swaminathan S, Hoelscher M, Zumla A. Tuberculosis--advances in development of new drugs, treatment regimens, host-directed therapies, and biomarkers. Lancet Infect Dis 2016;16(4):e34–e46. doi: https://doi.org/10.1016/S1473-3099(16)00070-0.
25. Kayukova LA, Berikova EA. Modern anti-tuberculosis drugs and their classification. Part I: first-line drugs. Pharm Chem J. 2020;54:555–63. https://doi.org/10.1007/s11094-020-02239-2.
26. WHO Library Cataloguing-in-Publication Data: Treatment of tuberculosis: guidelines—4th ed. https://apps.who.int/iris/bitstream/handle/10665/44165/9789241547833_eng.pdf?sequence=1
27. DR-TB STAT. Country updates. http://drtb-stat.org/country-updates/. Accessed 22 Dec 2020.
28. WHO. Antibacterial agents in clinical development: an analysis of the antibacterial clinical development pipeline, including tuberculosis. Geneva: WHO; 2017.
29. Lessem E, Low M. The tuberculosis treatment pipeline. In: Claydon P, Collins S, Frick M, et al., editors. 2016 pipeline report: HIV and TB, drugs, diagnostics, vaccines, preventive technologies, cure research, and immune-based and gene therapies in development. New York: Treatment Action Group; 2016. p. 129–42.
30. Tiberi S, D'Ambrosio L, De Lorenzo S, et al. Tuberculosis elimination, patients' lives and rational use of new drugs: revisited. Eur Respir J. 2016;47:664–7.
31. Working Group on New TB Drugs. Clinical pipeline. www.newtbdrugs.org/pipeline/clinical. Accessed 22 Dec 2020.
32. Li SY, Tasneen R, Soni H, et al. Bactericidal and sterilizing activity of a novel regimen with bedaquiline, pretomanid, moxifloxacin, and pyrazinamide in a murine model of tuberculosis. Antimicrob Agents Chemother. 2017;61:e00913–7.
33. Haagsma AC, Abdillahi-Ibrahim R, Wagner MJ, et al. Selectivity of TMC207 towards mycobacterial ATP synthase compared with that towards the eukaryotic homologue. Antimicrob Agents Chemother. 2009;53:1290–2.
34. Ndjeka N, Conradie F, Schnippel K, et al. Treatment of drug-resistant tuberculosis with bedaquiline in a high HIV prevalence setting: an interim cohort analysis. Int J Tuberc Lung Dis. 2015;19:979–85.
35. Falzon D, Schünemann HJ, Harausz E, et al. World Health Organization treatment guidelines for drug-resistant tuberculosis, 2016 update. Eur Resp J. 2017;49:1602308.
36. Matteelli A, D'Ambrosio L, Centis R, et al. Compassionate and optimum use of new tuberculosis drugs. Lancet Infect Dis. 2015;15:1131–2.
37. Bialvaei AZ, Rahbar M, Yousefi M, et al. Linezolid: a promising option in the treatment of gram-positives. J Antimicrob Chemother. 2017;72:354–64.
38. Zhang Z, Pang Y, Wang Y, et al. Beijing genotype of mycobacterium tuberculosis is significantly associated with linezolid resistance in multidrug-resistant and extensively drug-resistant tuberculosis in China. Int J Antimicrob Agents. 2014;43:231–5.
39. Shevchenko SY, Kulchavenya EV, Kholtobin DP. Method for evaluating the efficiency of treatment of urogenital tuberculosis. Urologiia. 2020;(4):10–3. Russian
40. Figueiredo AA, Lucon AM, Srougi M. Urogenital tuberculosis. Microbiol Spectr. 2017;5:1. https://doi.org/10.1128/microbiolspec.TNMI7-0015-2016.
41. Bansal P, Figueiredo A. Surgical treatment of urogenital tuberculosis. Version: 2020 08-12. In: Bjerklund Johansen TE, Wagenlehner FME, Matsumoto T, Cho YH, Krieger JN, Shoskes D, Naber KG, editors. Urogenital infections and inflammations. Berlin: German Medical Science GMS Publishing House; 2017. https://doi.org/10.5680/lhuii000051.
42. Urogenital Tuberculosis. Guidelines of Asian Association of UTI&STI. http://guidelines.aaus.info/aaus/index.php/Urogenital_tuberculosis

43. Suditu N, Negru D. Bacillus Calmette-Guérin. Therapy-associated granulomatous prostatitis mimicking prostate cancer on MRI: A case report and literature review. Mol Clin Oncol. 2015;3(1):249–51. Published online Sep 19, 2014. https://doi.org/10.3892/mco.2014.422.
44. Chuang AY, Tsou MH, Chang SJ, et al. Mycobacterium abscessus granulomatous prostatitis. Am J Surg Pathol. 2012;36:418–22.
45. Balasar M, Doğan M, Kandemir A, et al. Investigation of granulomatous prostatitis incidence following intravesical BCG therapy. Int J Clin Exp Med. 2014;7(6):1554–7. Published online Jun 15, 2014

Bacteriophage Therapy for Urinary Tract Infections

15

Matthew Dunne, Tamara S. Perepanova, and Truls E. Bjerklund Johansen

Take-Home Messages

- Bacteriophages (phages) are viruses that can specifically infect and kill bacteria.
- Phages demonstrate high specificity toward particular bacterial species, minimizing disruption to the commensal microbiome, unlike antibiotics.
- Phages have demonstrated excellent safety and tolerability profiles when used clinically.
- Combining phages in "phage cocktails" broadens their effective range while providing a way to mediate phage resistance development.
- Their different mechanisms of action enable synergistic co-administration of phages with certain antibiotics to enhance efficacy.
- Phages are versatile in terms of administration, with different routes, including oral and topical, demonstrating high effectiveness.
- Phages are effective against biofilm-forming uropathogens.
- Engineering of phage genomes can expand their therapeutic effectiveness, equipping them with unique capabilities in combating bacterial infections.

M. Dunne (✉)
Institute of Food Nutrition and Health, ETH Zurich, Zurich, Switzerland

Micreos GmbH, Wädenswil, Switzerland
e-mail: m.dunne@micreos.com

T. S. Perepanova
Department of Urinary Tract Infections and Clinical Pharmacology N. A. Lopatkin Scentific Research Institute of Urology and Interventional Radiology, Branch of the National Research Center for Radiology of the Ministry of Health of Russia, Moscow, Russia

T. E. Bjerklund Johansen
Institute of Clinical Medicine, University of Oslo, Oslo, Norway

Institute of Clinical Medicine, University of Aarhus, Aarhus, Denmark
e-mail: tebj@uio.no

T. E. Bjerklund Johansen, T. Cai (eds.), *Guide to Antibiotics in Urology*,
https://doi.org/10.1007/978-3-319-92366-6_15

15.1 Phages as Precision Antimicrobials

15.1.1 Introduction

Antibiotic resistance is a major concern for global health, with the latest estimations showing 1.27 million deaths were attributable to antibiotic resistance worldwide in 2019 [1]. A significant contributor to this issue is the uncontrolled and excessive use of antibiotics in various domains, including medicine, agriculture, and animal husbandry, since their introduction to the world in the 1940s. This misuse has, in turn, facilitated the proliferation of multiresistant bacteria harboring genes for resistance to common antibiotics such as β-lactams, fluoroquinolones, aminoglycosides, and chloramphenicol. This alarming trend poses a significant threat to the treatment of infectious diseases, particularly in the context of urological infections. Recognized global authorities, including the World Health Organization (WHO), the United Nations, and the Center for Disease Control (CDC), have declared antibiotic resistance a threat to global health [2, 3] that necessitates the exploration of alternative strategies. Bacteriophage (phage) therapy has reemerged as a compelling alternative solution, offering several advantages over antibiotics. These include their precision in targeting specific bacteria, the ability to self-replicate at infection sites, and their excellent safety and tolerability profiles when applied in humans, among others as described within [4].

Phages are viruses that infect bacterial cells with excellent specificity, typically down to the species- or strain-level. Phages are environmentally ubiquitous and the most abundant biological entities on Earth, having been identified in all environments amenable to bacterial life where they outnumber their bacterial hosts approximately tenfold [5, 6]. The phenomenon of phage-based lysis of bacterial cells was discovered separately by Frederick Twort and Felix d'Hérelle in 1915 and 1917 [7, 8]; however, given the submicroscopic size of phages (as shown in Fig. 15.1 for *Klebsiella* phage K1 and *E. coli* phage CM001 both being ~200 nm and ~180 nm in height, respectively), their very existence and viral lifestyle was a matter of dispute until phages could be observed by transmission electron microscopy (TEM) in the 1940s [9]. Over the last 80 years, a wide variety of phages have been isolated and visualized to unveil an incredible array of morphologies and sizes [10]. The vast majority (~95%) of phages investigated to date, and are lead candidates as therapeutic agents, are the tailed, double-stranded DNA (dsDNA) phages of the class *Caudoviricetes*. However, the genetic diversity of phages is remarkable, and other morphologies, e.g., polyhedral, filamentous, and pleomorphic, as well as single-stranded (ss)DNA, ssRNA, or dsRNA phages have been identified [11].

15.1.2 Availability of Phage Therapy

The use of phages to combat bacterial infections dates to the early twentieth century; however, it quickly declined in popularity with the advent and widespread use of antibiotics [13]. Nevertheless, phage therapy continued to be researched and used

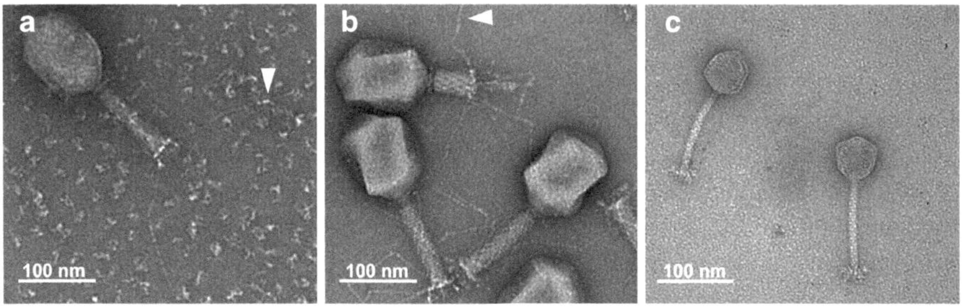

Fig. 15.1 Transmission electron microscopy (TEM) of therapeutic bacteriophages. TEM micrographs depict (**a**) *Klebsiella* phage UTI-K1 (GenBank OL870318) [12], (**b**) *Enterobacter cloacae* phage S10 (*unpublished*), and (**c**) *E. coli* phage CM001 (GenBank OM810255) [12]. Phages K1 and S10 exhibit a myoviral morphology and feature long tail fibers (LTFs), observable as fibrous extensions emanating from the baseplate at the end of the phage tail (white arrows). These fibers play a crucial role in probing the bacterial surface, binding to specific receptors, and facilitating adsorption to their bacterial hosts. In contrast, Phage CM001 displays a siphoviral morphology and uses bulky tailspike proteins, rather than fibers, to recognize bacteria. These tailspikes specifically target and depolymerize the capsules of particular *E. coli* bacteria, rendering the phage highly selective for encapsulated bacteria. Shown at the top of panel **b** is a contracted baseplate of a single S10 phage, demonstrating the syringe-like mechanism used to penetrate the outer membranes of bacterial cells. TEM micrographs were generated by Matthew Dunne at the ScopeM facility, ETH Zurich, Switzerland

in Eastern Europe, particularly in Poland, Georgia, and Russia [14]. Phage cocktails can be acquired as over-the-counter medication in Russia and Georgia for the treatment of bacterial infections of broad etiology, such as the Pyophage and Intestiphage cocktails produced by the Eliava Institute in Tbilisi [15]. As we confront the era of escalating antibiotic resistance, there has been a global shift in focus towards this overlooked therapy. With no licensed phage products available, physicians in different countries are resorting to invoking Article 37 (Unproven Clinical Practice Interventions) of the Declaration of Helsinki [16] to apply phage therapy to patients suffering from bacterial infections refractory to antibiotics. Countries are also developing or have already established national solutions to facilitate salvage (or rescue) therapy using phages. Examples include the emergency-use expanded access of investigational new drugs (eINDs) for individual patients in the USA; the Standardized Treatment and Monitoring Protocol for Adults and Pediatric Patients (STAMP), an open-label, single-arm trial investigating a standardized treatment and monitoring protocol for phage therapy use in Australia [17]; and the highly regarded magistral preparation pathway currently employed in Belgium [18]. Additionally, numerous clinical trials are currently underway, assessing the efficacy of both wild-type and genetically engineered phages as potential medicines of the future. Many of these trials, particularly those initiated in the last 5 years, are taking place in the USA [19], focusing on various indications and underlying pathogens for phage therapy.

15.1.3 What Makes Phages Precision Antimicrobials

The first stage of any phage infection is recognition of a suitable host bacterium. Phages have evolved an array of different receptor binding proteins (RBPs), classed as tail fibers or tailspikes [20, 21], capable of recognizing a diverse array of proteinaceous and/or saccharidic components of the bacterial cell surface. Tail fibers (e.g., the long tail fibers (LTFs) of phages K1 and S10 shown in Fig. 15.1a, b) initiate the infection process by binding to specific bacterial receptors in addition to facilitating the correct positioning of the phage particle to the bacterial surface prior to infection. Tailspikes (e.g., the bulky capsular depolymerase of *E. coli* phage CM001 (Fig. 15.1c) have enzymatic activity toward saccharidic components of the cell wall such as capsular polysaccharides (CPS) or lipopolysaccharides (LPS) and degrade these defensive barriers to enable the phage to adsorb to the bacterial outer membrane. Phages have also evolved different infection mechanisms of varying complexity [22–24] to penetrate the outer membrane and produce a conduit for genome ejection from the capsid and into the bacterial cytoplasm.

Phages and their RBPs are restricted to recognize and infect only bacteria possessing a complementary receptor. While this limits the antibacterial spectrum of phages compared to antibiotics, a clear benefit is that phages can be precisely targeted to specific pathogens without impacting the commensal and beneficial bacteria in our microbiomes. Importantly, when characterizing the targeting spectrum and activity of phages, assessment can be efficiently conducted within a relatively short timeframe using microbiological methods. These may include agar spot lysis testing (similar to an antibiogram), turbidity reduction assays, or more advanced and rapid approaches such as developing engineered reporter phage assays [25]. Furthermore, by adapting these methodologies, new phages can be easily isolated from the environment or, in some cases, be combined and selectively passaged against a refractory bacterial pathogen to evolve new phage variants with superior activity, e.g., the Appelmans Protocol [26]. As such, when therapeutically viable phages are not available, new phage variants can be easily isolated or generated through a personalized approach tailored to each individual case requiring phage therapy. Finally, the combination of a greater understanding of RBP structure and function, coupled with advances in genetic engineering, has led to the development of structure-guided strategies to reprogram and improve the host ranges of phages through RBP receptor-binding site modification [21, 27, 28].

15.1.4 Lytic or Temperate Phages as Therapeutic Candidates

Once inside the cell, the phage genome typically begins a lytic or lysogenic cycle (as well as pseudolysogeny as discussed here [29]) to replicate or exist within the host bacteria. Lytic phages hijack the host cell to generate the proteinaceous and genomic components of new phages, resulting in bacterial lysis and the release of infective viral progeny. A complete lytic cycle is phage-specific but typically takes ~40 min from phage adsorption to progeny phage release [30]. Temperate phages encode additional components that enable the phage to enter a lysogenic cycle and integrate its genome into the bacterial chromosome resulting in a prophage. Notably, prophages coexist with their bacterial hosts, refraining from bacterial destruction, and can even confer distinct advantages. This mutual relationship is indicative of a synergistic coevolution between phages and bacteria. Functioning as a "mobile gene bank," prophages can aid their bacterial hosts in swiftly adapting to environmental changes, be it shifts in nutrient availability, elevated temperatures, pressure, or exposure to chemicals. These genes may prove beneficial for the bacterial host, containing coding for virulence factors, metabolic genes, and even antibiotic resistance genes like resistance to β-lactamases [31]. Prophages possess the ability to detect specific signals or respond to cellular stress, triggering the excision of their genetic material and initiating the lytic cycle leading to progeny phage production, destruction of the bacterial host, and progeny phage release.

Typically, strictly lytic phages are desired for therapeutic purposes to circumvent the risk of prophage integration and the inherent variability in bacteriolytic activity associated with temperate phages. Nevertheless, progress in synthetic biology and the availability of new genetic engineering strategies has opened up the possibility of modifying lysogenic phages to render them suitable for therapeutic applications [32]. For instance, engineered strictly lytic variants of temperate phages have already proven effective in the clinic, such as for the treatment of a disseminated drug resistant *Mycobacterium abscessus* infection [33].

15.1.5 Phage Resistance and Its Clinical Relevance

The mechanism of action of phages differs significantly from that of small molecule antibiotics. While their orthogonal mode of action makes phages highly effective at treating multidrug-resistant bacteria, the fundamental challenge confronting phage therapy is the same as encountered with antibiotics: the emergence of phage resistance by the target bacteria. Bacteria and phages have coevolved for billions of years, leading to an impressive array of defensive and counter-defensive strategies evolved by bacteria and phages, respectively [34]. The most common types of phage resistance is the development of phage resistance by mutations and/or changes in the expression of genes encoding phage-binding receptors, including the loss or gain of barriers, such as the capsule [35]. However, many other mechanisms of phage resistance have been identified and continue to be discovered, for instance, prevention of phage DNA integration, cutting of the phage genome by restriction enzymes, action of CRISPR/Cas systems, and abortive infectious processes [36]. Nevertheless, internal resistances do not necessarily impede the development or use of phage therapy as these are less unlikely to evolve or adapt within clinically relevant timelines unlike surface and receptor modifications. Phages can also be prescreened prior to therapeutic use to ensure only those that can effectively kill a given bacterial patient isolate are used regardless of any preexisting internal defenses (whether they are identified or not).

A common strategy to counteract potential resistance development during phage therapy, and maintain treatment effectiveness, is to employ combinations of phages, often referred to as "phage cocktails." These cocktails consist of several phages from different families that recognize diverse receptors and utilize alternative infection mechanisms. As such, if one receptor mutates there is another phage present that can target an alternative set of receptors. The more phages the cocktail contains the less likely resistance to all phages will arise. Furthermore, by combining phages targeting different pathogenic species, a cocktail of broad activity can be used for different infecting species or polymicrobial infections [37]. Nevertheless, when considered from both a production and regulatory standpoint, the expansion of the number of phages within a cocktail may not always be advisable. This is due to the associated increase in production costs and regulatory requirements. Therefore, achieving the right balance in assembling a specific phage cocktail becomes crucial when contemplating the development of phages as medicinal products.

An alternative strategy to combat resistance development, which complements the use of phage cocktails, is employing genetic engineering to improve the host range and/or the antibacterial activity of individual phages.

15.1.6 Designer Phages and Genetic Engineering

The World Economic Forum recognized "designer phages" as one of the top ten emerging technologies in 2023 [38]. These are phages that have been genetically engineered to enhance or add new functionalities that can overcome therapeutic limitations associated with wild-type phages. Genetic engineering techniques, including synthetic genome assembly, homologous recombineering, bacteriophage recombineering of electroporated DNA (BRED), in vivo recombineering, the use of clustered regularly interspaced short palindromic repeats (CRISPR)/Cas-mediated counterselection, as well as yeast-based phage genome assembly and cell-free transcription/translation systems, have all been employed successfully to modify phage genomes by removing or inserting distinct genetic components [32]. For example, synthetic phages can be engineered to produce intracellular heterologous effector payloads, such as Cas9 or Cas3 [39–41], or produce extracellular heterologous effector payloads, such as bacteriocins and biofilm depolymerases, for release during phage infection to provide a two-pronged attack against bacteria or their biofilms [12, 42, 43].

Engineered phages are currently being evaluated for the treatment of various bacterial infections in patients, including UTIs. The Phase 2/3 ELIMINATE trial (NCT05488340) by Locus Biosciences (USA) is currently assessing a cocktail of CRISPR-enhanced phages, LBP-EC01, in combination with oral trimethoprim/sulfamethoxazole to treat female patients between 18 and 65 years of age who are suffering from UTIs caused by multidrug-resistant (MDR) *E. coli* and have a history of prior UTIs. The company plans to enroll approximately 800 patients across the US and the EU, with phages given by Intraurethral or Intravenous administration. SNIPR Biome (Denmark) have also developed a cocktail of four CRISPR-enhanced

E. coli phages that can selectively target and eliminate *E. coli* resistant to fluoroquinolones [39]. The SNIPR001 cocktail showed positive results in a phase I study (NCT05277350) with the treatment aimed at reducing the rate of infections in cancer patients with hematological malignancies at high risk of *E. coli* gut translocation that are vulnerable to bloodstream infections. In another case report, the *Mycobacterium smegmatis* phage, ZoeJ, was engineered using BRED to remove its repressor gene to produce a strictly lytic variant. This phage was combined with other phages and used to successfully treat a patient with a disseminated drug-resistant *Mycobacterium abscessus* in the UK [33].

The potential for enhancing and broadening the application of phage therapy through genetic engineering is vast. For more information on the enhancement of phage therapy through genetic engineering, we recommend the following reviews:

- Meile and Du et al. 2022. Current Opinion in Virology. *Engineering therapeutic phages for enhanced antibacterial efficacy* [44].
- Gibb et al. 2021. Pharmaceuticals. *The Many Applications of Engineered Bacteriophages-An Overview* [45].

15.1.7 Phage-Antibiotic Synergy

In biology, genetic trade-offs are a common observation, where organisms evolve one trait that enhances fitness while simultaneously experiencing reduced performance in another trait. Phage therapy is particularly intriguing in this context as it has been shown that while bacteria will evolve resistance to phages during therapeutic use, the same bacteria can develop greater sensitivity to antibiotics [46]. Moreover, when specific phages infect bacteria cultured in the presence of sublethal antibiotic doses, the sizes of phage plaques can significantly increase, a phenomenon known as phage-antibiotic synergy (PAS) [46–48]. However, further research is essential to identify optimal combinations of phages and antibiotics. Notably, some antibiotics, such as aminoglycosides, with mechanisms reliant on inhibiting bacterial protein synthesis machinery, have instead been found to exhibit antagonistic effects against phage therapy [49]. While the simultaneous use of phages and antibiotics shows promise in offering a dual attack to combat specific bacterial infections, this does not rule out the effectiveness of phages as a monotherapy.

15.1.8 Phage Targeting of Uropathogenic Biofilms

Bacteriuria and the presence of a catheter can significantly elevate the risk of biofilm formation as bacteria adhere to catheter surfaces, form complex polymicrobial communities, and lead to overall heightened resistance to antibiotics. Consequently, the exploration of novel treatments for biofilms in UTIs, particularly catheter-associated UTIs (CAUTIs), may offer solutions to address this challenge [12, 50]. Mono- and cocktail phage therapy has proven effective at targeting biofilm-forming uropathogenic strains in vitro [51, 52]; however, the development of phage resistance has also been observed that can lead to biofilm regrowth. Fu et al. investigated the effect of pretreating hydrogel-coated catheters with *Pseudomonas aeruginosa* targeting phages on subsequent in vitro biofilm development. A five-phage cocktail was shown highly effective, leading to significant delay and reduction in biofilm formation after 48 h and a reduction in phage resistance development by individual isolates [52]. Phage treatment of catheter surfaces has also proven effective in vitro against other mono- and poly-species biofilms [53, 54]. Phages with inherent activity against biofilm-producing strains can also be selectively isolated from the environment for potential therapeutic use. For instance, Chibeu et al. characterized biofilm formation in 253 uropathogenic *E. coli* (UPEC) strains and specifically isolated phages with an affinity for the most prolific biofilm producers. These phages were all capable of significantly reducing biofilms formed by these biofilm-producing strains [55]. While biofilms inherently present challenges for removal using conventional biological or chemical methods [56], innovative approaches have emerged that harness phages with intrinsic anti-biofilm activity or genetically engineer phages to inhibit biofilm formation and effectively eliminate preformed biofilms during treatment [57]. As an illustration of this concept, separate studies have successfully engineered *E. coli* phage T7 to express quorum-quenching enzymes, inhibiting biofilm formation [58] or to produce a biofilm-degrading enzyme, Dispersin-B, that hydrolyzes β-1,6-*N*-acetyl-D-glucosamine, a critical component of *Staphylococcus* and *E. coli* biofilms [42].

15.1.9 Interplay Between Phages, Bacteria, and the Host

Phage therapy is generally recognized as safe and well tolerated in studies to date, with very few and mostly transient adverse events (AEs) reported (although their association with the administered phages is generally unclear) [59]. Nevertheless, there is a need for more clinical and in vivo data informing human and animal host responses to phage therapy. This is particularly evident when considering the diverse genomic and morphological variation of phages that have or are currently being employed for therapeutic purposes, as well as the various routes of administration possible with phage therapy. After intravenous administration, it has been shown that phages rapidly localize in the liver, spleen, lungs, kidney, and urine [60, 61], as is the case also after oral administration [62] where protection against gastric acid has been shown to improve phage dissemination into the body [63]. One hour after oral administration in humans, phage particles have been detected in the blood, the bronchial content, and the cerebrospinal fluid, on the surface of burn wounds, and in urine. In healthy subjects, phages have been shown to be excreted from the body within 24 h; however, if there is an active infection, phages can replicate and can be identified in urine for up to 6–7 days [64]. Rectal administration may also be an efficient route of phage delivery. It was shown in rabbits and mice that it only takes a few minutes for phages to penetrate through the rectal wall into the circulation [65, 66]. The blood phage concentration after rectal administration may be twice as high as after oral administration, which may be due to a lack of phage inactivation by gastric acid. Phages have also proven to be highly effective in the urine environment and have proven to be well adapted to survive in the urinary tract niche that is characterized by low pH levels [25, 67, 68]. The efficacy of phage therapy can also be impacted by phage clearance through the immune system. Patients may even display low phage-specific antibody titers before treatment begins due to prior exposure, given our common and constant interaction with phages within our microbiome and in the environment [69]. However, the clinical significance of this phenomenon in determining the success or failure of therapy is currently unclear. This uncertainty arises because even with a robust anti-phage humoral response, success in phage therapy is not necessarily ruled out [70]. It is also possible that repeated administration of phages, increased phage concentration, or using different phages or a phage cocktail may counteract immunological clearance, simply the stimulation of the immune system by administered phages may also enhance treatment outcomes [71, 72]. Aleshkin et al. [73] studied anti-phage immunity in 42 patients in a neurointensive care unit using enzyme-linked immunosorbent assay (ELISA) before and after phage therapy. During the first course of phage therapy, phage activity was confirmed in 54–62.5% of cases; however, repeated courses with the same phage combinations did not result in significant eradication of the underlying pathogens. Anti-phage immunity following a single administration of the phage preparations was confirmed by the presence of IgG antibody titer. Neutralizing IgG antibodies appeared 2–3 weeks after the initial course of phage therapy and were also strain specific.

While phages were previously considered as bystanders that indirectly influenced the immune system by targeting their bacterial hosts, emerging evidence suggests that phages can have a direct impact on immunity, often in an anti-inflammatory manner [74], and can physically interact with our mucosal surfaces [75]. Although current data indicate the safety of using lytic phages, there is still much to explore regarding the broader implications of phage-mammalian interactions. For an in-depth exploration of the topic of phage pharmacokinetics and their interactions with the human immune system and its constituent components, we refer the reader to the following reviews:

- Krystyna Dąbrowska. 2019. Medicinal Research Reviews. *Phage therapy: What factors shape phage pharmacokinetics and bioavailability? Systematic and critical review* [60].
- Leo Kan and Jeremy J. Barr. 2023. Annual Review of Virology. *A Mammalian Cell's Guide on How to Process a Bacteriophage* [76].

15.2 Clinical Application of Phage Therapy to Treat UTIs

The following is a concise yet comprehensive overview of noteworthy clinical cases available at the time of writing that explore the utilization of phages in the treatment of urinary tract infections (UTIs). Articles were sourced from articles and books written in English or Russian through a literature search using PubMed, Medline, Embase, and the Cochrane database and keywords: bacteriophage, bacteriophage therapy, phages, and bacteriophage therapy for urinary tract infections. There were no restrictions on gender, age, or the type of clinical studies. For a complementary overview of phage therapy for the treatment of UTIs, we recommend the 2023 systematic review *Phage Therapy in the Management of Urinary Tract Infections: A Comprehensive Systematic Review* by Al-Anany et al. [77].

In 1971, researchers from a prominent medical institute in Bucharest reported the outcomes of phage treatment for a large cohort of 87 UTI patients [78]. Phage therapy was shown effective in treating acute UTIs, leading to rapid reduction in temperature and decreased leukocyturia. A synergistic effect was also observed when phages were combined with standard of care antibiotic treatments. Similar findings were reported by Russian physicians in 1995 [79]. In a cohort of 46 patients with acute or chronic urogenital inflammation, receiving local (direct administration into the bladder) and oral phage treatments targeting *P. aeruginosa*, *Proteus* sp., *Staphylococcus* spp., *E. coli*, or a combined pyobacteriophage (applied both independently and in combination with antibiotics), clinical improvement was noted in 92% of cases.

In 1994, Boratynska et al. [80] summarized the results of treating 15 patients (aged 24–77) who suffered from recurrent UTIs associated with chronic pyelocystitis, nephrolithiasis, vesicoureteral reflux, or floating kidney. Some patients had UTIs after receiving a kidney transplantation (KT). The UTIs were caused by various pathogens: *E. coli* ($n = 9$), *P. aeruginosa* ($n = 2$), *Klebsiella pneumoniae* ($n = 2$), *Proteus vulgaris* ($n = 2$), *Enterobacter aerogenes* ($n = 2$), and *S. aureus* ($n = 2$), all of which were resistant to available antibiotics. The treatment involved administering 10 mL of specific phages orally three to four times daily, after gastric acid neutralization. For patients who had received a KT ($n = 3$), antibiotics were given concurrently. The treatment duration ranged from 3 to 11 months, with an average of 5.4 months. Notably, five patients (including one with KT) experienced long-lasting symptom relief (12–36 months) and eradication of the pathogens. In three cases, remission occurred after 3–6 months. Phages were detected in some patients' urine, and no adverse changes were observed in blood parameters, serum proteins, electrolytes, or kidney and liver function.

In 2013, Zorkin and Shakhnovsky [81] reported the efficacy of bacteriophages compared to antibiotics in children with complicated UTIs due to congenital urinary tract abnormalities. Although this method cannot be considered entirely safe, the authors conducted local irrigation of the pelvicalyceal cavity, bladder cavity, or ureter lumen with 5–10 mL of phages, using a drainage clamp for 15–20 min for 5–7 days. Six to twelve months after urodynamics normalization, the combination of antibiotics with bacteriophages demonstrated the best clinical and bacteriological efficacy.

In 2019, Haddad et al. [82] presented a systematic review on devoted to phage therapy against multidrug-resistant ESKAPE pathogens in humans from 30 studies enrolling in total 1,152 patients. Most studies showed efficacy (87%) and safety (67%), with three publications reporting phage therapy of UTIs: (i) in 2011,

Khawaldeh et al. [83] presented the experience with a woman with a lower UTI who was given intravesicular phage therapy using Pyophage combined with intravenous meropenem and colistin. Following 21 days of treatment, the microbial count exhibited a reduction of 4 $\log_{10}$; (ii) in 1995, Perepanova et al. [79] reported 46 patients with acute and chronic urogenital infections. After determining the sensitivity, preparations of phages were administered orally or topically with clinical efficacy observed in 92% of patients; and (iii) in 2010, Letkiewicz et al. [84] treated 22 men with chronic bacterial prostatitis. Bacteriophage preparations were administered rectally, topically, or orally. Eradication of target bacteria was observed in 50% of cases.

In 2009, Letkiewicz et al. [85] provided detailed accounts of three cases of prostatitis treated with phages, resulting in successful pathogen eradication. Specific phage preparations, with activity shown against *Enterococcus faecalis* isolated from the patients, were administered rectally (10 mL twice daily) for a duration of 28–33 days. The treatment led to bacterial eradication, confirmed by two negative cultures of expressed prostatic secretion (EPS) conducted 7–17 weeks apart. Additionally, improvements were observed in the National Institutes of Health Chronic Prostatitis Symptom Index (NIH-CPSI), analyzed in two cases, along with a reduction in prostate size and pain. Notably, there were significant increases in the maximum urinary flow rate in all cases.

The most effective administration routes for phage preparations in 22 women with urogenital infections was found to be intravaginal and oral, both yielding a favorable treatment response in 50% of cases. A positive outcome following oral administration suggests that phages effectively reached the infection site after gastrointestinal absorption [86]. In a recent case report from Poland, intrarectal administration of phage-based preparations in combination with meropenem successfully treated a *K. pneumoniae* UTI in a 60-year-old kidney transplant recipient, who achieved symptom remission that was maintained for 5.5 years posttransplantation [87].

A number of reports also describe the use of phages to treat biofilms formed on urinary catheters [88–90]. A significant reduction of biofilm formation was detected after covering permanent catheters with bacteriophages specific for *P. aeruginosa*, *E. coli*, and *P. mirabilis*. Studies have shown that phages can reduce biofilms formed by uropathogenic *E. coli* regardless of the dose, which means that low titers of phages are as efficient as higher titers for the destruction of biofilms [55]; however, low doses of phages have also been shown to inversely stimulate the growth of biofilms on catheters [91], requiring further investigation.

In 2021, Terwilliger et al. [92] documented the treatment of a 56-year-old male liver transplant recipient experiencing recurrent prostate infections and UTIs caused by an extended-spectrum beta-lactamase (ESBL) UPEC strain. The patient underwent a 2-week treatment with an intravenous phage cocktail alongside concurrent ertapenem for 6 weeks. The UTI reverted to asymptomatic recurrent bacteriuria at 6 and 11 weeks post the conclusion of phage therapy, which did not necessitate further antibiotic treatment.

In 2020, Leitner et al. [93] reported on a randomized, placebo-controlled, double-blind clinical trial for intravesical phage therapy treatment of UTIs in patients undergoing transurethral resection of the prostate. The trial took place at the Alexander Tsulukidze National Centre of Urology, Tbilisi, Georgia, in men scheduled for transurethral resection of the prostate (TURP). Of 97 patients, 28 received Pyophage (a phage cocktail prepared by the Eliava Institute, Tbilisi, Georgia), 32 received placebo (bladder irrigation), and 37 received standard of care antibiotics. Success rates did not differ between the three groups, indicating that while in this study intravesical phage therapy was non-inferior to standard-of-care antibiotic treatment, it was also not shown superior to the bladder irrigation placebo treatment.

15.3 Future Perspectives

The rise of multidrug-resistant strains in uropathogenic bacteria underscores the need to explore non-antibiotic treatments for bacterial infections. Phage therapy, including natural phages, phage cocktails, engineered phages, and their combination with antibiotics, shows promise as a future option for the treatment of UTIs; however, broader clinical adoption requires evidence from validated clinical trials. Fortunately, an increasing number of trials have been initiated that are evaluating phage therapy, including the assessment of both wild-type phages (e.g., NCT05967130, NCT05537519, and NCT04287478) and engineered phages (e.g., NCT04191148 and NCT05488340) specifically for the treatment of UTIs, and undoubtedly more trials are yet to emerge in the coming years. This encouraging trend fosters optimism for the prospective integration of phage therapy as a standard and highly promising therapeutic choice for clinicians to further expand their array of options for addressing urogenital infections.

Acknowledgements The authors acknowledge the ScopeM facility at ETH Zurich for their support and assistance.

Competing Interests M.D. is an employee of Micreos, developing phage-based antimicrobials. The other authors declare no competing interests.

References

1. Antimicrobial Resistance Collaborators. Global burden of bacterial antimicrobial resistance in 2019: a systematic analysis. Lancet. 2022;399:629–55.
2. Ventola CL. The antibiotic resistance crisis. P T. 2015;40:277–83.
3. Talebi Bezmin Abadi A, Rizvanov AA, Haertlé T, Blatt NL. World Health Organization report: current crisis of antibiotic resistance. BioNanoSci. 2019;9:778–88.
4. Hatfull GF, Dedrick RM, Schooley RT. Phage therapy for antibiotic-resistant bacterial infections. Annu Rev Med. 2022;73:197–211.
5. Bergh O, Børsheim KY, Bratbak G, Heldal M. High abundance of viruses found in aquatic environments. Nature. 1989;340:467–8.

6. Ashelford KE, Norris SJ, Fry JC, Bailey MJ, Day MJ. Seasonal population dynamics and interactions of competing bacteriophages and their host in the rhizosphere. Appl Environ Microbiol. 2000;66:4193–9.
7. Twort FW. Further investigations on the nature of ultra-microscopic viruses and their cultivation. J Hyg (Lond). 1936;36:204–35.
8. D'Herelle F. On an invisible microbe antagonistic toward dysenteric bacilli: brief note by Mr. F. D'Herelle, presented by Mr. Roux. 1917. Res Microbiol. 2007;158:553–4.
9. Ackermann H-W. The first phage electron micrographs. Bacteriophage. 2011;1:225–7.
10. Ackermann H-W. 5500 phages examined in the electron microscope. Arch Virol. 2007;152:227–43.
11. Hendrix RW. Bacteriophages: evolution of the majority. Theor Popul Biol. 2002;61:471–80.
12. Du J, Meile S, Baggenstos J, Jäggi T, Piffaretti P, Hunold L, Matter CI, Leitner L, Kessler TM, Loessner MJ, et al. Enhancing bacteriophage therapeutics through in situ production and release of heterologous antimicrobial effectors. Nat Commun. 2023;14:4337.
13. Wittebole X, De Roock S, Opal SM. A historical overview of bacteriophage therapy as an alternative to antibiotics for the treatment of bacterial pathogens. Virulence. 2014;5:226–35.
14. Chanishvili N. Phage therapy—history from Twort and d'Herelle through Soviet experience to current approaches. Adv Virus Res. 2012;83:3–40.
15. Myelnikov D. An alternative cure: the adoption and survival of bacteriophage therapy in the USSR, 1922–1955. J Hist Med Allied Sci. 2018;73:385–411.
16. World Medical Association. World medical association declaration of Helsinki: ethical principles for medical research involving human subjects. JAMA. 2013;310:2191–4.
17. Khatami A, Foley DA, Warner MS, Barnes EH, Peleg AY, Li J, Stick S, Burke N, Lin RCY, Warning J, et al. Standardised treatment and monitoring protocol to assess safety and tolerability of bacteriophage therapy for adult and paediatric patients (STAMP study): protocol for an open-label, single-arm trial. BMJ Open. 2022;12:e065401.
18. Pirnay J-P, Verbeken G, Ceyssens P-J, Huys I, De Vos D, Ameloot C, Fauconnier A. The magistral phage. Viruses. 2018;10:64.
19. Hitchcock NM, Devequi Gomes Nunes D, Shiach J, Valeria Saraiva Hodel K, Dantas Viana Barbosa J, Alencar Pereira Rodrigues L, Coler BS, Botelho Pereira Soares M, Badaró R. Current clinical landscape and global potential of bacteriophage therapy. Viruses. 2023;15:1020.
20. de Jonge PA, Nobrega FL, Brouns SJJ, Dutilh BE. Molecular and evolutionary determinants of bacteriophage host range. Trends Microbiol. 2019;27:51–63.
21. Dunne M, Rupf B, Tala M, Qabrati X, Ernst P, Shen Y, Sumrall E, Heeb L, Plückthun A, Loessner MJ, et al. Reprogramming bacteriophage host range through structure-guided design of chimeric receptor binding proteins. Cell Rep. 2019;29:1336–1350.e4.
22. Degroux S, Effantin G, Linares R, Schoehn G, Breyton C. Deciphering bacteriophage T5 host recognition mechanism and infection trigger. J Virol. 2023;97:e0158422.
23. Guerrero-Ferreira RC, Hupfeld M, Nazarov S, Taylor NM, Shneider MM, Obbineni JM, Loessner MJ, Ishikawa T, Klumpp J, Leiman PG. Structure and transformation of bacteriophage A511 baseplate and tail upon infection of listeria cells. EMBO J. 2019;38:e99455.
24. Taylor NMI, van Raaij MJ, Leiman PG. Contractile injection systems of bacteriophages and related systems. Mol Microbiol. 2018;108:6–15.
25. Meile S, Du J, Staubli S, Grossmann S, Koliwer-Brandl H, Piffaretti P, Leitner L, Matter CI, Baggenstos J, Hunold L, et al. Engineered reporter phages for detection of Escherichia coli, enterococcus, and Klebsiella in urine. Nat Commun. 2023;14:4336.
26. Burrowes BH, Molineux IJ, Fralick JA. Directed in vitro evolution of therapeutic bacteriophages: the Appelmans protocol. Viruses. 2019;11:241.
27. Yehl K, Lemire S, Yang AC, Ando H, Mimee M, Torres MDT, de la Fuente-Nunez C, Lu TK. Engineering phage host-range and suppressing bacterial resistance through phage tail fiber mutagenesis. Cell. 2019;179:459–469.e9.
28. Ando H, Lemire S, Pires DP, Lu TK. Engineering modular viral scaffolds for targeted bacterial population editing. Cell Syst. 2015;1:187–96.
29. Łoś M, Węgrzyn G. Pseudolysogeny. Adv Virus Res. 2012;82:339–49.

30. Delbrück M. The growth of bacteriophage and lysis of the host. J Gen Physiol. 1940;23:643–60.
31. Fortier L-C, Sekulovic O. Importance of prophages to evolution and virulence of bacterial pathogens. Virulence. 2013;4:354–65.
32. Kilcher S, Loessner MJ. Engineering bacteriophages as versatile biologics. Trends Microbiol. 2019;27:355–67.
33. Dedrick RM, Guerrero-Bustamante CA, Garlena RA, Russell DA, Ford K, Harris K, Gilmour KC, Soothill J, Jacobs-Sera D, Schooley RT, et al. Engineered bacteriophages for treatment of a patient with a disseminated drug-resistant Mycobacterium abscessus. Nat Med. 2019;25:730–3.
34. Georjon H, Bernheim A. The highly diverse antiphage defence systems of bacteria. Nat Rev Microbiol. 2023;21:686–700.
35. Labrie SJ, Samson JE, Moineau S. Bacteriophage resistance mechanisms. Nat Rev Microbiol. 2010;8:317–27.
36. Egido JE, Costa AR, Aparicio-Maldonado C, Haas P-J, Brouns SJJ. Mechanisms and clinical importance of bacteriophage resistance. FEMS Microbiol Rev. 2022;46:fuab048.
37. Goodridge LD. Designing phage therapeutics. Curr Pharm Biotechnol. 2010;11:15–27.
38. Communications FS: Designer phages: world economic forum emerging technologies report—science & research news | Frontiers. 2023,
39. Gencay YE, Jasinskytė D, Robert C, Semsey S, Martínez V, Petersen AØ, Brunner K, de Santiago TA, Salazar A, Turcu IC, et al. Engineered phage with antibacterial CRISPR-Cas selectively reduce E. coli burden in mice. Nat Biotechnol. 2023.
40. Bikard D, Barrangou R. Using CRISPR-Cas systems as antimicrobials. Curr Opin Microbiol. 2017;37:155–60.
41. Bikard D, Euler CW, Jiang W, Nussenzweig PM, Goldberg GW, Duportet X, Fischetti VA, Marraffini LA. Exploiting CRISPR-Cas nucleases to produce sequence-specific antimicrobials. Nat Biotechnol. 2014;32:1146–50.
42. Lu TK, Collins JJ. Dispersing biofilms with engineered enzymatic bacteriophage. Proc Natl Acad Sci USA. 2007;104:11197–202.
43. Masuda Y, Kawabata S, Uedoi T, Honjoh K-I, Miyamoto T. Construction of leaderless-Bacteriocin-producing bacteriophage Targeting E. coli and neighboring gram-positive pathogens. Microbiol Spectr. 2021;9:e0014121.
44. Meile S, Du J, Dunne M, Kilcher S, Loessner MJ. Engineering therapeutic phages for enhanced antibacterial efficacy. Curr Opin Virol. 2021;52:182–91.
45. Gibb B, Hyman P, Schneider CL. The many applications of engineered bacteriophages—an overview. Pharmaceuticals (Basel). 2021;14:634.
46. Burmeister AR, Turner PE. Trading-off and trading-up in the world of bacteria–phage evolution. Curr Biol. 2020;30:R1120–4.
47. Diallo K, Dublanchet A. Benefits of Combined Phage–Antibiotic Therapy for the Control of Antibiotic-Resistant Bacteria: A Literature Review. Antibiotics (Basel). 2022;11:839.
48. Kim M, Jo Y, Hwang YJ, Hong HW, Hong SS, Park K, Myung H. Phage-antibiotic synergy via delayed lysis. Appl Environ Microbiol. 2018;84:e02085–18.
49. Kever L, Hardy A, Luthe T, Hünnefeld M, Gätgens C, Milke L, Wiechert J, Wittmann J, Moraru C, Marienhagen J, et al. Aminoglycoside antibiotics inhibit phage infection by blocking an early step of the infection cycle. mBio. 2022;13:e0078322.
50. Zalewska-Piątek B, Piątek R. Phage therapy as a novel strategy in the treatment of urinary tract infections caused by E. Coli Antibiotics (Basel). 2020;9:304.
51. Maszewska A, Zygmunt M, Grzejdziak I, Różalski A. Use of polyvalent bacteriophages to combat biofilm of Proteus mirabilis causing catheter-associated urinary tract infections. J Appl Microbiol. 2018;125:1253–65.
52. Fu W, Forster T, Mayer O, Curtin JJ, Lehman SM, Donlan RM. Bacteriophage cocktail for the prevention of biofilm formation by Pseudomonas aeruginosa on catheters in an in vitro model system. Antimicrob Agents Chemother. 2010;54:397–404.
53. Curtin JJ, Donlan RM. Using bacteriophages to reduce formation of catheter-associated biofilms by Staphylococcus epidermidis. Antimicrob Agents Chemother. 2006;50:1268–75.

54. Lehman SM, Donlan RM. Bacteriophage-mediated control of a two-species biofilm formed by microorganisms causing catheter-associated urinary tract infections in an in vitro urinary catheter model. Antimicrob Agents Chemother. 2015;59:1127–37.
55. Chibeu A, Lingohr EJ, Masson L, Manges A, Harel J, Ackermann H-W, Kropinski AM, Boerlin P. Bacteriophages with the ability to degrade uropathogenic Escherichia coli biofilms. Viruses. 2012;4:471–87.
56. Flores-Mireles AL, Walker JN, Caparon M, Hultgren SJ. Urinary tract infections: epidemiology, mechanisms of infection and treatment options. Nat Rev Microbiol. 2015;13:269–84.
57. Chegini Z, Khoshbayan A, Taati Moghadam M, Farahani I, Jazireian P, Shariati A. Bacteriophage therapy against Pseudomonas aeruginosa biofilms: a review. Ann Clin Microbiol Antimicrob. 2020;19:45.
58. Pei R, Lamas-Samanamud GR. Inhibition of biofilm formation by T7 bacteriophages producing quorum-quenching enzymes. Appl Environ Microbiol. 2014;80:5340–8.
59. Suh GA, Lodise TP, Tamma PD, Knisely JM, Alexander J, Aslam S, Barton KD, Bizzell E, Totten KMC, Campbell JL, et al. Considerations for the use of phage therapy in clinical practice. Antimicrob Agents Chemother. 2022;66:e0207121.
60. Dąbrowska K. Phage therapy: what factors shape phage pharmacokinetics and bioavailability? Systematic and critical review. Med Res Rev. 2019;39:2000–25.
61. Bogovazova GG, Voroshilova NN, Bondarenko VM. The efficacy of Klebsiella pneumoniae bacteriophage in the therapy of experimental Klebsiella infection. Zh Mikrobiol Epidemiol Immunobiol. 1991:5.
62. Reynaud A, Cloastre L, Bernard J, Laveran H, Ackermann HW, Licois D, Joly B. Characteristics and diffusion in the rabbit of a phage for Escherichia coli 0103. Attempts to use this phage for therapy. Vet Microbiol. 1992;30:203–12.
63. Smith HW, Huggins MB, Shaw KM. Factors influencing the survival and multiplication of bacteriophages in calves and in their environment. J Gen Microbiol. 1987;133:1127–35.
64. Lazareva EB. Bacteriophages for the treatment and prevention of infectious diseases (Russian). Antibiot Chemother. 2003;48:10.
65. Hoffmann M. Animal experiments on the mucosal passage and absorption viremia of T3 phages after oral, tracheal and rectal administration. Zentralbl Bakteriol Orig. 1965;198:371–90.
66. Sechter I, Touitou E, Donbrow M. The influence of a non-ionic surfactant on rectal absorption of virus particles. Arch Virol. 1989;106:141–3.
67. Tan D, Zhang Y, Cheng M, Le S, Gu J, Bao J, Qin J, Guo X, Zhu T. Characterization of Klebsiella pneumoniae ST11 isolates and their interactions with lytic phages. Viruses. 2019;11:1080.
68. Pereira S, Pereira C, Santos L, Klumpp J, Almeida A: Potential of phage cocktails in the inactivation of Enterobacter cloacae--An in vitro study in a buffer solution and in urine samples. Virus Res 2016, 211:199–208.
69. Federici S, Nobs SP, Elinav E. Phages and their potential to modulate the microbiome and immunity. Cell Mol Immunol. 2021;18:889–904.
70. Łusiak-Szelachowska M, Międzybrodzki R, Rogóż P, Weber-Dąbrowska B, Żaczek M, Górski A. Do anti-phage antibodies persist after phage therapy? A Preliminary Report. Antibiotics (Basel). 2022;11:1358.
71. Roach DR, Leung CY, Henry M, Morello E, Singh D, Di Santo JP, Weitz JS, Debarbieux L. Synergy between the host immune system and bacteriophage is essential for successful phage therapy against an acute respiratory pathogen. Cell Host Microbe. 2017;22:38–47.e4.
72. Maciejewska B, Olszak T, Drulis-Kawa Z. Applications of bacteriophages versus phage enzymes to combat and cure bacterial infections: an ambitious and also a realistic application? Appl Microbiol Biotechnol. 2018;102:2563–81.
73. Aleshkin AV, Sel'Kova EP, Ershova ON, Savin IA, Shkoda AS, Bochkareva SS, Mitrokhin SD, Kiseleva IA, Orlova OE, Rubal'Skiy EO, et al. Concept of personalized phage therapy for intensive care unit patients with healthcare-associated infections. Fund Clin Med. 2018;3:66–74.
74. Van Belleghem JD, Dąbrowska K, Vaneechoutte M, Barr JJ, Bollyky PL. Interactions between bacteriophage, bacteria, and the mammalian immune system. Viruses. 2018;11:10.

75. Barr JJ, Auro R, Furlan M, Whiteson KL, Erb ML, Pogliano J, Stotland A, Wolkowicz R, Cutting AS, Doran KS, et al. Bacteriophage adhering to mucus provide a non-host-derived immunity. Proc Natl Acad Sci USA. 2013;110:10771–6.
76. Kan L, Barr JJ. A mammalian cell's guide on how to process a bacteriophage. Annu Rev Virol. 2023;10:183–98.
77. Al-Anany AM, Hooey PB, Cook JD, Burrows LL, Martyniuk J, Hynes AP, German GJ. Phage therapy in the management of urinary tract infections: a comprehensive systematic review. Phage. 2023;4:112.
78. Zilisteanu C, Ionescu H, Ionescu-Dorohoi T, Mintzer L. Considerations sur le traitement des infections urinaires par l'association bacteriophage–autovaccin–antibiotiques. Arch Roum Path Exp Microbiol. 1971;30:195.
79. Perepanova TS, Darbeeva OS, Kotliarova GA, Kondrat'eva EM, Maĭskaia LM, Malysheva VF, Baĭguzina FA, Grishkova NV. The efficacy of bacteriophage preparations in treating inflammatory urologic diseases. Urol Nefrol (Mosk). 1995:14–7.
80. Boratynska M, Szewczyk Z, Weber-Dabrowska B. Kliniczna ocena bakteriofagow w leczeniu zakaz' 'en układu' moczowego (Polish). Post Med Klin Dos'w. 1994;3:7–11.
81. Zorkin SN, Shakhnovskiy DS. Possibilities of bacteriophage therapy in the treatment of patients with complicated urinary tract infection. Pediatr Pharmacol. 2013;10(4):132–8.
82. El Haddad L, Harb CP, Gebara MA, Stibich MA, Chemaly RF. A systematic and critical review of bacteriophage therapy against multidrug-resistant ESKAPE organisms in humans. Clin Infect Dis. 2019;69:167–78.
83. Khawaldeh A, Morales S, Dillon B, Alavidze Z, Ginn AN, Thomas L, Chapman SJ, Dublanchet A, Smithyman A, Iredell JR. Bacteriophage therapy for refractory Pseudomonas aeruginosa urinary tract infection. J Med Microbiol. 2011;60:1697–700.
84. Letkiewicz S, Międzvbrodzki R, Kłak M, Weber Dąbrowska B, Górski A. Poster 374: pathogen eradication by phage therapy in patients with chronic bacterial prostatitis. Eur Urol Suppl. 2010;9:140.
85. Letkiewicz S, Miedzybrodzki R, Fortuna W, Weber-Dabrowska B, Górski A. Eradication of Enterococcus faecalis by phage therapy in chronic bacterial prostatitis—case report. Folia Microbiol (Praha). 2009;54:457–61.
86. Międzybrodzki R, Borysowski J, Weber-Dąbrowska B, Fortuna W, Letkiewicz S, Szufnarowski K, Pawełczyk Z, Rogóż P, Kłak M, Wojtasik E, et al. Clinical aspects of phage therapy. Adv Virus Res. 2012;83:73–121.
87. Rostkowska OM, Międzybrodzki R, Miszewska-Szyszkowska D, Górski A, Durlik M. Treatment of recurrent urinary tract infections in a 60-year-old kidney transplant recipient. The use of phage therapy. Transpl Infect Dis. 2021;23:e13391.
88. Perepanova TS, Merenov DS, Kazachenko AV, Khazan PL, Malova YA. Prevention of infectious and inflammatory complications after percutaneous nephrolithotomy (Russian). Urologiia. 2020;3:44–51.
89. Al-Qahtani M, Safan A, Jassim G, Abadla S. Efficacy of anti-microbial catheters in preventing catheter associated urinary tract infections in hospitalized patients: a review on recent updates. J Infect Public Health. 2019;12(6):760–6.
90. Melo LDR, Veiga P, Cerca N, Kropinski AM, Almeida C, Azeredo J, Sillankorva S. Development of a phage cocktail to control Proteus mirabilis catheter-associated urinary tract infections. Front Microbiol. 2016;7:1024.
91. Perepanova TS, Golovanov SA, Merinov DS, Arustamov LD, Radzhabov UA. Metaphylaxis of infectious renal stones after percutaneous nephrolithotom (Russian). Exp Clin Urol. 2016;4:96–9.
92. Terwilliger A, Clark J, Karris M, Hernandez-Santos H, Green S, Aslam S, Maresso A. Phage therapy related microbial succession associated with successful clinical outcome for a recurrent urinary tract infection. Viruses. 2021;13:2049.

93. Leitner L, Ujmajuridze A, Chanishvili N, Goderdzishvili M, Chkonia I, Rigvava S, Chkhotua A, Changashvili G, McCallin S, Schneider MP, et al. Intravesical bacteriophages for treating urinary tract infections in patients undergoing transurethral resection of the prostate: a randomised, placebo-controlled, double-blind clinical trial. Lancet Infect Dis. 2021;21:427–36.

Part IV

Urethritis and Male Accessory Gland Infections

Treatment of Urethritis

16

Riccardo Bartoletti, Alessandro Perotti, Matteo Pacini, and Alessandro Zucchi

16.1 Background

Urethritis is a sexually transmitted disease (STD), and it is characterized by specific symptoms such as dysuria and/or urethral discomfort and urethral discharge.

It can be classified according to the microorganism involved in the inflammatory process as gonococcal urethritis (GU) and non-gonococcal urethritis (NGU).

This kind of classification based on the traditional Gram stain for diplococci found at patient's urethral discharge collection has been maintained in daily clinical practice, although the nucleic acid amplification test (NAAT) replaced the Gram stain in the identification of *Neisseria gonorrhoeae*, *Chlamydia trachomatis*, and other microorganisms involved in the infective process [1].

The "modern view" of urethritis also includes noninfectious etiologies due to external or iatrogenic factors, such as urethral inflammation that occurs after trauma or intraurethral inoculation of irritating compounds. Conversely, infectious urethritis can be caused by bacterial, viral, or parasitic pathogens and is in general sexually transmitted (STDs).

GU is sustained by *Neisseria gonorrhoeae* is the microrganism involved in the GU infection. This is a Gram-negative diplococci bacterium that is oxidase-positive, aerobic, and non-motile with survival capacity within neutrophils [2].

R. Bartoletti (✉)
Urology Unit, Department of Translational Research and New Technologies, University of Pisa, Pisa, Italy

Cisanello Hospital, Pisa, Italy
e-mail: riccardo.bartoletti@unipi.it

A. Perotti · M. Pacini · A. Zucchi
Urology Unit, Department of Translational Research and New Technologies, University of Pisa, Pisa, Italy
e-mail: a.perotti@studenti.unipi.it; m.pacini@studenti.unipi.it; alessandro.zucchi@unipi.it

T. E. Bjerklund Johansen, T. Cai (eds.), *Guide to Antibiotics in Urology*,
https://doi.org/10.1007/978-3-319-92366-6_16

Several microorganisms are responsible for NGU, in particular *Chlamydia trachomatis*, an obligate intracellular Gram-negative bacterium, ovoid in shape and non-motile; *Mycoplasma genitalium*, a small Gram-positive bacterium; and *Trichomonas vaginalis*, an anaerobic, flagellated protozoan parasite. However, recent studies demonstrated the contribution of *Ureaplasma urealyticum*, herpes simplex virus, and adenovirus to the etiology of NGU, owing in part to advancements in nucleic acid amplification tests (NAATs) for detection [3].

Prevalence of the most common pathogens isolated from patients with NGU	
• *Chlamydia trachomatis*	11–50%
• *Mycoplasma genitalium*	6–50%
• *Trichomonas vaginalis*	1–20%
• *Ureaplasmas*	5–26%
• Adenovirus	2–4%
• Herpes simplex virus	2–3%

Adapted from Horner et al. [4]

The 2016 annual report of the Center for Disease Control and Prevention (CDC) on the incidence of case of urethritis in the United States shows an increase of *Neisseria gonorrhoeae* and *Chlamydia trachomatis* infections with a peak of incidence in the age range 25 and 29 years [3].

Similarly, Sonneberg and other authors stated that urethritis was distributed heterogeneously in the British population, with an increasing incidence of the *Chlamydia* infection from 2010 to 2012. In addition, they found a higher incidence of *Neisseria gonorrhoeae* infection in patients positive for *Chlamydia* infection [5]. This connection can be explained by the fact that patients with risky sexual behavior are exposed to different pathogens [6]. Due to this reasons, gonococcal and non-gonococcal infections often coexist, generating an additional confounding factor and limiting the use of empirical treatments.

The epidemiology of urethritis in Europe has seen important changes during the last decade due to the recent increase of migratory streams from North Africa. The entrance of a large number of migrants to all the European countries has had relevant implications on the urethritis prevalence also increasing the risk diffusion among the youngsters.

Many risk factors coexist in the transmission of urethritis. Youth is a major risk factor due to multiple factors including multiple and simultaneous sexual partners, lack of consistent and proper use of condoms, and increased susceptibility to infection due to their limited immunocompetence. In homosexual and bisexual relationships (especially for men), having more than three different partners (within 3 months from the onset of the infections) seems to be a more important risk factor than age. Marriage seems to be a protective factor due to the lower possibility to have multiple sexual partners. Furthermore, alcohol abuse and/or consumption of other substances, such as drugs or pharmacological compounds, tends to occur or precede sexual risk behaviors among young people [6–8].

Previous urethritis or other sexually transmitted diseases (STDs) occurred during adolescence or human immunodeficiency virus (HIV) infections are other significant factors that could increase the risk of recurrent urethritis episodes [9].

Newbern conducted a cohort study comparing one group of adolescents with previous STDs to another with no previous STDs and found that the first group had a double risk of developing subsequent HIV infection [10]. Similarly, previous *Herpes genitalium* infection can increase the risk of developing subsequent urethritis episodes from *Chlamydia*, *N. gonorrhoeae* and HPV infections [11].

Risk factors for urethritis
• Young age • MSM (men who have sex with men) • Lack of condom • Multiple and simultaneous sexual partners • HIV • Alcohol abuse • Drug consumption

Historically, the term urethritis collects all those pathologies characterized by urethral discharge. However, recent literature has shown that urethritis is more often found in men without discharge but with symptoms such as itching, tingling or dysuria. Urethritis can also be asymptomatic [3].

In men with urethral symptoms, a proper objective examination involves the search for inguinal lymphadenopathy, ulcers, or urethral discharge. The urethra should be gently "milked" with palpation from the bottom to the distal end of the penis. Any discharge thus obtained should be tested with laboratory methods available for gonorrhea and chlamydia. Currently, urethritis is diagnosed by the presence of at least one of the following signs or symptoms: the presence of urethral discharge, a positive result of the leukocyte esterase test in the first-empty urine, or at least 10 white blood cells for high-power field in the first-urinary urine sediment [12]. In the absence of urethral discharge, the urine of the first void needs to be tested to document pyuria and DNA-based tests for *Chlamydia* and *Gonorrhea*. Scrotum palpation is necessary to highlight concomitant epididymitis or orchitis; rectal exploration is a useful evaluation in case of rectal pain. Other possible sites of sexual exposure, such as oropharynx and anus, should be evaluated.

If the clinical suspicion based on anamnesis (the patient reports severe dysuria, hematuria, nocturia, urgency in the absence of sexual exposure), examination (lack of discharge), or laboratory results (nitrite present in the urinalysis) points to a urinary tract infection, a medium-flow urine sample should be obtained [13].

According to the 2022 European guidelines, microscopic examination of urethral discharge in pyogenic urethritis is always recommended and should be performed with Gram stain. Validated nucleic acid amplification tests on first void urine sample should be otherwise performed [14].

The microscopic diagnosis of NGU is made when five or more polymorphonuclear leucocytes (PMNL) are observed in high-powered field (HPF), in the absence of intracellular diplococci in the urethra discharge. However, according to the latest CDC guidelines, this cut-off has been reduced to 2 PMNL, with an increase in diagnosis and, therefore, in resistance. A false urethritis diagnosis may also have an impact on interpersonal relationships. Harald and others studied this aspect and concluded that a standardization of urethral smear microscopy seems to be impossible [15].

16.2 Treatment

The aim of treatment is to reduce symptoms, prevent complications, and reduce sexual transmission of the microorganism involved in the inflammatory process.

Empirical treatments are no more recommended in the latest CDC and European guidelines, although a broad-spectrum antibiotic treatment can be initiated while waiting for the results from the urethral discharge microbiological characterization.

Microbiological characterization by NAATs through adequate urethral discharge collection to determinate the most appropriate and efficient medical treatment is always indicated and recommended.

The risk of developing infections by multiple microorganisms decreases the chance of obtaining successful empirical treatments.

16.2.1 Treatment of Gonococcal Urethritis

Due to the widespread high levels of cephalosporin resistance, first-line treatment consists of combined therapy using a single dose of ceftriaxone 250 mg–1 g IM plus azithromycin 1–2 g orally [12, 16, 17].

Azithromycin is preferred to doxycycline because of the convenience and compliance advantages of single-dose therapy and the substantially higher prevalence of gonococcal resistance to tetracycline than to azithromycin [18]. Therefore, this dual therapy will not entirely prevent emerging resistance [16].

Among other cephalosporins, only cefixime, in a 400–800 mg single oral dose, should be considered as an alternative to ceftriaxone, although it is not as effective due to less favorable pharmacodynamics [18].

In case of cephalosporin allergy, an alternative regimen that can be considered consists of oral gemifloxacin 320 mg plus oral azithromycin 2 g and dual treatment with single doses of intramuscular gentamicin 240 mg plus oral azithromycin 2 g [19]. Use of a single 2 g azithromycin oral dose could be an option to treat uncomplicated gonococcal urethritis if patients are allergic to cephalosporins or are diagnosed as being infected with an Azithromycin-sensitive strain [18, 20, 21].

Lastly, aminocyclitol spectinomycin, with or without other antibiotics, where available, can be a valid alternative to cephalosporin and macrolide combined therapy [22, 23].

Treatment of gonococcal urethritis
• Single-dose ceftriaxone 250 mg–1 g IM PLUS **azithromycin** 1–2 g orally • Alternative: **cefixime** 400–800 mg PLUS **azithromycin** 1–2 g orally OR **gemifloxacin** 320 mg orally PLUS oral **azithromycin** 2 g orally OR **gentamicin** 240 mg IM single dose plus azithromycin 2 g orally OR **azithromycin** 2 g orally OR **spectinomycin** 2 g IM

Adapted from Bachmann et al. [1]

16.2.2 Treatment of Non-gonococcal Urethritis

Men with severe symptoms should be treated immediately with broad-spectrum antibiotics according to the antibiogram after appropriate microbiological investigations. Antibiogram-oriented treatment after NAAT(s) should be considered as mandatory in men with mild symptoms and less significant urethral discharge. Sometimes, urethritis can resolve without treatment [24].

Appropriate antibiotic treatment should be able to determine microbiological eradication (at least in 95% of cases) with low impact on patient's quality of life. Persistence of inflammation may not indicate the persistence of infection and may persist for an unknown length of time, although microbiological investigations should be repeated at least 10 days after the antibiotic treatment interruption [24].

In the 2015 CDC guidelines, the association of *M. genitalium* and STDs was included among the "emerging issues" and is estimated to have an incidence between 6 and 50% in patients with NGU [3]. Among the reasons for this alarmism is the lack of international consensus on treatment, coinfection with HIV, and injudicious use of macrolide by community-acquired pneumonia and inadequate treatment adherence in patients and their partners. *M. genitalium* is devoid of peptidoglycan, and therefore, it is not possible to use antibiotics that act on the cell wall. If proved to be useful tetracyclines, macrolides and quinolones can be used. The dosage and the regimens used with these drugs differ in various parts of the world, giving rise to an increasing resistance to these antibiotics, in particular to macrolides and quinolones [25].

Similarly, *Chlamydia trachomatis* and *Ureaplasma* infections may be easily treated by azithromycin or doxycycline for a period of at least 7 days. Fluoroquinolones may be used as second-line treatment only in selected cases [24].

On the other hand, *Trichomonas vaginalis* male infection may be treated by metronidazole single dose [24].

- ***Chlamydia trachomatis***
  Single-dose **azithromycin** 1 g orally **OR doxycycline** 100 mg orally twice a day for 7 days [26]
  Alternative: **erythromycin** 500 mg orally four times a day for 7 days OR **erythromycin** 800 mg orally four times a day for 7 days OR **levofloxacin** 500 mg orally once daily for 7 days OR **ofloxacin** 300 mg orally twice a day for 7 days [27]
- ***Trichomonas vaginalis***
  Single-dose **metronidazole** or **tinidazole** 2 g orally in a [28]
  Alternative: **metronidazole** 4 g daily for 3–5 days, **doxycycline** 100 mg orally twice a day for 7 days [24, 28, 29]
- ***Ureaplasma urealyticum***
  Doxycycline 100 mg twice daily for 7 days OR a single 1 g dose of **azithromycin** [24, 30]
  Alternative: **clarithromycin** 500 mg bid for 7 days or **azithromycin** at a dose of 1 × 500 mg/6 days [27, 31, 32]
- ***Mycoplasma genitalium***
  Azithromycin 1 g orally OR **doxycycline** 400 mg daily for 7–14 days [2]
  Alternative: **josamycin** 500 mg 3 times a day for 10 days OR **pristinamycin** 1 g 4 times a day for 10 days OR **lymecycline** 300 bd for 10 days [24, 33–37]

16.2.3 Persistent or Recurrent Non-gonococcal Urethritis

Diagnosis of persistent or recurrent non-gonococcal urethritis should be made before considering additional antimicrobial therapy. It is estimated that 20–40% of NGU does not respond to first-line treatment, with up to 20% of men with chlamydial NGU and 30–50% of men with non-chlamydial NGU experiencing persistence/recurrence [24, 38]. The differential diagnosis for recurrence includes reinfection, nonadherence, drug resistance, a persistent post-infectious immunologic response, and complicated infection.

Treatment for persistent or recurrent non-gonococcal urethritis

- If azithromycin is used for initial episode: **moxifloxacin** 400 mg orally for 7 days
- If doxycycline is used for initial episode: **azithromycin** 1 g orally single dose

PLUS

- For men who have sex with women who live in areas where *T. vaginalis* is highly prevalent. **Metronidazole** 2 g orally single dose OR **tinidazole** 2 g orally single dose

16.2.4 Follow-Up and Management of Sexual Partner

To avoid reinfection, abstinence of at least 7 days should be observed from the start of the therapy. All sex partners of men with NGU within the preceding 60 days should be referred for evaluation, testing, and treatment with a drug regimen effective against *Chlamydia trachomatis*.

If *N. gonorrhea* or *T. vaginalis* is documented, all partners should be evaluated and treated properly.

Patients who have been diagnosed with a new STD should receive testing for other STDs, including syphilis and HIV [5, 6, 8, 24].

In case of *Chlamydia*, *N. gonorrhoeae*, or *Trichomonas* infections, partner services should be offered and partners instructed to return 3 months after treatment to repeat testing because of high rates of reinfection.

References

1. Bachmann LH, Manhart LE, Martin DH, Seña AC, Dimitrakoff J, Jensen JS, Gaydos CA. Advances in the understanding and treatment of male urethritis. Clin Infect Dis. 2015;61(Suppl 8):S763–9.
2. Murray P, Rosenthal K, Pfaller M. Medical microbiology. 8th ed. Elsevier; 2015. ISBN: 978032.
3. The 2016 annual report of the Center for Disease Control and Prevention. Atlanta: U.S. Department of Health and Human Services; 2015, pp. 1–177. www.ncsddc.org/wp-content/uploads/2017/09/CDC_2016_STDS_Report_for_508websep21_2017_1644.pdf
4. Horner P, Blee K, O'Mahony C, Muir P, Evans C, Radcliffe K. Clinical Effectiveness Group of the British Association for Sexual Health and HIV. 2015 UK National Guideline on the management of nongonococcal urethritis. Int J STD AIDS. 2016;27(2):85–96.
5. Sonnenberg P, Clifton S, Beddows S. Prevalence, risk factors, and uptake of interventions for sexually transmitted infections in Britain: findings from the National Surveys of Sexual Attitudes and Lifestyles. Lancet. 2013;382:1795–806.
6. Gilbert LK, Levandowski BA, Roberts CM. Characteristics associated with genital herpes testing among young adults: assessing factors from two national data sets. J Am Coll Heal. 2010;59:143–50.
7. Wu LT, Ringwalt CL, Patkar AA, Hubbard RL, Blazer DG. Association of MDMA/ecstasy and other substance use with self-reported sexually transmitted diseases among college-aged adults: a national study. Public Health. 2009;123:557–64.
8. Vivancos R, Abubakar I, Hunter PR. Foreign travel, casual sex, and sexually transmitted infections: systematic review and metanalysis. Int J Infect Dis. 2010;14:e842–51.
9. Bonar EE, Walton MA, Caldwell MT, Whiteside LK, Barry KL, Cunningham RM. Sexually transmitted infection history among adolescents presenting to the emergency department. J Emerg Med. 2015;49(5):613–22.
10. Newbern EC, Anschuetz GL, Eberhart MG, et al. Adolescent sexually transmitted infections and risk for subsequent HIV. Am J Public Health. 2013;103:1874–81.
11. Shiely F, Hayes K, Horgan M. Comparison of risk factors for prevalent sexually transmitted infections based on attendees at two genitourinary medicine clinics in Ireland. Int J STD AIDS. 2014;25(1):29–39.
12. Centers for Disease Control and Prevention. Sexually transmitted diseases treatment guidelines 2015: diseases characterized by urethritis and cervicitis. MMWR. 2015;64(3):51–2. http://www.cdc.gov/STD/t
13. Shahmanesh M, Moi H, Lassau F, Janier M. for IUSTI/WHO. 2009 European guideline on the management of male non-gonococcal urethritis. Int J STD AIDS. 2009;20(7):458–64.
14. Bonkat G, Bartoletti R, Bruyère F, Cai T, Geerlings SE, Koves B, Schubert S, Pilatz A, Veeratterapillay R, Wagenlehner F. EAU Guidelines on urinary infections; 2022.
15. Moi H, Hartgill U. Microscopy of stained urethral smear in male urethritis; which cutoff should be used? Sex Transm Dis. 2017;44(3):189–94.
16. Unemo M, Shafer WM. Antimicrobial resistance in Neisseria gonorrhoeae in the 21st century: past, evolution, and future. Clin Microbiol Rev. 2014;27:587–613.
17. Lewis DA, Sriruttan C, Muller EE, et al. Phenotypic and genetic characterization of the first two cases of extended-spectrum-cephalosporin-resistant *Neisseria gonorrhoeae* infection

in South Africa and association with cefixime treatment failure. J Antimicrob Chemother. 2013;68:1267–70.
18. Newman LM, Moran JS, Workowski KA. Update on the management of gonorrhea in adults in the United States. Clin Infect Dis. 2007;44(Suppl 3):S84–101.
19. Kirkcaldy RD, Weinstock HS, Moore PC, et al. The efficacy and safety of gentamicin plus azithromycin and gemifloxacin plus azithromycin as treatment of uncomplicated gonorrhea. Clin Infect Dis. 2014;59:1083–91.
20. Soda M, Ito S, Matsumaru N, Nakamura S, Nagase I, Takahashi H, Ohno Y, Yasuda M, Yamamoto M, Tsukamoto K, Itoh Y, Deguchi T, Kitaichi K. Evaluation of the microbiological efficacy of a single 2-gram dose of extended-release azithromycin by population pharmacokinetics and simulation in japanese patients with gonococcal urethritis. Antimicrob Agents Chemother. 2017;62(1). pii: e01409-17.
21. Yasuda M, Ito S, Hatazaki K, Deguchi T. Remarkable increase of Neisseria gonorrhoeae with decreased susceptibility of azithromycin and increase in the failure of azithromycin therapy in male gonococcal urethritis in Sendai in 2015. J Infect Chemother. 2016;22(12):841–3.
22. Kojima M, Masuda K, Yada Y, Hayase Y, Muratani T, Matsumoto T. Single-dose treatment of male patients with gonococcal urethritis using 2g spectinomycin: microbiological and clinical evaluations. Int J Antimicrob Agents. 2008;32(1):50–4.
23. Moran JS, Levine WC. Drugs of choice for the treatment of uncomplicated gonococcal infections. Clin Infect Dis. 1995;20(Suppl 1):S47–65.
24. Horner PJ, Blee K, Falk L, van der Meijden W, Moi H. 2016 European guideline on the management of non-gonococcal urethritis. Int J STD AIDS. 2016;27(11):928–37.
25. Tully JG, Taylor-Robinson D, Cole RM, Rose DL. A newly discovered mycoplasma in the human urogenital tract. Lancet. 1981;1(8233):1288–91.
26. Lau CY, Qureshi AK. Azithromycin versus doxycycline for genital chlamydial infections: a meta-analysis of randomized clinical trials. Sex Transm Dis. 2002;29:497–502.
27. Manhart LE, Gillespie CW, Lowens MS, et al. Standard treatment regimens for non gonococcal urethritis have similar but declining cure rates: a randomized controlled trial. Clin Infect Dis. 2013;56:934–42.
28. Seña AC, Bachmann LH, Hobbs MM. Persistent and recurrent Trichomonas vaginalis infections: epidemiology, treatment and management considerations. Expert Rev Anti-Infect Ther. 2014;12(6):673–85.
29. Nanda N, Michel RG, Kurdgelashvili G, Wendel KA. Trichomoniasis and its treatment. Expert Rev Anti-Infect Ther. 2006;4(1):125–35.
30. Skerk V. Azithromycin and doxycycline in the treatment of female patients with acute urethral syndrome caused by Ureaplasma urealyticum: significance of duration of clinical symptoms. Drugs Exp Clin Res. 2001;27(4):135–9.
31. Khosropour CM, Manhart LE, Gillespie CW, Lowens MS, Golden MR, Jensen NL, Kenny GE, Totten PA. Efficacy of standard therapies against Ureaplasma species and persistence among men with non-gonococcal urethritis enrolled in a randomized controlled trial. Sex Transm Infect. 2015;91(5):308–13.
32. Schwebke JR, Rompalo A, Taylor S, et al. Re-evaluating the treatment of nongonococcal urethritis: emphasizing emerging pathogens—a randomized clinical trial. Clin Infect Dis. 2011;52:163–70.
33. Mena LA, Mroczkowski TF, Nsuami M, Martin DH. A randomized comparison of azithromycin and doxycycline for the treatment of Mycoplasma genitalium-positive urethritis in men. Clin Infect Dis. 2009;48:1649–54.
34. Falk L, Fredlund H, Jensen JS. Tetracycline treatment does not eradicate Mycoplasma genitalium. Sex Transm Infect. 2003;79(4):318–9.
35. Bjornelius E, Anagrius C, Bojs G, et al. Antibiotic treatment of symptomatic Mycoplasma genitalium infection in Scandinavia: a controlled clinical trial. Sex Transm Infect. 2008;84(1):72–6.
36. Couldwell DL, Tagg KA, Jeoffreys NJ, Gilbert GL. Failure of moxifloxacin treatment in Mycoplasma genitalium infections due to macrolide and fluoroquinolone resistance. Int J STD AIDS. 2013;24(10):822–8.

37. Sethi S, Zaman K, Jain N. Mycoplasma genitalium infections: current treatment options and resistance issues. Infect Drug Resist. 2017;10:283–92. https://doi.org/10.2147/IDR.S105469. eCollection 2017. Review.
38. Moi H, Blee K, Horner PJ. Management of non-gonococcal urethritis. BMC Infect Dis. 2015;15:294.

Acute Bacterial Prostatitis

17

Paolo Verze, Massimiliano Creta, Gianluigi Califano, and Alessandro Palmieri

17.1 Acute Bacterial Prostatitis

Acute bacterial prostatitis (ABP, category I, NIH classification [1]) is an acute bacterial infection of the prostate gland that causes urinary tract symptoms and pain in men [1] (Table 17.1). ABP is a serious condition, requiring a timely and adequate treatment, due to the risk of developing life-threatening complications, such as urosepsis, or of evolving into chronic bacterial prostatitis (CBP, category II) or into chronic prostatitis/chronic pelvic pain syndrome (CP/CPPS, category III).

Patients with acute bacterial infection of the prostate gland may present systemic symptoms, such as fever, chills, nausea, emesis, and general malaise, that should prompt physicians to determine if patients meet clinical criteria for sepsis [2].

Diagnosis is predominantly made based on clinical history, physical examination, and urine cultures. Any patient at risk should be screened for sexually transmitted infections. Clinicians should investigate urogenital disorders, new sexual contacts, and recent transurethral manipulation procedures or transrectal prostate biopsy. Physical examination focus on lower abdomen, genitalia, and rectum. Digital rectal examination (DRE) of the prostate is not recommended due to the risk of causing bacteriemia, but if done gently, the gland is swollen, tender, warm, and painful. Prostatic massage is contraindicated. A midstream urine culture should be

P. Verze (✉)
Department of Medicine and Surgery, Scuola Medica Salernitana, University of Salerno, Fisciano, Italy
e-mail: pverze@unisa.it

M. Creta · G. Califano · A. Palmieri
Department of Neurosciences, Reproductive Sciences, Odontostomatology—Urology Unit, University of Naples, Federico II, Naples, Italy
e-mail: massimiliano.creta@unina.it; gianluigi.califano@unina.it; alessandro.palmieri@unina.it

T. E. Bjerklund Johansen, T. Cai (eds.), *Guide to Antibiotics in Urology*,
https://doi.org/10.1007/978-3-319-92366-6_17

Table 17.1 Lower urinary tract symptoms and sites pain correlate to acute bacterial prostatitis. Data from the 2017 EAU guidelines

LUTS		Sites of pain
Irritative	Obstructive	Prostate/perineum
Dysuria	Hesitancy	Testes/scrotum
Urinary frequency	Incomplete voiding	Penis
Urinary urgency	Straining to urinate	Urinary bladder
	Weak stream	Lower back

obtained in all patients who are suspected of having ABP for diagnosis and targeted treatment planning. Urinalysis may be useful. Blood cultures are sometimes necessary to detect the septic spread of the disease [3].

Most ABP infections are community acquired, due to ascending urethral infection or intraprostatic reflux, but some occur after invasive maneuvers on the low genitourinary tract, such as urethral catheterization, cystoscopy, or transrectal prostate biopsy.

Most infections are due to aerobic gram-negative bacilli, and *E. coli* cause 50–80% of cases. In sexually active men, *Neisseria gonorrhoeae* and *Chlamydia trachomatis* should be considered [4].

Management of ABP should be based on clinical condition, risk factors, and culture results. The choice of an appropriate antibiotic treatment is central for the treatment of bacterial infections of the prostate. Initial empiric antibiotic therapy is based on the suspected mode of infection and the presumed infecting organism [2]. Antibiotic therapy should be reviewed as soon as culture and antibiogram results are available. Until defervescence and normalization of infection parameters, for systemically ill patients, parenteral administration of high doses of bactericidal antimicrobials is recommended [5] (Table 17.2, a). Clinically stable patients may be treated with oral therapy (Table 17.2, b). Usually, the duration of therapy varies from 2 to 4 weeks.

Table 17.2 shows the complete list of antibiotics used in the management of ABP, according to the EAU guidelines for 2017. It is advisable to repeat urine culture 1 week after the suspension of antibiotic therapy, to verify the complete eradication of the infection [4].

The treatment of bacterial prostatitis is complicated by the difficulty of antibacterial agents to reach the infected prostate tissue [6]. Therefore, the choice of the most appropriate antibiotic treatment must first concentrate on the evaluation of the pharmacokinetic characteristics of the different molecules. *Fluoroquinolones* are recognized as drugs of choice for this clinical indication; compared with concentrations in plasma, drug levels are generally higher in urine, similar in seminal fluid and prostatic tissue, and lower (albeit therapeutic) in prostatic fluid [6, 7]. The increase in resistance to fluoroquinolones is a source of great concern and requires the use of other molecules such as a third-generation cephalosporin (e.g., ceftazidime or ceftriaxone) or a carbapenem (e.g., imipenem or ertapenem). *Cephalosporins* can attain therapeutic levels in prostatic fluid or tissue. *Aztreonam*, *Imipenem*, and

Table 17.2 Recommendations forP the disease management of acute bacterial prostatitis (EAU guidelines, urological infections, 2017)

(a) Acute febrile bacterial prostatitis with symptoms and fever					
Antimicrobial	Daily dose		LE	GR	
Levofloxacin	500 mg/day		2	B	
Ciprofloxacin	500 mg twice daily		2	B	
Ceftriaxone	2 g/day		2	B	
Piperacillin/tazobactam	4.5 g/three times day		2	B	
Cefepime	2 g twice daily		2	B	
(b) Acute afebrile bacterial prostatitis with symptoms or after defervescence					
Antimicrobial	**Daily dose**	**Duration of therapy**	**LE**	**GR**	**Comments**
Levofloxacin	500 mg/day	2–4 weeks	2	B	
Ciprofloxacin	500 mg twice daily or 1000 mg/day	2–4 weeks	2	B	
Trimethoprim	200 mg twice daily	2–4 weeks	2	B	
Co-trimoxazole	960 mg twice daily	2–4 weeks	2	B	
Doxycycline	100 mg twice daily	10 days	2	B	Only for *Chlamydia trachomatis* or *mycoplasma* infections

some aminoglycosides can attain levels in prostatic tissue that exceed the minimum inhibitory concentration of most *Enterobacteriaceae*. *Erythromycin*, *Clindamycin*, and *Trimethoprim* can develop high prostate concentrations.

17.2 Chronic Bacterial Prostatitis

17.2.1 Antibiotic Treatment of Chronic Bacterial Prostatitis: General Principles

Etiological determinants of chronic bacterial prostatitis (CBP, category II, NIH classification [1]) include a wide range of bacteria, yeasts, and cryptic microorganisms. Traditional pathogens include the following: *Enterobacteriaceae* such as *Escherichia coli*, *Klebsiella* spp., *Proteus* spp., *and Pseudomonas* spp. Other microorganisms, such as *Enterococcus* spp. and *Staphylococcus* spp., and unusual pathogens, such as *Chlamydia trachomatis*, *Trichomonas vaginalis*, and *Mycoplasma*, are found to be causative pathogens in CBP less frequently [8]. *M. tuberculosis*, *Candida* spp., and rare pathogens, such as *Coccidioides immitis*, *Blastomyces dermatitidis*, and *Histoplasma capsulatum* may cause CBP in patients with immune deficiency [9]. Anaerobic bacteria have been proposed to play a pathogenic role in CBP, although their role may be underestimated as they are not routinely cultured.

Treatment of CBP primarily involves the use of antibiotics [10]. Adequate concentrations of these agents are required at the site of infection, i.e., prostatic ducts and prostatic secretions [10]. Consequently, antibiotics should travel across both capillary and prostatic epithelia. Unlike acute prostatitis, several barriers hamper the penetration of most antimicrobial agents into a chronically inflamed prostate and into prostatic secretions. Indeed, capillaries are non-fenestrated, and the prostatic epithelium lacks an active transport mechanism facilitating drug uptake within it [7–13]. Moreover, some bacteria involved in CBP, such as *Escherichia coli*, *Staphylococci*, and *Enterococci*, may generate biofilms that allow them to survive in a protected milieu, thus causing resistance to therapy and persistence of infection [10, 11, 14]. Prostatic calcifications, commonly found in CBP patients, have been associated with bacterial biofilms [10]. Additionally, agents such as *Ureaplasma* spp. and *Chlamydia trachomatis* may infect prostate cells and act intracellularly [10, 11].

The European Association of Urology guidelines recommend the following antimicrobial agents: fluoroquinolones, tetracyclines, trimethoprim, or co-trimoxazole (Table 17.3) [9]. Further, antimicrobial agents potentially active in patients suffering from CBP include aminoglycosides and fosfomycin-tromethamine. Combination antibiotic protocols have also been evaluated with promising results [10, 15]. Treatment with intraprostatic injection of antibiotics is supported by only anecdotal reports and therefore is not recommended [16].

Table 17.3 Antibiotic regimens recommended by EAU guidelines

Antimicrobial	Daily dose	Duration of treatment	Comments	Level of evidence	Grade of recommendation
Quinolones					
Levofloxacin	500 mg every day	4–6 weeks		3	B
Ciprofloxacin	500 mg twice daily or 1000 mg every day	4–6 weeks		3	B
Tetracyclines					
Doxycycline	100 mg twice daily	10 days	Only for *Chlamydia trachomatis* or mycoplasma infections	2	B
Co-trimoxazole	960 mg twice daily	4–6 weeks		3	B
Trimethoprim	200 mg twice daily	4–6 weeks		3	B

17.2.2 Fluoroquinolones

Fluoroquinolones are recommended as first-line agents for CBP, except in cases of confirmed or strongly suspected resistance [6, 9]. These agents are active against most usual and atypical pathogens and are available as both oral and intravenous formulations [6]. The main advantage of fluoroquinolones is their good prostate penetration. Indeed, the pH of prostatic fluid in patients with CBP is often alkaline, and fluoroquinolones achieve adequate concentrations in prostatic secretion and seminal fluid, mainly thanks to their amphoteric nature [17]. Moreover, fluoroquinolones are active on biofilms. The following fluoroquinolones have been evaluated for the treatment of CBP: ciprofloxacin, levofloxacin, lomefloxacin, ofloxacin, and prulifloxacin [15]. Although plasma concentrations and penetration rates into prostatic secretion and seminal fluid vary according to the type of fluoroquinolone, current evidences failed to demonstrate significant differences in clinical or microbiological efficacy or in the rate of adverse effects [15, 17]. Overall, microbiological eradication rates for ciprofloxacin, levofloxacin, prulifloxacin, lomefloxacin, and ofloxacin have been reported to be 77%, 75%, 71%, 80%, and 67%, respectively [8, 15, 16, 18–24]. Eradication rates are higher in CBP due to *Escherichia coli* and other members of the family *Enterobacteriaceae*, with respect to *P. aeruginosa* and *Enterococci*. Guidelines recommend a treatment duration with fluoroquinolones of 4–6 weeks [9]. This length of therapy is based on experience and expert opinion and is supported by many clinical studies. A major concern with these agents is the growing problem of resistance. Fluoroquinolone resistance rates in Europe and North America range from ~10% to >30% [25, 26].

17.2.3 Tetracyclines

Tetracyclines are recommended in patients with CBP if intracellular bacteria have been detected or are suspected [9]. These agents are characterized by good penetration into prostatic tissue and secretions. Skerk V. evaluated the efficacy of doxycycline 100 mg twice daily for 28 days in 125 adult patients with CBP due to *Chlamydia trachomatis* [20]. Microbiological eradication rate and clinical cure rate at 4–6 weeks after the end of therapy were 76.6% and 69.7%, respectively [20]. In patients with CBP due to by *Ureaplasma urealyticum*, the microbiological eradication rate and clinical cure rate at 4–6 weeks after the end of therapy with doxycycline 100 mg twice daily for 21 days were 74.1% and 67.7%, respectively [27]. Limits of tetracyclines include absence of activity against *Pseudomonas* and limited activity against many *Enterobacteriaceae* and *Enterococci* [6].

17.2.4 Macrolides

Macrolides are considered alternatives to tetracyclines in patients with CBP if intracellular bacteria have been detected or are suspected [9]. These agents characterized by a good penetration into prostatic tissue and fluids and have a wide spectrum of activity that includes a variety of gram-positive, gram-negative, and anaerobe pathogens [10]. Moreover, macrolides are characterized by high intracellular accumulation [10]. Beyond direct antibacterial activity, pharmacodynamics of macrolides includes nonantibiotic pharmacological properties, such as biofilm inhibition and immunomodulatory actions [10]. The efficacy of macrolides in CBP patients has been evaluated in the context of both monotherapy and combination therapy protocols [20, 21, 23, 28, 29].

As single agent, macrolides showed higher microbiological and clinical cure rates compared to fluoroquinolones in patients with CBP caused by obligate intracellular pathogens [15].

The efficacy of azithromycin (500 mg once daily for three consecutive days for 3 weeks) and ciprofloxacin (500 mg twice daily for 20 days) for the treatment of CBP caused by *C. trachomatis* was compared in a prospective, comparative randomized study [10, 28]. Significantly higher eradication rates and clinical cure rate were achieved in the group of patients receiving azithromycin 4–6 weeks after completion of therapy (80% vs 38.6% and 68.9% vs 34.1%, respectively) [10, 28]. Bacteriological eradication rates and clinical cure rates achieved by azithromycin in patients with CBP caused by *C. trachomatis* and *U. urealyticum* have been reported to be similar to that achieved by doxycycline [10, 20, 27].

The fluoroquinolone-macrolide combination has been effectively administered in patients with CBP caused by both common and uncommon pathogens [10, 30, 31]. Theoretically, the addiction of a macrolide as a highly effective agent against biofilms may translate into improved microbiological eradications [10, 22]. Smelov V. showed that the combination of azithromycin with pefloxacin resulted in increased eradication rates, compared to single-agent regimens in CBP patients presenting with chlamydial infection [10, 32]. The combination of azithromycin and ciprofloxacin has been reported to be effective in eradicating both traditional uropathogens and unusual pathogens infecting the prostate gland, with similar and high eradication rates (traditional uropathogens, 75–84%; unusual uropathogens, 82%) [10, 30, 31]. Pathogen eradication achieved with azithromycin-ciprofloxacin combination was characterized by a rapid symptom decrease and by low rates of clinical relapse/reinfection [10, 33]. Magri V. retrospectively compared the microbiological and clinical findings of two treatment schemes for CBP based on the combination of azithromycin (500 mg, thrice weekly) with a once daily 500 or 750 mg dose of ciprofloxacin [34]. Combined administration of azithromycin with ciprofloxacin at the rate of 750 mg day for 4 weeks rather than at 500 mg day for 6 weeks increased the eradication rates from 62.35% to 77.32% and the total bacteriological success from 71.76% to 85.57% [34].

17.2.5 Trimethoprim and Co-Trimoxazole

Trimethoprim, whether or not combined with sulfamethoxazole (co-trimoxazole), was the mainstay of treatment until the mid-1980s, achieving pathogen eradication in approximately 30–65% of cases [10]. The resistance rate to co-trimoxazole in *E. coli* CBP is 24% [35, 36]. This drug is now indicated as a last-resource agent in case of fluoroquinolone resistance or when first-choice agents are contraindicated [8, 10].

17.2.6 Aminoglycosides

Positive evidence is available about the distribution of certain aminoglycosides to the sites of chronic infection in the prostate. Amikacin can reach concentrations into prostatic fluids higher than β-lactams, tetracyclines, or fluoroquinolones, although the latter show higher prostatic fluid-to-serum ratio [37]. Magri V. evaluated the efficacy of netilmicin (4.5 mg/kg, once daily, intramuscular), combined or not with a β-lactam antibiotic for 4 weeks in patients affected by fluoroquinolone-resistant CBP or excluded from fluoroquinolone therapy due to various contraindications [25]. Follow-up visits were scheduled 6 and 12 months after the end of treatment [25]. Fifty-five out of 70 patients (78.6%) showed eradication of the causative pathogen and a significant reduction of the NIH-Chronic Prostatitis Symptom Index (NIH-CPSI) total score from a baseline median value of 21 to 14 at the end of therapy and to 9 and 8 at 6-month and 12-month follow-up assessments, respectively [25].

17.2.7 Fosfomycin-Tromethamine

Fosfomycin has recently been proposed as an attractive alternative for the treatment of prostatitis because of its high oral bioavailability and ability to attain therapeutic levels in prostatic tissue. The antibiotic concentration in semen has been reported to be higher than the minimal inhibitory concentration against the etiological agent [38]. Fosfomycin-tromethamine has broad-spectrum antimicrobial activity and is useful for treating lower UTIs caused by extended-spectrum β-lactamase-producing *Enterobacteriaceae* [35]. However, microbiological negativization is not always correlated with favorable clinical outcomes [38]. Fosfomycin-tromethamine may be considered an alternative treatment for CBP in patients with multidrug-resistant *Enterobacteriaceae* infection based on susceptibility results and discussion with local microbiologists and resistance or side effects to first-line drugs [23, 35].

References

1. Krieger JN, Nyberg L Jr, Nickel JC. NIH consensus definition and classification of prostatitis. JAMA. 1999;282(3):236–7.
2. Coker TJ, Dierfeldt DM. Acute bacterial prostatitis: diagnosis and management. Am Fam Physician. 2016;15;98(2):114-20
3. Cai T, Bjerklund Johansen TE, et al. Prostatitis and its management. Springer; 2016.

4. Brede CM, Shoskes DA. The etiology and management of acute prostatitis. Nat Rev Urol. 2011;8(4):207–12.
5. Wagenlehner FM, et al. Bacterial prostatitis. World J Urol. 2013;31:711.
6. Lipsky BA, Byren I, Hoey CT. Treatment of bacterial prostatitis. Clin Infect Dis. 2010;50(12):1641–52.
7. Naber KG, Sorgel F. Antibiotic therapy–rationale and evidence for optimal drug concentrations in prostatic and seminal fluid and in prostatic tissue. Andrologia. 2003;35:331–5.
8. Magri V, et al. Fluoroquinolone-macrolide combination therapy for chronic bacterial prostatitis: retrospective analysis of pathogens eradication rates, inflammatory findings and sexual dysfunction. Asian J Androl. 2011 Nov;13(6):813–27.
9. Bonkat G, Pickard R, Bartoletti R, Bruyère F, Geerlings SE, Wagenlehner F, Wullt B. EAU guidelines on urological infections; 2017.
10. Perletti G, Skerk V, Magri V, Markotic A, Mazzoli S, Parnham MJ, Wagenlehner FM, Naber KG. Macrolides for the treatment of chronic bacterial prostatitis: an effective application of their unique pharmacokinetic and pharmacodynamic profile (review). Mol Med Rep. 2011;4(6):1035–44.
11. Soto SM, Smithson A, Martinez JA, Horcajada JP, Mensa J, Vila J. Biofilm formation in uropathogenic Escherichia coli strains: relationship with prostatitis, urovirulence factors and antimicrobial resistance. J Urol. 2007;177(1):365–8.
12. Barza M, Cuchural G. The penetration of antibiotics into the prostate in chronic bacterial prostatitis. Eur J Clin Microbiol. 1984;3(6):503–5.
13. Perletti G, Wagenlehner FM, Naber KG, Magri V. Enhanced distribution of fourth-generation fluoroquinolones in prostatic tissue. Int J Antimicrob Agents. 2009;33:206–10.
14. Mazzoli S. Biofilms in chronic bacterial prostatitis (NIH-II) and in prostatic calcifications. FEMS Immunol Med Microbiol. 2010;59(3):337–44.
15. Perletti G, Marras E, Wagenlehner FM, Magri V. Antimicrobial therapy for chronic bacterial prostatitis. Cochrane Database Syst Rev. 2013;(8):CD009071.
16. Naber KG. Antimicrobial treatment of bacterial prostatitis. Eur Urol Suppl. 2003;2:23–6.
17. Wagenlehner FM, Weidner W, Sörgel F, Naber KG. The role of antibiotics in chronic bacterial prostatitis. Int J Antimicrob Agents. 2005;26(1):1–7.
18. Bundrick W, Heron SP, Ray P, Schiff WM, Tennenberg AM, Wiesinger BA, Wright PA, Wu SC, Zadeikis N, Kahn JB. Levofloxacin versus ciprofloxacin in the treatment of chronic bacterial prostatitis: a randomized double-blind multicenter study. Urology. 2003;62(3):537–41.
19. Zhang ZC, Jin FS, Liu DM, Shen ZJ, Sun YH, Guo YL. Safety and efficacy of levofloxacin versus ciprofloxacin for the treatment of chronic bacterial prostatitis in Chinese patients. Asian J Androl. 2012;14:870–4.
20. Skerk V, Krhen I, Lisić M, Begovac J, Roglić S, Skerk V, Sternak SL, Banaszak A, Strugar-Šulca J, Vuković J. Comparative randomized pilot study of azithromycin and doxycycline efficacy in the treatment of prostate infection caused by Chlamydia trachomatis. Int J Antimicrob Agents. 2004;24(2):188–91.
21. Skerk V, Schönwald S, Krhen I, Markovinović L, Barsić B, Mareković I, Roglić S, Zeljko Z, Vince A, Cajić V. Comparative analysis of azithromycin and clarithromycin efficacy and tolerability in the treatment of chronic prostatitis caused by Chlamydia trachomatis. J Chemother. 2002;14(4):384–9.
22. Magri V, Marras E, Skerk V, Markotić A, Restelli A, Garlaschi MC, Perletti G. Eradication of Chlamydia trachomatis parallels symptom regression in chronic bacterial prostatitis patients treated with a fluoroquinolone-macrolide combination. Andrologia. 2010;42(6):366–75.
23. Rees J, Abrahams M, Doble A, Cooper A, Prostatitis Expert Reference Group (PERG). Diagnosis and treatment of chronic bacterial prostatitis and chronic prostatitis/chronic pelvic pain syndrome: a consensus guideline. BJU Int. 2015;116(4):509–25.
24. Giannarini G, Mogorovich A, Valent F, Morelli G, De Maria M, Manassero F, Barbone F, Selli C. Prulifloxacin versus levofloxacin in the treatment of chronic bacterial prostatitis: a prospective, randomized, double-blind trial. J Chemother. 2007;19(3):304–8.

25. Magri V, Montanari E, Marras E, Perletti G. Aminoglycoside antibiotics for NIH category II chronic bacterial prostatitis: a single-cohort study with one-year follow-up. Exp Ther Med. 2016;12(4):2585–93.
26. Dalhoff A. Global fluoroquinolone resistance epidemiology and implictions for clinical use. Interdiscip Perspect Infect Dis. 2012;2012:976273.
27. Skerk V, Mareković I, Markovinović L, Begovac J, Skerk V, Barsić N, Majdak-Gluhinić V. Comparative randomized pilot study of azithromycin and doxycycline efficacy and tolerability in the treatment of prostate infection caused by Ureaplasma urealyticum. Chemotherapy. 2006;52(1):9–11.
28. Skerk V, Schönwald S, Krhen I, Banaszak A, Begovac J, Strugar J, Strapac Z, Vrsalovic R, Vukovic J, Tomas M. Comparative analysis of azithromycin and ciprofloxacin in the treatment of chronic prostatitis caused by Chlamydia trachomatis. Int J Antimicrob Agents. 2003;21(5):457–62.
29. Nickel JC, Patel M, Cameron M. Chronic prostatitis/chronic pelvic pain syndrome: finding a way forward in the United Kingdom: report from the first United Kingdom symposium on chronic prostatitis, January 30, 2008, London, United Kingdom. Rev Urol. 2008;10(2):160–3; Spring.
30. Magri V, Trinchieri A, Pozzi G, Restelli A, Garlaschi MC, Torresani E, Zirpoli P, Marras E, Perletti G. Efficacy of repeated cycles of combination therapy for the eradication of infecting organisms in chronic bacterial prostatitis. Int J Antimicrob Agents. 2007;29(5):549–56.
31. Magri V, Trinchieri A, Ceriani I, Marras E, Perletti G. Eradication of unusual pathogens by combination pharmacological therapy is paralleled by improvement of signs and symptoms of chronic prostatitis syndrome. Arch Ital Urol Androl. 2007;79(2):93–8.
32. Smelov V, Gorelov A, Smelova N, Krylova T. Single-drug or combined antibacterial therapy in the treatment of patients with chronic prostatitis and Chlamydia trachomatis? Int J Antimicrob Agents. 2004;23(Suppl 1):S83–7.
33. Magri V, Trinchieri A, Montanari E, Del Nero A, Mangiarotti B, Zirpoli P, de Eguileor M, Marras E, Ceriani I, Vral A, Perletti G. Reduction of PSA values by combination pharmacological therapy in patients with chronicprostatitis: implications for prostate cancer detection. Arch Ital Urol Androl. 2007;79(2):84–92.
34. Magri V, Montanari E, Škerk V, Markotić A, Marras E, Restelli A, Naber KG, Perletti G. Fluoroquinolone-macrolide combination therapy for chronic bacterial prostatitis: retrospective analysis of pathogen eradication rates, inflammatory findings and sexual dysfunction. Asian J Androl. 2011;13(6):819–27.
35. Los-Arcos I, Pigrau C, Rodríguez-Pardo D, Fernández-Hidalgo N, Andreu A, Larrosa N, Almirante B. Long-term fosfomycin-tromethamine oral therapy for difficult-to-treat chronic bacterial prostatitis. Antimicrob Agents Chemother. 2015;60(3):1854–8.
36. Cai T, Mazzoli S, Meacci F, Boddi V, Mondaini N, Malossini G, Bartoletti R. Epidemiological features and resistance pattern in uropathogens isolated from chronic bacterial prostatitis. J Microbiol. 2011;49(3):448–54.
37. Goto T, Makinose S, Ohi Y, Yamauchi D, Kayajima T, Nagayama K, Hayami H. Diffusion of piperacillin, cefotiam, minocycline, amikacin and ofloxacin into the prostate. Int J Urol. 1998;5(3):243–6.
38. Heras-Cañas V, Gutiérrez-Soto B, Almonte-Fernández H, Lara-Oya A, Navarro-Marí JM, Garrido-Frenich A, Vázquez-Alonso F, Gutiérrez-Fernández J. Antibiotic activity and concentrations in clinical samples from patients with chronic bacterial prostatitis. Actas Urol Esp. 2017;41(10):631–8.

Treatment of Epididymitis and Orchitis 18

José Medina-Polo

18.1 Introduction and Epidemiology

Epididymitis consists of an acute or chronic inflammation affecting the epididymis. If the clinical condition lasts less than 6 weeks, it is considered acute epididymitis; chronic epididymitis is considered when the symptoms are present longer than 3 months. The infection may spread from the epididymis to the testicle, which is then called epididymo-orchitis. Acute epididymitis is the most common cause for seeking emergency medical care due to scrotal pain in adults, and one of the most frequent urological infectious conditions in men [1, 2]. It is estimated that the incidence rate ranges from 25 to 65 cases per 10,000 adult males per year [3]. Among men younger than 50 years old, epididymitis represents 0.29% of ambulatory office visits, reaching up to 600,000 cases per year in the United States [1].

18.2 Etiology and Pathophysiology

The most common causes of epididymitis and orchitis are secondary to sexually transmitted infections (STIs) or *Enterobacteriaceae* that cause other types of urinary tract infections, such as *Escherichia coli* (*E. coli*), *Klebsiella* spp., and *Proteus mirabilis* [4]. *Neisseria gonorrhoeae* and *Chlamydia trachomatis* are the most common etiology for sexually transmitted epididymitis. *E. coli* may be the cause for acute epididymitis in men with sexual transmission from anal intercourse [5]. Although, traditionally, the cutoff age of 35 years has been proposed for a sexually transmitted origin in young patients, several studies stated that age should not be considered as the primary parameter for the suspicion of a sexually transmitted infection (STI) [6].

J. Medina-Polo (✉)
Department of Urology, Health Research Institute i+12, Hospital Universitario 12 de Octubre imas12, Madrid, Spain
e-mail: jose.medina@salud.madrid.org

T. E. Bjerklund Johansen, T. Cai (eds.), *Guide to Antibiotics in Urology*,
https://doi.org/10.1007/978-3-319-92366-6_18

Apart from sexually transmitted infections and *Enterobacteriaceae*-mediated epididymo-orchitis, other causes such as systemic infections, secondary to urinary manipulation, congenital abnormalities, enterovirus or mumps virus orchitis/epididymitis, tuberculous epididymitis, urinary reflux into the vas deferens, and trauma have been described. Despite the fact that it is a rare condition, epididymo-orchitis secondary to viral sources might be associated with direct viral infection or postinfectious immunologic epididymal reaction secondary to adenoviruses, enteroviruses, BK viruses, and Epstein-Barr [7–9]. (The etiology and risk factors for acute epididymitis is summarized in Table 18.1).

Although microorganisms might reach the epididymis by systemic pathways, the main mechanism implicated in the pathophysiology of the infection is a canalicular route from the urethra ascending through the vas deferens. Therefore, symptoms related to urethritis or a urinary tract infection might precede the diagnosis of epididymo-orchitis by anything from days to weeks. However, in patients where the disease is related to *C. trachomatis*, urethral discharge is not usually reported [10]. Even though the ascending canalicular route is also confirmed in men with an indwelling urinary catheter into the lower urinary tract, the infection can appear in men who have previously undergone a vasectomy [1, 11].

The infection is usually localized in the epididymis, and the testicle is not affected. The testis has a higher resistance to the infection due to an abundant blood and lymphatic supply; severe epididymitis can extend to the testicle, causing epididymal-orchitis. However, if an adequate therapy is not prescribed, it is estimated that the infection will spread from the epididymis to the testis within a couple of days [6].

Table 18.1 Etiology for epididymo-orchitis

Etiology for epididymo-orchitis	
Acute infectious epididymitis	Sexually transmitted infection *Neisseria gonorrhoeae* *Chlamydia trachomatis* *Enterobacteriaceae* infection No risk factors Urinary manipulation Catheter-associated epididymitis
Epididymitis secondary to mumps virus	Prior salivary gland enlargement and viral symptoms
Viral epididymitis (prior respiratory tract infection)	Direct viral infection of the epididymis Immunological epididymal reaction
Epididymitis due to congenital abnormalities	Ectopic ureter meatus
Epididymitis due to urinary reflux into the seminal vesicles and vas deferens	
Epididymitis secondary to scrotal trauma	
Infectious chronic epididymitis	Tuberculous epididymitis (associated with immunosuppression) *Brucella* and *Candida*

The main histological characteristics of the epididymitis include inflammatory reaction, numerous leucocytes, and an abscess in advanced cases. The infection spreads from the inferior to the superior part of the epididymis. The testicle and the vaginal may be affected and a reactional hydrocele or even a pyocele may be presented [12].

18.3 Symptoms and Signs

The main reason for seeking medical care is unilateral scrotal pain irradiating toward the inguinal and lumbar region with an onset from hours to days. Fever may also be present in up to one-third of patients [6]. In severe cases, the patient may present with sepsis symptoms. Those older than 65 years old, with a history of diabetes mellitus and fever, are associated with a more severe clinical presentation [13]. Mumps epididymo-orchitis should be suspected in cases with unilateral and painful enlargement of the testis occurring 1–2 weeks after parotiditis [14].

Physical exploration reveals pain, swelling, tenderness, and increased temperature of the epididymis, the testis, and the spermatic cord. The inflammation starts from the tail of the epididymis and extends to the head of the epididymis and the testis. The affected part of the epididymis is usually indurated. In early stages, the cremasteric reflex is presented. Therefore, the contraction of cremasteric muscle produces testis elevation. Moreover, the pain in the scrotum decreases when the testis is elevated (Prehn's sign). Although physical examination and Prehn's sign are useful in the differential diagnosis of testicular torsion, the primary diagnostic tool for differentiating both entities is a scrotal ultrasound [15].

The scrotal skin may be involved with edema and erythema. A reactional hydrocele may be associated with orchitis and epididymis. The size of the testis is increased by doubling or tripling the standard dimensions. Especially, attention is required about signs related to severe disease and sepsis such as fever or tachycardia [13, 16].

According to the original paper by Campbell in 1927, rectal examination might be recommended to exclude prostatic abscess as the canalicular ascending route is the main origin of the infection [12].

18.4 Diagnostic Evaluation

The most important differential diagnosis to rule out is testicular torsion, more frequent in children and young men.

The medical history should include information about sexual history, inguinal or scrotal surgery, and previous urethral instrumentation such urinary catheter or cystoscopy.

The following studies are useful in the diagnostic workup:

- Urine analysis: Hematuria, leucocytes, and nitrites in urine suggest an infection of the urinary tract. Although no alterations in urine analysis are common in patients with epididymitis and orchitis, leukocyturia and positive nitrites are reported in up to 80% and 30% of patients, respectively [6, 17].
- The urine culture may reveal the microorganism responsible for the infection. All microbiological cultures should be collected before initiating antibiotic treatment to ensure adequate isolation and detection of the microorganisms involved. Both the urine culture and urethral smear should be performed to identify *Enterobacteriaceae*, *C. trachomatis*, or *N. gonorrhoeae* when sexually transmitted infections are suspected. As sexually transmitted diseases are responsible for many cases considered idiopathic in patients with no risk factors, diagnostic studies including *C. trachomatis*, *N. gonorrhoeae,* and *Mycoplasma* are recommended in all sexually active patients [7]. The diagnosis of gonococcal infection is confirmed by the presence of white blood cells containing intracellular Gram-negative diplococci. *N. gonorrhoeae*, *Mycoplasma,* and *Chlamydia* isolation are assessed in first-void urine, urethral smear, or by a nucleic acid amplification test (NAAT) using chain reaction-based methods depending on local availability [1, 2].
- A blood sample is useful to rule out leukocytosis, an increase in the neutrophils, and a decrease in the percentage of lymphocytes. Leukocytosis is reported in up to 70%, and elevated levels of C-reactive protein are frequently found. In severe cases of systemic reaction and sepsis, the blood test might reveal thrombocytopenia and abnormalities in coagulation. Other tests such as semen cultures are not recommended [6].
- Scrotal ultrasound: It is the principal imaging study evaluation for all scrotal conditions. The epididymis and testicles are evaluated for size, inflammation signs, and possible neoplasms. Furthermore, an abscess or areas of testicular infarction may be diagnosed in severe cases. If a hydrocele is present, the ultrasound may reveal characteristics of a complicated hydrocele. Finally, the differential diagnosis of testicular torsion and infectious conditions may be assessed by Doppler ultrasound of the vascular supply of the testicle. In case of epididymitis, scrotal Doppler ultrasound demonstrated epididymal hyperperfusion, which also affects the testes in case of orchitis [16]. In cases where the diagnosis of epididymo-orchitis is clear in physical examination, and there is no diagnostic doubt, scrotal ultrasound is not required [6]. Scrotal ultrasound is mandatory in case of no response to treatment, severe disease, an unclear diagnosis, and a large reactive hydrocele [1, 2].
- A mumps infection diagnosis relies on serology with positive immunoglobulin M (IgM) and negative or positive immunoglobulin G (IgG) [14].
- Functional studies of the urinary tract are advised for pediatric patients with recurrent episodes to rule out underlying abnormalities [8].

Table 18.2 Differential diagnosis of acute epididymo-orchitis

	Acute epididymitis	Testicular torsion	Appendix testis torsion
Duration of symptoms	1–4 days	Hours	Days
Pain intensity	Moderate	Severe	Moderate
Age	From boys to old men	Adolescents, young adults	Children
Other associated symptoms	Urinary symptoms, fever	Nausea/vomiting	
Swelling	Spread from the tail of the epididymis to the head of the testis	High-riding, transversally oriented testis	Epididymal head
Physical examination	Epididymis induration	Testes elevated and transversally positioned	Palpable nodule with a blue dot sign on the upper pole
Cremaster reflex	Present in mild forms	Usually absent	Present
Prawn's sign	Positive (pain relief with testis elevation)	Negative (pain exacerbation with testis elevation)	–
Urine analysis	Pyuria, leukocytosis	No alterations	No alterations
Ultrasound	Increased perfusion	Absent/decreased perfusion	Normal/increased perfusion in the epididymal head

18.5 Differential Diagnosis

The differential diagnosis required in cases with acute scrotal pain and swelling is summarized in Table 18.2.

Testicular Torsion: It constitutes a urological emergency, and surgical treatment is required. Testicular torsion mainly affects young men and is characterized by a sudden onset of testicular pain. A scrotal evaluation may reveal an ascended and horizontalized testicle. In some cases, the torsion in the cremasteric cord is palpated. Doppler ultrasound confirms the diagnosis with a reduced or absent testicular vascular supply. Doppler ultrasound has reported a sensitivity of 90% and a specificity of 97% to diagnose testicular torsion [15].

Torsion in the appendix testis is presented as a painful nodule in the upper pole of the testicle and occurs in children. Examination may reveal a blue color in the region where the torsion is located [8].

Testicular Tumor: It usually appears as a painless mass in the testicle in men aged between 15 and 50 years old. Inflammations signs are absent, and the epididymis is not affected in localized cases. Scrotal ultrasound constitutes the primary diagnostic tool. Blood analysis should be performed as the levels of tumor markers alpha-fetoprotein (AFP) and beta-human chorionic gonadotropin (HCG) can be elevated [6].

Hydrocele: It is defined as the pathologic accumulation of liquid into the scrotum surrounding the testicle. A scrotal ultrasound is required in order to rule out any testicular pathology such trauma, orchitis, or tumor.

Varicocele: It is defined as a pathologic enlargement of the pampiniform venous plexus in the scrotum. The main clinical presentation is chronic scrotal pain without inflammatory signs.

Inguinal hernia and **testicular trauma** are also included in the differential diagnosis in patients with acute scrotal pain.

18.6 Disease Management

General Principles in the Treatment of Infectious Epididymitis and Orchitis:

- Relative rest and avoid any effort.
- Scrotal elevation and tight underwear.
- Local cooling.
- Pain and inflammation are managed with nonsteroidal anti-inflammatories drugs.
- Avoid sexual intercourse until the infection is completely cured and information about the risk factors for sexually transmitted infections has been shared with the patients and their sexual partners.

Antibiotics: Empirical antimicrobial treatment is chosen according to the suspected source of the infection (STI or urinary tract infection), local susceptibility patterns, and the penetration properties into the epididymis and the testis. The empirical management should be effective against *C. trachomatis* and *Enterobacteriaceae* such as quinolones. Currently, fluoroquinolones with activity against *C. trachomatis* are considered the first choice when *N. gonorrhoeae* is not suspected [3]. Although quinolones are a group of antibiotics with a high penetration into the testicular parenchyma, high resistance rates are reported in some regions, for instance, in the South of Europe [4, 18]. It should bear in mind that ciprofloxacin, which is frequently prescribed, is not effective in the treatment of *C. trachomatis* [19]. In case of epididymitis, treatment of 10–14 days is recommended and 3 weeks in case of orchitis. Doxycycline and tetracyclines constitute an alternative in the treatment of *C. trachomatis*. When. *N. gonorrhoeae* is suspected, a single parenteral dose with third-generation cephalosporin is advisable [6].

An essential point in the treatment of acute epididymitis secondary to a sexually transmitted infection (STI) is that sexual partners should also be treated to prevent reinfection and avoid transmission of the disease. The rate of infection in sexual partners has been reported in 50%–80% of cases with Epididymitis secondary to *Chlamydia*, and the infection may be asymptomatic [10, 11, 19]. Antibiotic recommendations for empirical management of epididymitis and orchitis are summarized in Table 18.3.

Most of the patients are managed on an outpatient basis. For patients with high fever, systemic inflammatory response syndrome, and sepsis, hospitalization and

Table 18.3 Antibiotic management of epididymitis and orchitis

Management of epididymitis and orchitis	
Antibiotics effective against *C. trachomatis* and *Enterobacteriaceae* if gonorrhea is not suspected	Fluoroquinolones such as levofloxacin 500 mg once a day or ofloxacin 300 mg twice a day for 10–14 days
	Doxycycline: Initial dose with 200 mg plus 100 mg twice a day for 10–14 days PLUS Antibiotic active against *Enterobacteriaceae* for 10–14 days such as third-generation cephalosporins
	Tetracyclines 500 mg orally every 6 h for 10 days PLUS Antibiotic active against *Enterobacteriaceae* for 10–14 days such as third-generation cephalosporins
If gonorrhea is suspected: combination of antibiotics active against *N. gonorrhoeae* and *C. trachomatis*	Single dose of ceftriaxone 500 mg intramuscularly plus 10–14 days doxycycline (initial dose with 200 mg plus 100 mg twice)

parenteral treatment management can be required, following the same principles described in the management of sepsis.

If a testicular or epididymal abscess is diagnosed, surgical drainage is recommended, although in small and selected cases, conservative therapy may achieve complete resolution [7]. Surgical treatment consisting of epididymectomy and orchiectomy is seldom necessary but is indicated whether testicular infarction and scrotal abscess or phlegmon [16].

18.7 Chronic Epididymitis/Orchitis

Chronic epididymitis is defined as cases where complete resolution is not achieved or the clinical symptoms last at least 6 weeks and significantly interfere with the daily activities. The patient usually reports uni- or bilateral discomfort or pain in the scrotum. It is necessary to rule out some less frequent causes of infectious epididymitis and orchitis such as granulomatous reactions, including tuberculous epididymitis, brucellosis, and sarcoidosis. Other etiologies that cause chronic epididymo-orchitis are obstruction (post vasectomy), postinfectious inflammatory reactions, induced by drugs (amiodarone), and associated with Behçet's disease [20, 21].

The evaluation of the epididymis usually reveals an increase in the epididymal volume and consistency. Pain during palpation is the main sign. Epididymal and testicular tumors are the leading differential diagnosis, and a scrotal ultrasound is recommended. Other diseases to rule out are hydrocele, painful varicocele, and chronic pain syndrome [6].

Chronic epididymitis can obstruct the epididymis, and the semen quality can deteriorate, which can include a decrease in sperm count and mobility. Moreover, the seminal analysis might show an increasing number of peroxidase-positive white blood cells and elevated levels of inflammatory markers such as interleukin 6 (IL-6) and IL-8. Other abnormalities in sperm are atypical staining of flagella, alterations in DNA integrity, increased granulocyte elastase, and decreased α-glucosidase [22].

The management of chronic epididymo-orchitis is frequently a challenging task. Several treatments have been proposed ranging from conservative treatment to surgery. Local heat, scrotal elevation, and avoiding activities that worsen symptoms are included among conservative recommendations with variable outcomes. Medical treatment includes nonsteroidal anti-inflammatory agents, antibiotics, phytotherapy, anxiolytics, narcotic analgesic, acupuncture and injection with steroid, anesthetic drugs for spermatic cord blockage, or onabotulinumtoxin A [6, 21]. Therefore, empiric antibiotic treatment with quinolones for 2–4 weeks and pain management with nonsteroidal anti-inflammatory agents are recommended as first-choice therapy. In men with refractory pain, drugs such as amitriptyline at an initial dose of 10–20 mg at night, gabapentin 300 mg three times a day, or pregabalin 75–150 mg once a day are advised. Tatem and Kovac reported a technique for spermatic cord blockage with an injection at the level of the pubic tubercle consisting of 10–20 cc of a 50:50 mixture with 2% lidocaine and 0.25% bupivacaine [23].

Surgical treatment with epididymectomy and microdenervation of the spermatic cord (MDSC) are alternatives in cases refractory to more conservative treatments, with better results in patients with a previous vasectomy or epididymal cysts. MDSC consists of division of all structures in the spermatic cord sparing only arteries, lymphatics, and vas deferens (if required). Impaired sperm quality and alterations in testicular blood supply are the main possible adverse events associated with epididymectomy. Both medical and surgical treatment reported a pain relief rate between 30% and 82%, with better results in patients with structural abnormalities in the epididymis. Finally, orchiectomy has also been proposed as the last surgical option, with a cure rate ranging from 55% to 73% in selected cases [23–26].

Tuberculous epididymitis: It is characterized by a subacute onset with swelling affecting one or both epididymis or testes and may be associated with systemic symptoms. The infection spreads from the epididymis to the testicle. Prostatic tuberculosis should be considered in cases with bilateral involvement. Other signs in advanced cases are scrotal thickening and cutaneous fistula [21]. A compromised immune system is a risk factor for tuberculosis, and genitourinary infection leads to infertility. The diagnosis relies on the results of an acid-fast bacilli culture and a nucleic acid amplification test (NAAT) for *Mycobacterium tuberculosis* DNA. The development of chronic epididymo-orchitis following treatment with intravesical instillation with bacillus Calmette-Guérin (BCG) has also been described [27, 28]. Antimicrobiological treatment includes a combination of antituberculosis drugs. One of the regimens proposed for tuberculous epididymo-orchitis consists of a 2-month treatment with a combination of isoniazid, rifampicin, pyrazinamide, and ethambutol, followed by a 4- to 6-month treatment with isoniazid and rifampicin [28]. Epididymectomy or orchiectomy is indicated in case of an abscess, medical treatment failure, or difficulties in the differential diagnosis with a testicular tumor [29].

18.8 Follow-Up After Epididymitis and Orchitis

In case of complete recovery after infectious epididymitis and orchitis, no additional studies are required. Semen quality may be impaired during the infection or due to obstructive azoospermia. Sperm disorders are more common in cases of recurrent chronic epididymo-orchitis [22]. Nevertheless, in most of the cases with a single acute infection, no alteration in semen parameters is reported after following successful treatment [3].

Vaccination against parotiditis is the main measure to prevent mumps epididymo-orchitis as mumps may affect the testicles and induce impaired spermatogenesis in up to 13% of patients. It is estimated that testicular atrophy occurs in 30%–50% of affected testes. In young patients with a suspicion of mumps infections, the vaccination status should be assessed [14].Conflict of InterestsThe author of the manuscript has not any conflict of interest regarding this paper.

References

1. 2015 STD Treatment Guidelines [Internet]. [cited 2017 Nov 13]. https://www.cdc.gov/std/tg2015/default.htm
2. Sexually transmitted diseases: summary of 2015 CDC treatment guidelines. J Miss State Med Assoc. 2015;56(12):372–5.
3. EAU Guidelines on Urological infections 2017 [Internet]. [cited 2017 Nov 5]. http://uroweb.org/wp-content/uploads/19-Urological-infections_2017_web.pdf
4. Eickhoff JH, Frimodt-Møller N, Walter S, Frimodt-Møller C. A double-blind, randomized, controlled multicentre study to compare the efficacy of ciprofloxacin with pivampicillin as oral therapy for epididymitis in men over 40 years of age. BJU Int. 1999;84(7):827–34.
5. Redfern TR, English PJ, Baumber CD, McGhie D. The aetiology and management of acute epididymitis. Br J Surg. 1984;71(9):703–5
6. Çek M, Sturdza L, Pilatz A. Acute and chronic epididymitis. Eur Urol Suppl. 2017;16(4):124–31.
7. Pilatz A, Hossain H, Kaiser R, Mankertz A, Schüttler CG, Domann E, et al. Acute epididymitis revisited: impact of molecular diagnostics on etiology and contemporary guideline recommendations. Eur Urol. 2015;68(3):428–35.
8. Gkentzis A, Lee L. The aetiology and current management of prepubertal epididymitis. Ann R Coll Surg Engl. 2014;96(3):181–3.
9. Pilatz A, Kaiser R, Mankertz A, Schuppe H-C, Weidner W, Wagenlehner F. 139 Viral epididymitis and orchitis—myth or reality? Eur Urol Suppl. 2015;14(2):e139.
10. Robinson AJ, Grant JBF, Spencer RC, Potter C, Kinghorn GR. Acute epididymitis: why patient and consort must be investigated. Br J Urol. 1990;66(6):642–5.
11. Pearson RC, Baumber CD, McGhie D, Thambar IV. The relevance of *Chlamydia trachomatis* in acute epididymitis in young men. Br J Urol. 1988;62(1):72–5.
12. Campbell MF. Gonococcus epididymitis: observations in three thousand cases from the urological service of Bellevue hospital. Ann Surg. 1927;86(4):577–90.
13. Hongo H, Shinojima T, Yazawa S, Kanao K, Morita S, Kosaka T, et al. MP16-18 development of an algorithm for predicting severe acute epididymitis. J Urol. 2014;191(4):e160.

14. Tae BS, Ham BK, Kim JH, Park JY, Bae JH. Clinical features of mumps orchitis in vaccinated postpubertal males: a single-center series of 62 patients. Korean J Urol. 2012;53(12):865–9.
15. Yu K-J, Wang T-M, Chen H-W, Wang H-H. The dilemma in the diagnosis of acute scrotum: clinical clues for differentiating between testicular torsion and epididymo-orchitis. Chang Gung Med J. 2012;35(1):38–45.
16. Pilatz A, Wagenlehner F, Bschleipfer T, Schuppe H-C, Diemer T, Linn T, et al. Acute epididymitis in ultrasound: results of a prospective study with baseline and follow-up investigations in 134 patients. Eur J Radiol. 2013;82(12):e762–8.
17. Kaver I, Matzkin H, Braf ZF. Epididymo-orchitis: a retrospective study of 121 patients. J Fam Pract. 1990;30(5):548–52.
18. Sadahira T, Wada K, Araki M, Ebara S, Watanabe M, Watanabe T, et al. 162 Pharmacokinetics of fluoroquinolones into human epididymis. Eur Urol Suppl. 2016;15(3):e162.
19. Drury NE, Dyer JP, Breitenfeldt N, Adamson AS, Harrison GSM. Management of acute epididymitis: are European guidelines being followed? Eur Urol. 2004;46(4):522–5.
20. Strebel RT, Schmidt C, Beatrice J, Sulser T. Chronic scrotal pain syndrome (CSPS): the widespread use of antibiotics is not justified. Andrology. 2013;1(1):155–9.
21. Nickel JC, Siemens DR, Nickel KR, Downey J. The patient with chronic epididymitis: characterization of an enigmatic syndrome. J Urol. 2002;167(4):1701–4.
22. Haidl G, Allam JP, Schuppe H-C. Chronic epididymitis: impact on semen parameters and therapeutic options. Andrologia. 2008;40(2):92–6.
23. Tatem A, Kovac JR. Chronic scrotal pain and microsurgical spermatic cord denervation: tricks of the trade. Transl Androl Urol. 2017;6(S1):S30–6.
24. Calleary JG, Masood J, Hill JT. Chronic epididymitis: is epididymectomy a valid surgical treatment? Int J Androl. 2009;32(5):468–72.
25. Sweeney P, Tan J, Butler MR, McDermott TE, Grainger R, Thornhill JA. Epididymectomy in the management of intrascrotal disease: a critical reappraisal. Br J Urol. 1998;81(5):753–5.
26. Levine L. Chronic orchialgia: evaluation and discussion of treatment options. Ther Adv Urol. 2010;2(5–6):209–14.
27. Hoag N, Pommerville PJ, Kibsey PC, Cavers DJ, Eddy RJ. Tuberculous epididymitis following intravesical Bacillus Calmette-Guérin immunotherapy. Can J Urol. 2009;16(2):4589–91.
28. Kulchavenya E, Naber K, Bjerklund Johansen TE. Urogenital tuberculosis: classification, diagnosis, and treatment. Eur Urol Suppl. 2016;15(4):112–21.
29. Gómez García I, Gómez Mampaso E, Burgos Revilla J, Molina MR, Sampietro Crespo A, Buitrago LA, et al. Tuberculous orchiepididymitis during 1978-2003 period: review of 34 cases and role of 16S rRNA amplification. Urology. 2010;76(4):776–81.

Part V

Antibiotic Prophylaxis and Treatment of Infectious Complications After Urological Procedures

Principles of Antibiotic Prophylaxis in Urology: Why, When and How

19

Lars Fredrik Qvigstad, Tommaso Cai, José Medina-Polo, Zafer Tandogdu, and Truls E. Bjerklund Johansen

19.1 Introduction

The aim of antibiotic prophylaxis (AP) is to avoid nosocomial infections. Before the introduction of antibiotic prophylaxis, most surgical procedures were open surgery and postoperative infections were common. To counteract infections, surgeons adhered carefully to classical principles such as anatomical dissection, avoidance of unnecessary bleeding and cautery, reducing damage to superficial structures by limiting pressure from retractors, containing spillage of gastrointestinal contents and

L. F. Qvigstad (✉)
Department of Urology, Oslo University Hospital, Oslo, Norway
e-mail: larqvi@ous-hf.no

T. Cai
Department of Urology, Santa Chiara Regional Hospital, Trento, Italy

Institute of Clinical Medicine, University of Oslo, Oslo, Norway
e-mail: tommaso.cai@apss.tn.it

J. Medina-Polo
Department of Urology, Health Research Institute i+12, Hospital Universitario 12 de Octubre imas12, Madrid, Spain
e-mail: jose.medina@salud.madrid.org

Z. Tandogdu
Department of Urology, University College London Hospital, London, UK

University College London, Medical School, London, UK
e-mail: z.tandogdu@ucl.ac.uk

T. E. B. Johansen
Department of Urology, Oslo University Hospital, Oslo, Norway

Institute of Clinical Medicine, University of Oslo, Oslo, Norway

Institute of Clinical Medicine, University of Aarhus, Aarhus, Denmark
e-mail: t.e.b.johansen@medisin.uio.no

T. E. Bjerklund Johansen, T. Cai (eds.), *Guide to Antibiotics in Urology*,
https://doi.org/10.1007/978-3-319-92366-6_19

urine, ensuring proper drainage, prioritizing delayed primary closure in high-risk situations, early evacuation of hematomas, and generally keeping operation times to a minimum. Urologists avoided the abdominal approach as much as possible in order not to spread infected urine to the abdominal cavity. It was a conventional wisdom that the best surgeons had the fewest infections.

The introduction of antibiotic prophylaxis lead to a significant reduction in postoperative infections and made the development of modern medicine possible. Transplantation surgery, intensive care medicine, neonatal medicine, oncology, etc. would not have been possible without effective AP. Urologists converted from the retroperitoneal approach to the transabdominal route, as the minimally invasive techniques developed. Bleeding could now be reduced by increasing the abdominal pressure and more extensive use of cautery. Application of non-resorbable foreign bodies also emerged as means to ligate vessels. Long-lasting procedures became more common, as for example, robot-assisted radical cystectomy with urinary reconstruction. In the modern era of surgical training, the concept of contamination categories, and the classical surgical principles for reducing infectious complications have become less emphasized.

Gradually, we have realized that the period of available effective antibiotic prophylaxis and treatment might soon end. Due to increasing antimicrobial resistance, current antibiotics are losing efficacy. Without new antibiotics in the pipelines of pharmaceutical companies, the prospects are poor. Antibiotic resistance is taking its toll in the form of increasing number of deaths, longer hospital stays, and increasing costs for healthcare providers. We have witnessed the development of a new concept called antibiotic stewardship that aims to preserve the antibiotics we currently have as long as possible. The situation threatens the basis of modern medicine and urological surgeons have to reassess their antibiotic prophylaxis policy: why we use it, when we use it, and how we use it.

19.2 Material and Methods

The present review is based on EAU guidelines on urinary tract infection 2000–2021, cross-references in guidelines and relevant published papers identified by the authors during the same period. We searched for papers addressing the principles of antibiotic prophylaxis in urology. Our aim is to provide the reader with a broad understanding of why, when, and how to administer antibiotic prophylaxis in an era of antimicrobial stewardship.

19.3 WHY Shall We Give Antibiotic Prophylaxis?

19.3.1 Prevention of Hospital-Acquired Infections

A postoperative infection is per definition a hospital-acquired infection (HAI), also called nosocomially acquired infection (NAUTI), after the Greek word for hospital.

Urinary tract infections are the most common type of HAIs (HAUTI or NAUTI). The prevalence of HAUTI in urology is about 10%, with significant variations according to hospital, country, region, and continent. The prevalence rate varies with the type of surgery, prophylaxis policy, and antimicrobial resistance. As regards types of HAUTIs, asymptomatic bacteriuria is not routinely regarded as a postoperative infection, and in recent years, there has been an increase in the rate of urosepsis. The consequences of HAUTI are prolonged hospitalization, deaths, and increased healthcare-related costs [1].

In urological patients, Enterobacteriaceae is the most common cause of HAUTIs, with *E. coli* being the predominant microorganism. Resistance rates against fluoroquinolones are registered as high as 35% and 57% in Northern Europe and Asia, respectively, according to the GPIU surveillance study. It has been shown that adherence to correct use of antibiotic prophylaxis in a urology department can reduce costs and decrease common resistance patterns [2].

19.3.2 Types of Infective Complications in Urology

In order to understand the rationale for AP, urologists need to know the rate of infective complications without AP. Data are available from the pre-AP period and from placebo arms in early comparative studies on AP. In order to assess the severity of infective complications and to tailor prophylactic measures, it is also essential to know the type and severity of each type of infection. Traditionally, infective complications have been classified according to the anatomical site of the infection (Table 19.1).

A more detailed classification of urinary tract infections is the EAU/ESIU severity grading (Table 19.2), which is recommended for UTI in general, but also

Table 19.1 Anatomical site of postoperative infections [3]

Site of infection	Minor	Major
Surgical wound incision/ surgical site infection (SSI)	Superficial wound infection	Deep wound infection Wound rupture (abdominal dehiscence) Deep abdominal or surgical site abscess
UTI or organ-specific infection Catheter-associated UTI	Asymptomatic bacteriuria (bacterial colonization) Symptomatic lower UTI (cystitis)	Febrile UTI Pyelonephritis Renal abscess Perirenal abscess
Blood stream	Bacteremia without signs of systemic response	Sepsis with signs of systemic response (SIRS)
Male accessory gland infection	Epididymitis Orchitis	Acute bacterial prostatitis (type I)
Other sites		Septic embolism Pneumonia Secondary bone infection

Table 19.2 Types and severity grades of urinary tract infections

Acronym	Clinical diagnosis	Clinical symptoms
CY-1	Cystitis	Dysuria, frequency, urgency, suprapubic pain, sometimes unspecific symptoms
PN-2	Mild and moderate pyelonephritis	Fever, flank pain, CVA tenderness, sometimes unspecific symptoms with or without symptoms of CY
PN-3	Severe pyelonephritis	As PN-2, but in addition nausea and vomiting with or without symptoms of CY
US-4	Urosepsis (simple)	Temperature >38 °C or <36 °C Heart rate >90 beats/min Respiratory rate >20 breaths/min or $PaCO_2$ <32 mmHg (<4.3 kPa) WBC >12,000 cells/mm^3 or <4000 cells/mm^3 or >19% immature (band) forms With or without symptoms of CY or PN
US-5	Severe urosepsis	As US-4, but in addition associated with organ dysfunction hypoperfusion or hypotension. Hypoperfusion and perfusion abnormalities may include, but are not limited to, lactic acidosis, oliguria, or an acute alternation of mental status
US-6	Uroseptic shock	As US-4 og US-5, but in addition with hypotension despite adequate fluid resuscitation along with the presence of perfusion abnormalities, that may include, but are not limited to lactic acidosis, oliguria, or an acute alteration in mental status. Patient who are on inotropic or vasopressor agents may not be hypotensive at the time that perfusion abnormalities are measured.

relevant for postoperative UTIs [4]. While the lowest severity grades can be treated with oral antibiotics in an outpatient setting, infections of higher severity grades require intravenous antibiotics and hospitalization, often in intensive care units. Nowadays, urosepsis accounts for about 25% of HAUTIS. Severe urosepsis and septic shock carry a significant risk of mortality in the immediate postoperative period as well as for several months afterward.

19.3.3 Rates of Infective Complications Without AP

The rate of infectious complications depends on the type of the surgical procedure. Without antibiotic prophylaxis PCNL (percutaneous nephrolithotripsy), implantation of prosthetic devices and cystectomy have the highest reported rates of infective complications with figures up to 25%. Few data are available on the rates of sepsis. Details are displayed in Table 19.3.

Transrectal prostate biopsy without AP has the highest rate of infective complications of all elective urological procedures with bacteremia rates up to 70% and fever rates up to 48% (Table 19.4).

Table 19.3 Rate of infectious complications without AP, modified from Naber et al. [4]

Procedure	Febrile/symptomatic UVI/SSI
Cystoscopy	1–5%
Urodynamic studies	23%[a]
TURB	No data
TURP	5–10%
ESWL	5.7% (median probability)
Ureteroscopy (standard)	No data
Percutaneous stone extraction and difficult ureterorenoscopy	4–25%
Open/lap. nephrectomy	SSI ≤5% (higher reported)
Open/lap/robotic total prostatectomy	SSI ≤5%
Cystectomy and bladder substitution	SSI 10–15%
Scrotal surgery	SSI 3–9%
Implantation of prosthetic devices	1–16.7%

[a]Rates of bacteriuria including asymptomatic bacteriuria

Table 19.4 RCTs on prostate biopsy (modified after Bootsma et al. (2008). Courtesy of Kurt Naber)

Author	Study type	Population	Intervention	Outcome	AB	No AB
Kapoor et al. (1998)	RCT, double blind	*N* = 457 230/227	• Ciprofloxacin 500 mg p.o. SD • Placebo	Bacteriuria Sympt. UT.	3% 3%	8% 5%
Aron et al. (2000)	RCT, patient blinded	*N* = 457 75/79/77	• Ciprofloxacin 500 mg p.o. SD + tinidazole 600 mg p.o. • Ciprofloxacin 500 mg p.o. bid + tinidazole 600 mg p.o. bid 3 days • Placebo	Bacteriuria Fever Bacteremia	5–8% 3% 0–1%	19% 7% 3%
Isen et al. (1999)	RCT	*N* = 110 23/42/45	• Ofloxacin 400 mg p.o. SD • TMP/SMX 160/800 mg p.o. SD • No AB	Bacteriuria	5–7%	26%
Ruebush et al. (1979)	RCT	*N* = 89	• TMP/SMX • Placebo	Bacteriuria Fever Bacteemia	0%	21% 18% 70%
Melekos et al. (1990)	RCT	*N* = 38 16/22	• Piperacillin 2 g i.v. bid • No AB	Bacteriuria Bacteremia	9% 14%	31% 38%
Crawford et al. (1982)	RCT, patient blinded	*N* = 48 25/23	• Carbenicillin 3 days • Placebo	Bacteriuria Fever Bacteremia	9% 17% 22%	36% 48% 16%
Brown et al. (1981)	RCT	*N* = 19 9/10	• Gentamicin 80 mg i.v. • No AB	Bacteriuria Fever Bacteremia	20% 50% 20%	44% 22% 44%

19.3.4 Key Arguments for AP

The main objective of AP is to prevent postoperative infective complications of all types after urological procedures, diagnostic and therapeutic procedures alike. Severe complications may cause significant harm to patients and increase costs for healthcare providers. Additionally, AP should contribute to antibiotic stewardship in reducing the need for longer antibiotic treatment courses in the postoperative period.

19.4 WHEN Shall We Give Antibiotic Prophylaxis?

The planned urological procedure in itself is not the only risk factor to consider for prevention of a postoperative infection. The urologist must evaluate each patient individually as regards the risk of infective complications. An infection develops if the balance between the host defense mechanisms and the bacterial intruder tips in favor of the intruders. Like all other prescriptions, the administration of antibiotic prophylaxis should be based on evidence that demonstrate a clinically significant benefit.

19.4.1 Patient-Related Risk Factors for Infection

The most important risk factors for infection are those who increase the likelihood of presence of bacteria, such as urinary catheters or stents. Previous use of antibiotics, recent hospitalization, and travel to endemic regions increase the risk of carriership of resistant pathogens. Risk factors that affect the host defense mechanisms are comorbidities and treatments that negatively influence the immune response. A pragmatic classification of patient-related risk factors, modified from EAU Guidelines 2015 [3], is presented in Table 19.5.

The ORENUC phenotyping is a more detailed and comprehensive classification of risk factors, also developed by EAU (Table 19.6). The classification is relevant for development of UTIs in general and hence also for assessment of the risk of postoperative UTIs.

The importance of risk factors is that they can become arguments for AP in procedures, where AP is not routinely recommended, and they can be used to tailor an individual prophylactic regimen to a given patient.

Table 19.5 Patient-related risk factors, modified from EAU Guidelines 2015 [3]

General factors	ASA score 1–5, older age, diabetes mellitus, impaired immune system, malnutrition, overweight, smoking, coexisting infection at a remote site
Endogenous factors	History of UTI/urogenital infection, colonization (intestinal and urinary), urinary obstruction, urinary stone, previous hospitalization, prior treatment with fluoroquinolones [5]
Exogenous factors	Indwelling catheter, nephrostomy tube, double j-stent

Table 19.6 Host risk factors in urinary tract infections categorized according to the ORENUC system [6]

Category of risk factor	Examples of risk factors	Phenotype
NO known risk factor	Otherwise healthy premenopausal women	***O***
Risk factors for **R**ecurrent UTI, but no risk of more severe outcome	Sexual behavior (frequency, spermicide) Hormonal deficiency in postmenopause Secretor type of certain blood groups Well-controlled diabetes mellitus	***R***
Extra-urogenital risk factor with risk of more severe outcome	Prematurity, newborn Pregnancy Male gender Badly controlled diabetes mellitus Relevant immunosuppression (not well-defined)	***E***
Nephropathic disease with risk of more severe outcome	Relevant renal insufficiency (not well-defined) Polycystic nephropathy Interstitial nephritis, e.g., due to analgetics	***N***
Urological risk factors with risk of more severe outcome, which can be resolved during therapy	Ureteral obstruction due to a ureteral stone Well controlled neurogenic bladder disturbances Transient short-term external urinary catheter Asymptomatic bacteriuria[a]	***U***
Permanent urinary **C**atheter and non-resolvable urological risk factors with risk of more severe outcome	Long-term external urinary catheter Non-resolvable urinary obstruction Badly controlled neurogenic bladder disturbances	***C***

[a] Only under certain circumstances in combination with other risk factors, e.g., pregnancy, urological intervention

19.4.2 Procedure-Related Risk Factors

The concept of contamination categories was developed during WW II as part of patient triage. In 2010, the system was adapted to urology by the EAU guidelines panel [4], presented in Table 19.7. The "clean-contaminated" category was divided into two subgroups, depending on whether the urinary tract or the intestinal tract was entered. The new subcategories were introduced to make a distinction between procedures where AP is not recommended and those where AP is recommended. As a general rule, AP is not given before procedures belonging to the clean and clean-contaminated IIa categories, while AP is always given before surgery in contamination category III. Whenever it is necessary to perform a surgical procedure in category IV, the patient should receive antibiotic treatment that extends beyond the period of prophylaxis. This leaves category IIb in a situation where the risk of spillage, the duration of the procedure, and patient-related risk factors are decisive for whether or not to give AP.

Table 19.7 Surgical contamination categories in urology

Contamination grades	Description	Examples of procedures
I. Clean	Uninfected surgical site No evidence of inflammation No break in technique	Simple nephrectomy Planned scrotal surgery Cystoscopy?
IIa. Clean-contaminated (urinary tract)	Urogenital tract (UT) entered with no or little (controlled) spillage. No break in technique	Pelvic-ureteric junction repair Nephron-sparing tumor resection Total prostatectomy Bladder surgery, partial cystectomy
IIb. Clean-contaminated (bowel)	Gastrointestinal tract (GIT) entered with no or little (controlled) spillage. No break in technique	Urine diversion (small intestine) Orthotopic bladder replacement
III. Contaminated	UT and/or GIT entered, spillage of GI content; inflammatory tissue Presence of bacteriuria (UT) Major break in technique Open, fresh accidental wounds	Urine diversion (large intestine) Spillage (small and large intestine) Concomitant GI disease Trauma surgery
IV. Infected	Preexisting infection; viscera perforation Old traumatic wound	Drainage of abscess Large dirty trauma surgery

19.4.3 What Is a Clinically Significant Benefit of AP?

Antibiotic prophylaxis does have side effects on both a patient level and a society level. Even a single dose of an antibiotic may put the patient at up to 50% risk of developing antimicrobial-resistant strains in the host microbiome. In addition, antibiotic prophylaxis puts the patient at risk of developing subsequent UTI. Every prophylaxis and every course of antibiotic treatment exerts collateral effects by increasing the general resistance rates in the population. Only clinically significant benefits of AP will outweigh the side effects. We used to think that asymptomatic bacteriuria was an infection, but we don't think like that anymore. Avoiding a low risk UTI, which can be treated successfully with a 3–5 days' course of oral antibiotics, can hardly be regarded a significant benefit. Avoiding severe urosepsis is, however, a significant benefit. Unfortunately, there is very little high-level evidence that AP prevents severe infections. The French Urological Association has turned the reasoning upside down and has advised against antibiotic prophylaxis in procedures where there is no evidence demonstrating a significant benefit for the patient.

19.4.4 Key Points About When to Give Antibiotic Prophylaxis

AP is indicated before procedures, where there is a significant risk of infective complications without prophylaxis. The risk assessment is based on the contamination category and duration of the procedure and is influenced by patient-related risk factors. Urologists should bear in mind that AP can never compensate for poor hygiene or surgical technique.

19.5 HOW to Give Antibiotic Prophylaxis

The objective of AP is to counteract contamination during surgery, both at the surgical site and systemically. The selection of the antibiotic agent and the duration of prophylaxis must be in accordance with well-established medical principles.

19.5.1 Core Principles

The antibiotic agent must be present at the surgical site in the required concentration for the required period. The presence depends on the pharmacokinetics of the drug, which refers to its bioavailability, distribution, metabolism, and excretion. The required concentration depends on the pharmacodynamics of the drug, which refers to the relationships between drug concentration and effect. Traditionally, AP should provide protection against infections for 24 h. Another principle is not to use the most potent antibiotics for prophylaxis but instead reserve them for treatment.

19.5.2 Pathogens and Resistance

Antibiotics must be effective against the most likely pathogens and their resistance profile. The types of pathogens vary with the type of hospital, type of procedure, and patient-related risk factors, such as previous antibiotics, recent hospitalization, and recent travel. Most HAIs occur in spite of AP, and causative microorganisms may stem from the patient or from the hospital ward. Infections may occur if the selection of the prophylactic antibiotic is not based on local resistance data, or if the patients are not properly screened for resistant pathogens.

Pooled data for all pathogens causing HAIs in urology show a resistance rate of about 70% for the most commonly used antibiotics in certain regions. Imipenem is the only antibiotic with a resistance rate below 20% (Fig. 19.1).

Pooled figures must be interpreted with caution as they represent average data from patients where AP either failed or was not given at all. Development of local prophylaxis protocols should be based on national or local susceptibility and resistance data and should also consider the most likely type of infective complication after a given procedure. This is a complex exercise, which can be facilitated with mathematical modeling.

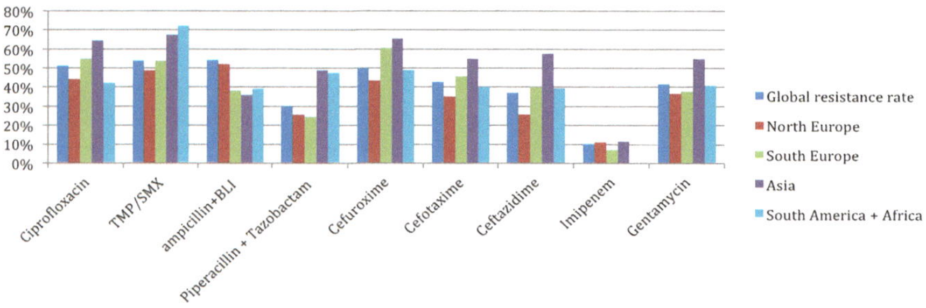

Fig. 19.1 Global and regional antibiotic resistance rates of all pathogens in patients with HAUTIs from the GPIU study during the period of 2003–2010. Reproduced with permission from [7]

19.5.3 Finding the Right Antibiotic

The considerations on how to find prophylactic antibiotics with the best coverage are the same as the considerations to find antibiotics with the highest likelihood of being effective as empirical treatment against severe urinary tract infections. Most hospitals register the spectrum and resistance rates of pathogens, but this information alone is of limited value without considering which bacteria is most likely to cause the infection and which clinical type of infection is most likely to occur. Before selecting an antibiotic, or a combination of antibiotics, one needs to know the probability for each antibiotic to provide coverage against the most likely pathogen that will cause the most likely infection. Luckily, this complex set of probabilities can be expressed by means of a single figure called the WISCA score (weighted incidence syndromic combination of antibiotics). To make this figure more clinically relevant, the information included in the WISCA score can be modeled by means of Bayesian mathematics to an estimate that includes confidence intervals. This gives the clinicians a more reliable background for decisions on prophylaxis as well as treatment. Figure 19.2 gives an example of Bayesian WISCA of antibiotic choices in European urology departments based on pooled, international resistance data.

The clinical relevance of WISCA will increase further if local data, instead of pooled international data, on pathogens and resistance are used to inform the modeling (Fig. 19.3).

19.5.4 Critical Levels of Coverage

After identification of the alternative prophylactic antibiotics, the final step is to decide where to put the threshold for acceptable likelihood of antibiotic coverage or risk of failure. Traditionally, a resistance rate of the most likely pathogens has been set at 10–20%. According to the global data shown above, there are very few antibiotics left to be used for prophylaxis, especially if the most potent antibiotic shall be reserved for treatment in case infectious complications do occur. This is a very big dilemma in modern medicine.

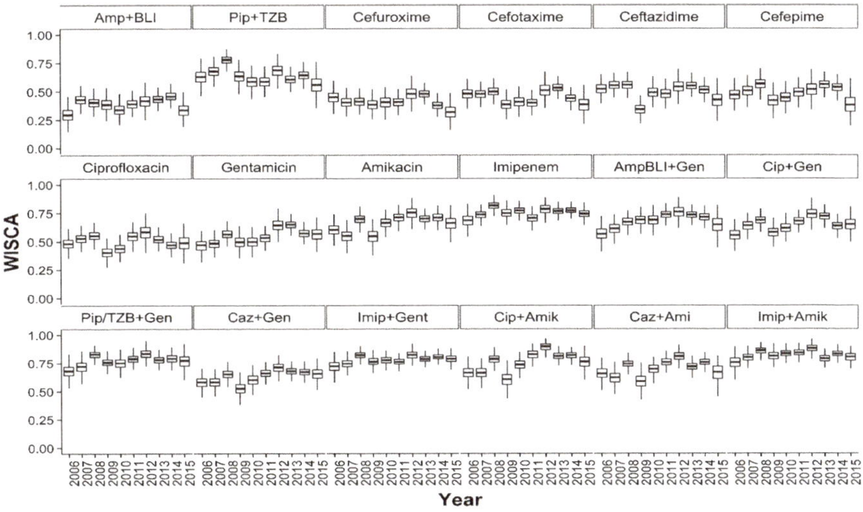

Fig. 19.2 Estimated Bayesian WISCA (informative prior) of antibiotic choices in HAUTIs reported in European urology departments from 2006 to 2015 [8]

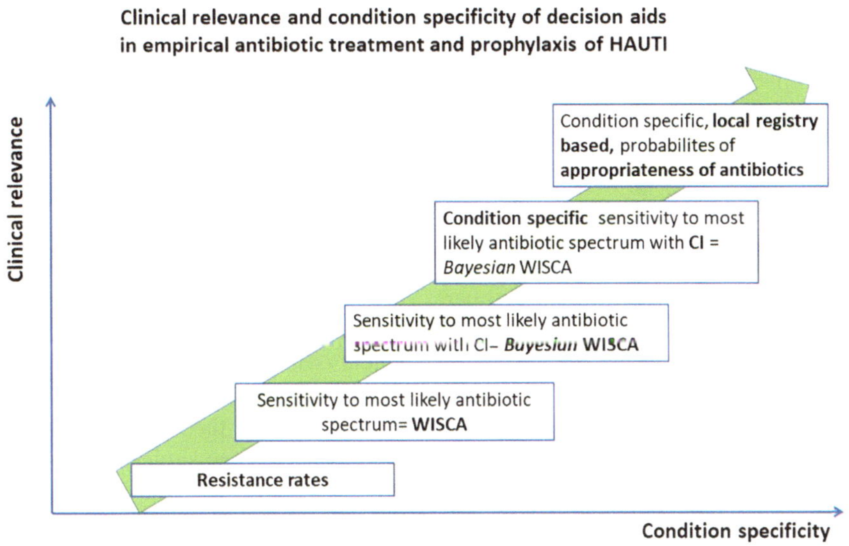

Fig. 19.3 Means to improve the coverage of antibiotic prophylactic regimens. "Condition" refers to severity types of UTI. Courtesy of Truls E. Bjerklund Johansen

19.5.5 Available Evidence for Effect of Antibiotic Prophylaxis

Unfortunately, high-level evidence proving significant benefit of antibiotic prophylaxis is missing for the most common urological operations—particularly when it comes to reduction of postoperative sepsis. For transurethral resection of the prostate (TURP) and transrectal prostate biopsies, however, there is evidence in favor of antibiotic prophylaxis from well-designed studies [9]. Therefore, most guidelines elicit a strong recommendation for AP in TURP. The systematic review and meta-analysis of Berry and Barratt from 2002 is frequently cited and included 32 RCTs investigating the use of AP in men undergoing TURP with preoperative sterile urine [10]. The results indicated that the incidence of bacteriuria and post-operative sepsis decreased from 26% to 9.1% and 4.4% to 0.7%, respectively. In 2005, Qiang et al. included 28 RCTs, and the analysis resulted in a similar conclusion. As regards transurethral resection of bladder tumor (TURB), there are only two well-designed RCTs, Delavierre et al. [11] and MacDermott et al. [12], which include 61 and 91 patients, respectively. The results demonstrated nonsignificant decreases in postoperative bacteriuria. Only Delavierre et al. included symptomatic UTI as an outcome parameter, but there were no symptomatic events reported in either group.

A systematic review of RCTs from 2015 on diagnostic cystoscopy demonstrate conflicting evidence whether symptomatic UTI is reduced or not by AP if one is to consider studies with a low risk of bias [13]. Some of the studies report only bacteriuria as an outcome parameter [14, 15], despite bacteriuria usually being a transient phenomenon with uncertain clinical significance. The low incidence of bacteriuria and symptomatic UTI after cystoscopy and urodynamic investigation does not indicate AP [13].

Stone surgery, regardless of modality, represents procedures where both endogenous and exogenous risk factors apply. Indwelling stents, infection stones, obstruction, etc. have greater impact on the indication for AP than the procedure itself. This reflects the complexity of analyzing study for this patient group and explains the paucity of clear recommendations. For ESWL, the incidence of post-procedural bacteriuria and febrile UTI seems to be low ($\leq 1\%$), regardless of the administration of AP, indicating that AP is unnecessary [16]. Ureterorenoscopy is the modality with the most heterogeneous surgical factors, considering stone location and the need for both preoperative and/or postoperative indwelling ureteral stents and catheters. A subgroup analysis of these factors is lacking, but a systematic review of the studies on AP in patients with preoperative, sterile urine indicates a general reduction in postoperative pyuria and bacteriuria but not in the rate of febrile UTI when AP is given [17, 18]. However, there is a consensus-based recommendation for AP in expected complicated stone surgery. AP is routinely administered before percutaneous nephrolithotripsy (PNL) due to potentially colonized large, stone masses, and use of irrigation fluid in a high-pressure setting. The only RCT on the subject is by Fourcade et al. 1990 grouping URS and PNL together, with small individual group sizes and nonsignificant results regarding postoperative fever, but collectively favoring AP in reducing postoperative bacteriuria [19].

The traditional method of transrectal ultrasound-guided prostate biopsy (TRPBx) involves passage of a biopsy needle from the contaminated bowel into the prostate. Meta-analysis of 22 RCTs analyzing antibiotic prophylaxis versus no treatment demonstrated significant risk reduction of postbiopsy bacteremia, fever, UTI and hospitalization when antibiotic prophylaxis was utilized [20]. Rectal cleansing with povidone-iodine is effective in reducing infectious complications in TRPBx. Prebiopsy screening with rectal swab culture enables targeted antibiotic prophylaxis. The method does reduce infections but needs further validation [21]. In despite of this, we have seen increasing rates of postbiopsy infections during the last decades due to the emergence of fluoroquinolone resistance [22]. As a result, the European Commission has banned the use of fluoroquinolones for antibiotic prophylaxis in TRPBx, because of a negative risk-benefit balance. Hence, urologists must find other antibiotic agents for prophylaxis. Also, urologists must adhere to the principle of antimicrobial stewardship and reduce the prescription of broad spectrum antibiotics.

Switching from transrectal to transperineal biopsy reduces the contamination category of the biopsy procedure [23]. By avoiding the GI tract, the contamination category of the procedure changes from contaminated (grade III) to clean-contaminated (grade IIa). Hopefully, this approach will reduce the need for AP. So far, a systematic review and meta-analysis of three RCTs and four case-control studies did not show statistically significant differences between the TR and TP biopsy route in regard to complications, but the methodological quality of the included studies is questioned [24]. In the past, TPPBx was performed in the setting of mapping or saturation biopsies and usually needed general anesthesia. The feasibility of targeted TPPBx in local anesthesia has now been demonstrated [25], and a trend to abandon the transrectal route is evident [26–28].

19.5.6 Practical Recommendations on Antibiotic Prophylaxis

For the majority of urological procedures, we don't have compelling evidence for a benefit of antibiotic prophylaxis. We must therefore rely on individualized prophylactic regimens based on the concepts of contamination categories, endogenous and exogenous risk factors, local resistance data, and pharmacokinetic and pharmacodynamic properties of available antibiotics. Antimicrobial stewardship has become an important navigation point. While local guidelines should be developed by a multidisciplinary group consisting of microbiologists, infectious disease specialists, and urologists, global recommendations of alternative antibiotics are still needed (Table 19.8).

Table 19.8 Alternative antibiotics for prophylaxis in urological procedures

Diagnostic procedure	Antibiotic prophylaxis	Remarks	Antimicrobial products[a]	References
Cystoscopy (+/− biopsy and/or diathermy/laser fulguration), urodynamic investigation	No			
Diagnostic ureterorenoscopy (+/− minor biopsy)	No			
Transperineal biopsy of the prostate	Unknown	Recommended route of biopsy Perineal cleansing	Trimethoprim-sulfamethoxazole	
Transrectal biopsy of the prostate	Yes	Rectal swab or stool culture to guide targeted prophylaxis should be considered. Rectal povidone-iodine preparation recommended	3rd-generation cephalosporin (e.g., ceftriaxone 1 g i.m.) Fosfomycin trometamol (3 g p.o. before and 3 g 24–48 h after biopsy) Aminoglycoside (e.g., gentamicin 3 mg/kg i.v.)	EAU Guidelines 2021 [29] Kranz et al. (2021) [30]
Endourology and stone surgery	**Antibiotic prophylaxis**	**Remarks**	**Antimicrobial products[a]**	
ESWL	No			
Ureterorenoscopy with distal/uncomplicated stone treatment	No			
Ureterorenoscopy with treatment of proximal/impacted stone or urothelial tumor	Yes		Trimethoprim Trimethoprim-sulfamethoxazole 1st-generation cephalosporin (e.g., cefazolin 2 g i.v.) Aminopenicillin + β-lactamase inhibitor	EAU Guidelines 2021 [29] SFAR 2018[b]
Percutaneous nephrolithotomy	Yes			
TURP	Yes			
TURB	In selected cases	Large necrotic tumors, high-risk patients		
Open and laparoscopic/robot-assisted surgery	**Antibiotic prophylaxis**	**Remarks**	**Antimicrobial products[a]**	

Clean operation	No			
Clean-contaminated IIa (opening of urinary tract)	Only in selected cases	High-risk patients, exogenous factors	Trimethoprim Trimethoprim-sulfamethoxazole 1st-generation cephalosporin (e.g., cefazolin 2 g i.v.)[c] Aminopenicillin + β-lactamase inhibitor[c]	EAU Guidelines 2021 [29] AUA Best Practice Statement 2019 [31]
Clean-contaminated IIb (use of bowel segments)	Yes	Use of large bowel: Add Metronidazole 1 g	1st-generation cephalosporin (e.g., cefazolin 2 g i.v.)[c] Aminopenicillin + β-lactamase inhibitor[c]	AUA Best Practice Statement 2019 [31] SFAR 2018[b]
Implant of prosthetic devices	Yes		2nd-generation cephalosporin (e.g., cefoxitin 2 g i.v.) Aminopenicillin + β-lactamase inhibitor	SFAR 2018[b]

[a]Duration of therapy is always in the form of a single dose, unless stated otherwise. Administration is recommended 2 h or 30 min preoperatively for enteral or parenteral use, respectively

[b]The French Society of Anesthesia and Intensive Care Medicine recommendations for antibiotic prophylaxis [32]

[c]Antibiotic which require repeat dosing if the operative time exceeds 2–4 h, depending on the half-life of the actual product

19.6 Discussion

19.6.1 Clinical Implications

Although there are few well-designed prospective studies that provide evidence to guide clinical practice, there is overwhelming experience that modern medicine is largely dependent on effective antibiotic prophylaxis and effective antibiotic treatment. It is, however, also clear that use of antibiotic prophylaxis has a downside, which doctors must discuss with the patients beforehand. The informed consent given by patients before surgical procedures should include a specific consent to AP. Surgeons used to decide AP without discussing this issue with the patient. Due to the collateral effects of AP, the healthcare providers and political leadership should also have a word. Recently, even international organizations like EMA (European Medical Agency) have issued regulations on the use of antibiotic prophylaxis in urology. This is a sign that AP receives increased attention in the era of antimicrobial stewardship. Therefore, we must bring the classical principles for prevention of infections to light and teach them to young urologists. Clinicians should establish teams with local microbiologists and infectious disease specialists to monitor infection rates and antimicrobial resistance as a basis for local prophylaxis protocols.

19.6.2 Lessons from Prostate Biopsy

Ever since the introduction of transrectal ultrasound probes and the technique of transrectal prostate biopsy about 40 years ago, urologists have been aware of the very high risk of infections and the need for effective prophylaxis. Sadly, it took many years before we realized that the complications of prostate biopsy outweighed the benefits of diagnosis and treatment of prostate cancer in terms of patient life years. The rates of infectious complications after transrectal biopsies with time-consuming image fusion technique reached 10%, and a mortality rate of 1 per 1000 biopsies was confirmed before we reacted. In some places, infections were kept low by broad-spectrum antibiotics and extended prophylaxis. Recently, it turned out that prostate biopsies can be performed safely via the transperineal route as an outpatient procedure and hopefully, without the need for AP. The story tells us that for decades, we overlooked the principle of contamination categories and violated the principles of antimicrobial stewardship. Practice did not change until registry data made us think different.

19.6.3 Future Research

There is a significant lack of research data in the field of AP. We need to know more about the optimal duration of prophylaxis, the potential of tailored prophylaxis according to patient-related risk factors and when AP is not needed at all. We need better routines for preoperative assessment of the patients' microbiome, and we need to explore the use of vaccines against the most common pathogens. While clinical quality can be improved by means of local registries, important research questions is better answered through prospective studies embedded in international registries.

19.7 Conclusions

AP has largely been based on good intentions and not on evidence. Antibiotic stewardship demands urologists to rethink current practice and highlight classical hygienic principles as part of prophylaxis policies.

Current rates of HAI of about 10% from urology departments that do give AP are not acceptable. Obviously, the prophylactic antibiotics are not able to combat bacteria in the surgical field. This might be due to suboptimal pharmacokinetic and pharmacodynamic properties and antimicrobial spectrum of the drugs used, as well as high bacterial resistance and load at the site of surgery. We urgently need more research to provide a better evidence base for development of antibiotic prophylaxis protocols.

References

1. Wagenlehner F, Tandogdu Z, Bartoletti R, Cai T, Cek M, Kulchavenya E, et al. The global prevalence of infections in urology (GPUI) study: a worldwide surveillance study in urology patients. Eur Urol Focus. 2016;2(4):345–7.
2. Cai T, Verze P, Brugnolli A, Tiscione D, Luciani LG, Eccher C, et al. Adherence to European Association of Urology guidelines on prophylactic antibiotics: an important step in antimicrobial stewardship. Eur Urol. 2016;69(2):276–83.
3. Grabe M, Bartoletti R, Bjerklund Johansen TE, Cai T, Cek M, Köves B, et al. EAU Guidelines on Urological Infections. European Association of Urology Guidelines 2015 Edition. Arnhem, The Netherlands: European Association of Urology Guidelines Office. p. 2015.
4. Naber KG, Scaeffer AJ, Heyns CF, Matsumoto T, Shoskes DA, Johansen TEB. Urogenital infections. European Association of Urology—International Consultation on Urological Diseases; 2010.
5. Cai T, Cocci A, Coccarelli F, Ruggera L, Lanzafame P, Caciagli P, et al. Infectious complications after laser vaporization of urinary stones during retrograde intrarenal surgery are not associated with spreading of bacteria into irrigation fluid but with previous use of fluoroquinolones. Eur Urol Focus. 2021;7(1):190–7.
6. Johansen TE, Botto H, Cek M, Grabe M, Tenke P, Wagenlehner FM, et al. Critical review of current definitions of urinary tract infections and proposal of an EAU/ESIU classification system. Int J Antimicrob Agents. 2011;38(Suppl):64–70.
7. Tandogdu Z, Cek M, Wagenlehner F, Naber K, Tenke P, van Ostrum E, et al. Resistance patterns of nosocomial urinary tract infections in urology departments: 8-year results of the global prevalence of infections in urology study. World J Urol. 2014;32(3):791–801.
8. Tandogdu Z, Kakariadis ETA, Naber K, Wagenlehner F, Bjerklund Johansen TE. Appropriate empiric antibiotic choices in health care associated urinary tract infections in urology departments in Europe from 2006 to 2015: a Bayesian analytical approach applied in a surveillance study. PLoS One. 2019;14(4):e0214710.

9. Bootsma AM, Laguna Pes MP, Geerlings SE, Goossens A. Antibiotic prophylaxis in urologic procedures: a systematic review. Eur Urol. 2008;54(6):1270–86.
10. Berry A, Barratt A. Prophylactic antibiotic use in transurethral prostatic resection: a meta-analysis. J Urol. 2002;167(2 Pt 1):571–7.
11. Delavierre D, Huiban B, Fournier G, Le Gall G, Tande D, Mangin P. The value of antibiotic prophylaxis in transurethral resection of bladder tumors. Apropos of 61 cases. Prog Urol. 1993;3(4):577–82.
12. MacDermott JP, Ewing RE, Somerville JF, Gray BK. Cephradine prophylaxis in transurethral procedures for carcinoma of the bladder. Br J Urol. 1988;62(2):136–9.
13. Carey MM, Zreik A, Fenn NJ, Chlosta PL, Aboumarzouk OM. Should we use antibiotic prophylaxis for flexible cystoscopy? A systematic review and meta-analysis. Urol Int. 2015;95(3):249–59.
14. Rané A, Cahill D, Saleemi A, Montgomery B, Palfrey E. The issue of prophylactic antibiotics prior to flexible cystoscopy. Eur Urol. 2001;39(2):212–4.
15. Johnson MI, Merrilees D, Robson WA, Lennon T, Masters J, Orr KE, et al. Oral ciprofloxacin or trimethoprim reduces bacteriuria after flexible cystoscopy. BJU Int. 2007;100(4):826–9.
16. Hsieh CH, Yang SS, Chang SJ. The effectiveness of prophylactic antibiotics with oral levofloxacin against post-shock wave lithotripsy infectious complications: a randomized controlled trial. Surg Infect. 2016;17(3):346–51.
17. Lo CW, Yang SS, Hsieh CH, Chang SJ. Effectiveness of prophylactic antibiotics against post-Ureteroscopic lithotripsy infections: systematic review and meta-analysis. Surg Infect. 2015;16(4):415–20.
18. Deng T, Liu B, Duan X, Cai C, Zhao Z, Zhu W, et al. Antibiotic prophylaxis in ureteroscopic lithotripsy: a systematic review and meta-analysis of comparative studies. BJU Int. 2018;122(1):29–39.
19. Fourcade RO. Antibiotic prophylaxis with cefotaxime in endoscopic extraction of upper urinary tract stones: a randomized study. The Cefotaxime Cooperative Group. J Antimicrob Chemother. 1990;26(Suppl A):77–83.
20. Lu Yang LG, Chen Y, Tang Z, Liu L, Han P, Zeng H, Li X, Wei Q. Prophylactic antibiotics in prostate biopsy: a meta-analysis based on randomized controlled trials. Surg Infect. 2015;16(6):733–47.
21. Pilatz A, Veeratterapillay R, Köves B, Cai T, Bartoletti R, Wagenlehner F, et al. Update on strategies to reduce infectious complications after prostate biopsy. Eur Urol Focus. 2019;5(1):20–8.
22. Nam RK, Saskin R, Lee Y, Liu Y, Law C, Klotz LH, et al. Increasing hospital admission rates for urological complications after transrectal ultrasound guided prostate biopsy. J Urol. 2010;183(3):963–9.
23. Pilatz A, Dimitropoulos K, Veeratterapillay R, Yuan Y, Omar MI, MacLennan S, et al. Antibiotic prophylaxis for the prevention of infectious complications following prostate biopsy: a systematic review and meta-analysis. J Urol. 2020;204(2):224–30.
24. Shen PF, Zhu YC, Wei WR, Li YZ, Yang J, Li YT, et al. The results of transperineal versus transrectal prostate biopsy: a systematic review and meta-analysis. Asian J Androl. 2012;14(2):310–5.
25. Jacewicz M, Günzel K, Rud E, Lauritzen PM, Galtung KF, Hinz S, et al. Multicenter transperineal MRI-TRUS fusion guided outpatient clinic prostate biopsies under local anesthesia. Urol Oncol. 2020;39:432.e1.
26. Pilatz A, Veeratterapillay R, Dimitropoulos K, Omar MI, Pradere B, Yuan Y, et al. European Association of Urology position paper on the prevention of infectious complications following prostate biopsy. Eur Urol. 2021;79(1):11–5.
27. Johansen TEB, Zahl P-H, Baco E, Bartoletti R, Bonkat G, Bruyere F, et al. Antibiotic resistance, hospitalizations, and mortality related to prostate biopsy: first report from the Norwegian patient registry. World J Urol. 2020;38(1):17–26.
28. Grummet J, Gorin MA, Popert R, O'Brien T, Lamb AD, Hadaschik B, et al. "TREXIT 2020": why the time to abandon transrectal prostate biopsy starts now. Prostate Cancer Prostatic Dis. 2020;23(1):62–5.

29. Bonkat G, Bartoletti R, Bruyére F, Cai T, Geerlings SE, Köves B, et al. EAU Guidelines on urological infections 2021. https://uroweb.org/guideline/urological-infections/. Accessed 12 May 2021.
30. Kranz J, Schneidewind L, Pilatz A, Wagenlehner FRA. Antibiotic prophylaxis for endourological interventions considering antibiotic stewardship. Urologe A. 2021;60(3):383–92.
31. Lightner DJ, Wymer K, Sanchez J, Kavoussi L. Best practice statement on urologic procedures and antimicrobial prophylaxis. J Urol. 2020;203(2):351–6.
32. Martin C, Auboyer M, Boisson H, Dupont D, Fletcher R, Gauzit M, et al. Antibioprophylaxie en chirurgie et médecine interventionnelle (patients adultes) Update 2018. https://sfar.org/mise-a-jour-de-la-rfe-antibioprophylaxie-2017/. Accessed 12 May 2021.

Prevention and Treatment of Urinary Tract Infections After Radical Cystectomy, Diversion, and Reservoirs

20

Mauro Gacci, Sergio Serni, and Jacopo Frizzi

Radical cystectomy (RC) is a morbid operation, with a complication rate between 55% and 67% within 90 days of surgery [1].

The infectious complication rate is between 8% and 61%, and the wound or soft tissue event rate is between 12% and 15% [2] with an average infection rate of 11.2% [3].

These patients are particularly susceptible in the early postoperative period to febrile urinary tract infections (UTIs), which increase patients' morbidity, impair their quality of life, and increase social and health costs.

Wound and infectious complications are the most expensive complications during the hospitalization time, especially for patients subjected to intestinal replacement for urinary reconstruction [3].

Complications significantly increase the costs for patient during post-intervention recovery or after readmission. The cost is about $7175 for each infectious event and $6510.74 for the complication of wound and soft tissue, while the predicted average cost for readmission due to a complication is $20,697. For any readmission, a base readmission cost is assumed of $5599.47 [3].

Perioperative care is more important than antimicrobial prophylaxis (AMP) for the prevention of perioperative infections. The preoperative hospitalization should be short. In urological surgery, urinalysis and urine culture are fundamental for the diagnosis of preoperative UTIs. Patients with inveterate UTIs, such as catheter-indwelling UTIs and infectious stones, should be treated with antimicrobials from 1 or 2 days before the operation. Hair removal should be avoided; if necessary, it should be done using electric clippers immediately before the operation. During the procedure, aseptic techniques, effective hemostasis, irrigation of the surgical field

M. Gacci (✉) · S. Serni · J. Frizzi
Department of Urological Minimally Invasive, Robotic Surgery and Kidney Transplantation, Careggi Hospital, University of Florence, Florence, Italy

Department of Experimental and Clinical Medicine, University of Florence, Florence, Italy
e-mail: sergio.serni@unifi.it

T. E. Bjerklund Johansen, T. Cai (eds.), *Guide to Antibiotics in Urology*,
https://doi.org/10.1007/978-3-319-92366-6_20

and surgical wound, and a closed drainage system should be used. The surgical wound should be covered with a sterile dressing for 48–72 h. The urethral catheter or drain should be removed as early as possible. The dressing should be changed with aseptic procedures, such as hand hygiene or the use of sterile gloves and equipment. Patients with infections caused by drug-resistant bacteria should be visited lastly [4].

For every type of surgery, the risk factors for perioperative infections can be separated into two groups: intrinsic patient-related characteristics and extrinsic environmental factors or procedure-related characteristics [5].

Predisposing factors for perioperative infectious complications in radical cystectomy are smoking history, history of chemotherapy, poor nutrition [6], higher BMI [7], prolonged operative time [8], diabetes, perioperative blood transfusion (PBT) [9], and patients undergoing continent diversion [10].

Improving nutrition [11], encouraging smoking cessation [12], and supporting exercise [13] should be promoted prior to surgery. An important role can play in immunonutrition before the procedure; it would improve the immune response of those who will be undergoing surgery [14].

In this surgery, the different risk of infections is closely related to the type of urinary diversion [9].

Patients undergoing diversion with orthotopic neobladder have an increased risk of UTI relative to conduit diversion (OR 1.21) [10].

Ureterocutaneostomy has a lower operating time, lower complication rate, a lower stay in intensive care, and a shorter length of hospital stay than ileal conduit, but previous clinical data suggest that ureter stenosis at cutaneous anastomosis and ascending UTI are more frequent in UCS diversion.

The causes and dynamics of infection are different in patients submitted to the incorporation of intestinal segments with the urinary tract according to the types of diversion that are classified in the following: noncontinent urinary diversion, continent nonorthotopic diversion, and orthotopic urinary diversion.

Studies in noncontinent urinary diversion and in continent nonorthotopic urinary diversion indicate an ascending infection pathway through the stoma for the bacterial skin population, which colonizes the conduit during the initial 10-day period of postoperative antibiotic therapy.

They form a mixed population of gram-positive bacteria (*Streptococcus* sp., *Staphylococcus epidermidis*) and resident intestinal flora as enterococci and gram-negative organisms (*Escherichia coli* and *Proteus*, *Pseudomonas*, and *Klebsiella* species). The distal part of the conduit showed less frequent growth than urine sampled from the stoma [15].

If the urinary diversion is anatomically intact without ureteral strictures, bacterial colonization of the conduit is not associated with renal scarring [16].

Reflux is an important risk factor for pyelonephritis that it may dependent by two factors:

1. High intraluminal pressure of the conduit
2. Construction of the ureterointestinal anastomosis

Theoretically, these conduits have low endoluminal pressure, and antireflux would be considered superfluous. However, some studies show that severe renal scarring and bacteriuria in the upper urinary tract are more common in refluxing ureterointestinal anastomoses with high intraluminal pressure.

In these cases, antireflux anastomosis is important for preventing ascending infections and renal scarring [17].

Furthermore, the application of urostomy to the skin promotes bacterial growth and reflux from the collecting device [18].

In continent nonorthotopic urinary diversion with ureterosigmoidostomy and its variations, rectal urine of all patients have rich bacterial flora. In fact, these derivations are associated with severe complications, including pyelonephritis IRC [19], metabolic acidosis [20], and tumor development at the ureterocolonic anastomotic site [21].

Patients with intestinal pouches have chronic bacteriuria. *E. coli* is the most common bacteria, followed by gram-negative *Enterobacteriaceae* and other gram-positive bacteria [22].

Also in pouches, the antireflux prevents clinical episodes of pyelonephritis.

Orthotopic bladder substitution is the standard of care in urinary diversion [23].

Radical cystectomy and reconstruction of neobladder with bowel change the anatomy and function of the lower urinary tract, altering the natural defenses against urinary tract infections (UTIs) [24].

Mucus plays an important role in the host bowel defense, preventing microbial attachment to the enterocytes also in ileal conduits and continent cecal urinary reservoirs [25, 26].

The mucus layer contains specific receptors bound by proteins expressed on *E. coli*'s pili [27, 28].

Moreover, the binding of *E. coli* to microvillus membranes of the enterocytes is found to be inhibited by purified mucin of goblet cell origin [29, 30]. These observations suggest that the binding of bacteria to mucus may prevent their adhesion to the enterocyte surface [30].

Normally, in bowel, the mucus luminal layer is moved away by digestion and peristalsis. In neobladder with high urine post-void residual, mucus may be stored and not washed out.

In fact, the complete and regular emptying of the urinary bladder constitutes a potent antibacterial defense [31].

Studies have shown that even a few residual urine increases the growth of bacteria at high densities, despite regular emptying [32, 33]. Patients with a neobladder full emptying have significantly lower rates of bacteriuria or higher rates of sterile urine, than those with larger volumes of residual urine that have significantly higher rates of febrile UTIs [24]. These data indicate that a postoperative education for emptying the neobladder is strongly recommended and the post-void residuals have to be monitored over the time.

These patients also lose the natural neuromuscular functions as a proper relaxation of the pelvic floor and reduction of abdominal tensions involved in micturition and voiding with an increased risk of post-void residual.

In men after cystoprostatectomy, the absence of the prostate and its antibacterial secretions can contribute to decrease the protections against ascending infections [26].

The intestinal mucosa has antibacterial properties, probably through the production of antibacterial peptides, or defensins, like immunoglobulins, that also are secreted by the bowel mucosa of excluded intestinal segments incorporated into the urinary tract.

Secretory IgA plays a protective role on the intestinal surface from bacterial colonization and invasion by pathogenic organisms. Anyhow, bacteriuria can be increased by a defect in the host response determined by the intrinsic qualities of the interposed intestinal mucosa [34–36].

Patients with neobladder have very low levels of IL-6 in urine, unlike patients with normal urinary tract and febrile urinary tract infection and pyelonephritis, which have high local and systemic IL-6 concentrations. This may indicate a reduced host response of the intestinal tissue to infective insults compared to the urothelium, predisposing the patient to infections [37].

In addition, reservoir urine has a different and altered composition than normal urine, which may promote microbial growth.

Urine in contact with intestinal mucosa contains many microbial nutrients, including carbohydrates and serum proteins. The oligosaccharides of the mucins are the substrates for the growth of some anaerobes [38], while the urea concentration is lower in the reservoir [39].

Also, the type of intestine interposed can change the presence of bacteriuria. Mixed flora is more frequent in ileal reservoir than in colonic conduits, while monocultures are more common in urine from colonic continent reservoirs and conduits [16–40].

In ileal neobladders with complete or almost complete emptying, there may be bacteriuria, while colonic ones often have sterile urine.

The most common cause of UTI in patients with neobladder is *E. coli*, responsible for 59% of monobacterial infections. Other microorganisms are the species *Klebsiella*, *Proteus mirabilis*, *Enterococcus*, *Pseudomonas*, and *Citrobacter* [41].

A large difference between the normal urinary tract and the reconstructed one is the type of bacteriuria made up by several strains [24] in continent urinary diversion, with only few strains prevailing for long periods [42]. Limited data suggest that differences in microbial distribution and the percentage of infectious events among patients with neobladder may be correlated with proper perioperative antibiotic antibacterial prophylaxis (AMP), administration times, predisposing factors, and already responsible bacteria. Enterococcus is the most common cause of infection in the early postoperative period, probably due to its incomplete sensitivity to the second-generation cephalosporin commonly used by surgeons [8].

A particular focus should be paid to the incidence of *Clostridium difficile* infections (CDI) in patients undergoing radical cystectomy. Some studies identify an increased risk of infection with CDI (1.7%), compared to patients undergoing radical prostatectomy (0.02%) or nephrectomy (0.23%) [43].

However, this rate is comparable to colorectal procedures (1.5%) [44]. The infection rate is increased in high-volume centers with a risk of 7.2% within 30 days from the surgery [45].

All the infective complications and, in particular, the CDI ones may be related to the abuse of AMP in urologic surgery. Infectious complications may also be related to the abuse of antimicrobial prophylaxis in urologic surgery, variability in practice patterns among providers, and suboptimal compliance with clinical guidelines [46].

Only 14.9% of patients received a regimen based on the guidelines and with discontinuation of antibiotics within 24 h after surgery [47].

Antimicrobial exposure is the most commonly risk factor for CDI development in surgical patients, and the risk increases with a longer duration of exposure [48, 49], particularly over 7 days, and it is greater during therapy and in the first month after exposure to antibiotics [50].

Correct antibiotic stewardship programs have been shown to decrease overall CDI rates [51, 52].

Limiting the use of preoperative antimicrobials, minimizing antimicrobial exposure, and following appropriate prophylaxis guidelines should be a priority to reduce CDI. The use of gastric acid reducers, such as histamine-2 antagonists or proton pump inhibitors, has been suggested as a potential risk factor for the development of CDI (53, 54).

AUA and EAU recommend AMP for urological surgery, especially if there is a reconstructive phase involving the intestine [55]. These recommendations are based on the general and colorectal surgery literature, but the experience is limited for urological surgery [56].

According to EAU Guidelines 2017, cystectomy with urine deviation has a high risk of perioperative infections, and they recommend an AMP with large spectrum against aerobic and anaerobic pathogens, such cefuroxime or aminopenicillin/betalactamase inhibitor + metronidazole (LE 2a GR B).

Single-shot or one-day dosage AMP is recommended, although prolonged operation and other morbidity risk factors may support the use of preemptive antimicrobial treatment, which should be less than 72 h [57].

The AMP should be started 30 min before the beginning of the operation. Additional doses are needed when the operation lasts for more than 3 h [4].

The data report that patients have the best results after an AMP coverage administered for less than 24 h, active against skin bacteria, genitourinary, and enteric gram-positive and gram-negative ones.

A second–/third-generation cephalosporin, as recommend by AUA and EAU guidelines, is the most commonly administered class, but it has a lesser coverage against gram-positive bacteria than first-generation cephalosporins and penicillins [58, 59].

Ampicillin/sulbactam and piperacillin/tazobactam are penicillins with a b-lactamase inhibitor that demonstrate excellent gram-positive, gram-negative, and anaerobic coverage with a reduction of 66% in the probability of infectious events. These antibiotics are also effective against enterococci, which remain an important cause of postoperative infections [7–60].

It is important to carefully evaluate gentamicin therapy in patients undergoing a neoadjuvant cisplatin-based chemotherapy [47].

Some studies report that the rate of uropathogenic bacteria in the neobladder is lower in those who received AMP than in untreated patients. The treatment may reduce bacterial colonization [24].

The microbiology of these infections describes polymicrobial infections in 38.1%, drug-resistant organisms in 18.6%, and fungal infections in 23.9% of cases.

The most common bacteria-causing infections after radical cystectomy are gram-negative organisms (65–91% of isolates) [60, 61].

Enterococcus is also frequent in the early postoperative period, even in patients with permanent ureteral stents (24%–51%), while *Candida* sp. is identified on the surface of 12% of stents, mainly in diabetic patients who have an increased risk of fungal UTIs [62].

A recent study demonstrates that a change in perioperative antibiotic prophylaxis from cefoxitin to ampicillin-sulbactam, gentamicin, and fluconazole resulted in a significant decrease in overall postoperative infections as well as in fungal infections [7].

For laparoscopic or robot-assisted surgery, there are poor and few studies. According to EAU, the laparoscopic procedures have to be treated in the same manner as their corresponding open procedures. In fact, laparoscopic surgery and robot-assisted surgery are approaches in great expansion, but specific urological data about antibiotic prophylaxis are lacking. Laparoscopic surgery is less invasive, and the incidence of surgical side infection (SSI) in this procedure should be lower than in open procedures, especially in clean-contaminated and contaminated ones. In general surgery, the infection rates are significantly lower with laparoscopic procedures than with open ones [63]. Moreover, the incidence of systemic inflammatory response syndrome (SIRS) in laparoscopic surgery compared to open procedures is significantly lower in the laparoscopic approach than in the open ones [64].

The incidence of UTI after urinary diversion is between 8.5% and 39% within 3 months of surgery [8]. The difference can also be correlated with the different diagnostic criteria for UTI in each study. Infections become sporadical after 1 year. The decreasing of UTIs after this period probably depends on the mutation of some risk factors during the maturation of the neobladder (lower mucus production, a better emptying, and an improvement of urodynamics indices).

P. aeruginosa and *E. coli* are the bacteria most often involved in late UTIs [47].

Some data on 1200 patients have reported an increased risk of UTI of about twice in those who receive a urinary continent diversion [8]. Bacteria more easily colonize the bowel epithelium than the urothelium, and bacteriuria in the urine from neobladder patients varies considerably in clinical reports from 3% [66] to 30% [67]. Other studies report an incidence of between 78% and 85% [61–67]. The rates of symptomatic UTI and urosepsis are substantially lower, from 0% to 39% and 0% to 12%, respectively. Serious life-threatening neobladder-associated UTIs have been reported from 0% to 12% of patients [68–70]. The risk of in-hospital mortality is high in patients who develop sepsis after radical cystectomy [71]. All episodes of urosepsis require hospitalization, rigorous monitoring, and intravenous antibiotic treatment for a minimum of 7 days.

Patients with urosepsis should always be evaluated for an underlying ureteroileal anastomotic stricture [72], or for other risk factors such as reflux.

Although the antireflux system does not have a significant impact on the development of symptomatic UTIs, many surgeons suggest the incorporation of an antireflux mechanism to avoid microbial colonization of the upper urinary tract [41], and although some reports indicate the benefits of active treatment of bacteriuria in the ileal neobladder lacking reflux protection, there has been no prospective study performed to determine if low-dose prophylactic antibiotic therapy reduces the risk of a future episode of pyelonephritis [22].

Recurrent pyelonephritis is a risk factor for renal impairment after RC [73], and in the case of sepsis, every hour of delay in the initiation of effective antimicrobial coverage leads to an increased risk of death [74].

In the case of high post-void urinary residual, the intermittent self-catheterization could be suggested [8].

The treatment of bacteriuria in the absence of risk factors is controversial.

Several studies have not shown benefits in the treatment of bacteriuria, and its screening is not recommended.

Treatment is recommended only if patients have recurrent symptomatic UTI [57] or when patients have subjective signs of local infection and/or involvement of the upper urinary tract [22].

In the case of recurrent UTIs, the presence of pathological conditions for infections has to be investigated and treated.

The asymptomatic presence of persistent bacteriuria promoted by uropathogenic growth in patients with bowel neobladder reflects a silent colonization of the intestinal tissues on how it happens in patients with bacteriuria and intact urinary tract. So, in this case, there is no indication for an active treatment or for prophylactic antibiotic therapy [24].

Studies show that prophylactic antibiotic therapy does not influence the rate of bacteriuria but only perioperative bacterial growth.

The growth of *E. coli* in urine occurs frequently after the treatment of bacteriuria.

Surprisingly, according to some reports, bacteriuria promoted by specific bacterial strains can protect the patient from the symptomatic UTI [75, 76].

In case of complicated UTIs, recurrent UTIs, or urosepsis, the treatment recommendations are the same as reported in the EAU or AUA guidelines. It is important to exclude any surgical complications that could cause infection such as ureteral stenosis, hydronephrosis, fistulae, etc. [22]

A particular infective complication in continent non-orthotopic diversion or noncontinent diversion is pouchitis, a rare infectious complication caused by infection of the intestinal pouch. It manifests itself with a sudden and important loss of urine through the continence mechanism, if it is a continent diversion, associated with pain in the region of the pouch.

In this infection, there is an increased mucus production with a high pouch hypercontractility.

Excessive production of mucus can contribute to the persistence of infections, which must be treated with antibiotic therapy for at least 10 days [41].

References

1. Lavallee LT, Schramm D, Witiuk K, et al. Perioperative morbidity associated with radical cystectomy in a multicenter database of community and academic hospitals. PLoS One. 2014;9(10):e111281. https://doi.org/10.1371/journal.pone.0111281. eCollection 2014.
2. Clark PE, Agarwal N, Biagioli MC, et al. Bladder cancer. J Natl Compr Cancer Netw. 2013;11:446–75.
3. Mossanen M, Krasnow R, et al. Associations of specific postoperative complications with costs after radical cystectomy. BJU Int. 2017;121:428. https://doi.org/10.1111/bju.14064.
4. CDC. Healthcare Infection Control Practices Advisory Committee. Guidelines for prevention of catheter-associated urinary tract infections; 2009.
5. Anderson DJ, Podgorny K. Strategies to prevent surgical site infections in acute care hospitals: 2014 update. Infect Control Hosp Epidemiol. 2014;35(Suppl 2):S66–88.
6. Hu M, Jacobs BL, Montgomery JS, He C, Ye J, Zhang Y, et al. Sharpening the focus on causes and timing of readmission after radical cystectomy for bladder cancer. Cancer. 2014;120(9):1409–16.
7. Pariser JJ, Anderson BB, Pearce SM, et al. The effect of broader, directed antimicrobial prophylaxis including fungal coverage on perioperative infectious complications after radical cystectomy. Urol Oncol. 2016;34(3):121.e9–14. https://doi.org/10.1016/j.urolonc.2015.10.007.
8. Parker WP, Tollefson MK, Heins C, et al. Characterization of perioperative infection risk among patients undergoing radical cystectomy: results from the national surgical quality improvement program. Urol Oncol. 2016;34(12):532.e13–9. https://doi.org/10.1016/j.urolonc.2016.07.001.
9. Parker WP, Toussi A, Tollefson MK, et al. Risk factors and microbial distribution of urinary tract infections following radical cystectomy. Urology. 2016;94:96–101. https://doi.org/10.1016/j.urology.2016.
10. van Hemelrijck M, Thorstenson A, Smith P, et al. Risk of inhospital complications after radical cystectomy for urinary bladder carcinoma: population-based follow-up study of 7608 patients. BJU Int. 2013;112(8):1113–20. https://doi.org/10.1111/bju.12239.
11. Tobert CM, Hamilton-Reeves JM, Norian LA, Hung C, Brooks NA, Holzbeierlein JM, et al. Emerging impact of malnutrition on surgical patients: literature review and potential implications for cystectomy in bladder cancer. J Urol. 2017;198(3):511–9. https://doi.org/10.1016/j.juro.2017.01.087.
12. Bassett JC, Gore JL, Chi AC, Kwan L, McCarthy W, Chamie K, et al. Impact of a bladder cancer diagnosis on smoking behavior. J Clin Oncol. 2012;30(15):1871–8.
13. Moran J, Guinan E, McCormick P, Larkin J, Mockler D, Hussey J, et al. The ability of prehabilitation to influence postoperative outcome after intra-abdominal operation: a systematic review and meta-analysis. Surgery. 2016;160(5):1189–201.
14. Hamilton-Reeves JM, Bechtel MD, Hand LK, Schleper A, Yankee TM, Chalise P, et al. Effects of immunonutrition for cystectomy on immune response and infection rates: a pilot randomized controlled clinical trial. Eur Urol. 2016;69:389–92. https://doi.org/10.1016/j.eururo.2015.11.019.
15. Mansson W, Ahlgren G, White T. Glomerular filtration rate up to 10 years after urinary diversion of different types. A comparative study of ileal and colonic conduit, refluxing and antirefluxing ureteral anastomosis and continent caecal reservoir. Scand J Urol Nephrol. 1989;23:195–200.
16. Husmann DA, McLorie GA, Churchill BM. Nonrefluxing colonic conduits: a long-term lifetable analysis. J Urol. 1989;142:1201–3.

17. Kristjansson A, Bajc M, Wallin L, Willner J, Mansson W. Renal function up to 16 years after conduit (refluxing or anti-reflux anastomosis) or continent urinary diversion. Renal scarring and location of bacteriuria. Br J Urol. 1995;76:546–50.
18. Stewart W, Cass AS, Matsen JM. Variation in bacteriuria with intestinal loop urinary diversions. J Urol. 1974;111:117–9.
19. Mottaz AE, Zingg EJ, Studer UE. Ureterosigmoidostomy in adults: long term results. Prog Urol. 1996;6:87–92.
20. Hall MC, Koch MO, McDougal WS. Metabolic consequences of urinary diversion through intestinal segments. Urol Clin NorthAm. 1991;18:725–35.
21. Husmann DA, Spence HM. Current status of tumor of the bowel following ureterosigmoidostomy: a review. J Urol. 1990;144:607–10.
22. Wullt B, Agace W, Mansson W. Bladder, bowel and bugs—bacteriuria in patients with intestinal urinary diversion. World J Urol. 2004;22:186–95.
23. Hautmann RE. Urinary diversion: ileal conduit to neobladder. J Urol. 2003;169:834–42.
24. Wullt B, Holstb E, Stevenc K, Carstensenc J, et al. Microbial flora in ileal and colonic neobladders. Eur Urol. 2004;45:233–9.
25. Bruce AW, Reid G, Chan RC, Costerton JW. Bacterial adherence in the human ileal conduit: a morphological and bacteriological study. J Urol. 1984;132:184–8.
26. Carlen B, Willen R, Mansson W. Mucosal ultrastructure of continent cecal reservoir for urine and its ileal nipple valve: 9 years after construction. J Urol. 1990;143:372–6.
27. Laux DC, McSweegan EF, Williams TJ, Wadolkowski EA, Cohen PS. Identification and characterization of mouse small intestine mucosal receptors for *Escherichia coli* K-12(K88ab). Infect Immun. 1986;52:18–25.
28. Mouricout MA, Julien RA. Pilus-mediated binding of bovine enterotoxigenic *Escherichia coli* to calf small intestinal mucins. Infect Immun. 1987;55:1216–23.
29. Drumm B, Roberton AM, Sherman PM. Inhibition of attachment of *Escherichia coli* RDEC-1 to intestinal microvillus membranes by rabbit ileal mucus and mucin in vitro. Infect Immun. 1988;56:2437–42.
30. Mack DR, Sherman PM. Mucin isolated from rabbit colon inhibits in vitro binding of *Escherichia coli* RDEC-1. Infect Immun. 1991;59:1015–23.
31. Cox CE, Hinman F Jr. Factors in resistance to infection in the bladder. The eradication of bacteria by vesical emptying and intrinsic defense mechanisms. In: Kass EH (ed) 1965 Progress in pyelonephritis. FA Davies, Philadelphia.
32. Gordon DM, Riley MA. A theoretical and experimental analysis of bacterial growth in the bladder. Mol Microbiol. 1992;6:555–62.
33. O'Grady F, Cattel WR. Kinetics of urinary tract infection in upper urinary tract. Br J Urol. 1966;38:156.
34. Iwakiri J, Freiha FS, Shortliffe LM. Prospective study of urinary tract infections and urinary antibodies after radical prostatectomy and cystoprostatectomy. Urol Clin North Am. 2002;29:251–8.
35. Mansson W, Colleen S, Low K, Mardh PA, Lundblad A. Immunoglobulins in urine from patients with ileal and colonic conduits and reservoirs. J Urol. 1985;133:713–6.
36. Trinchieri A, Braceschi L, Tiranti D, Dell'Acqua S, Mandressi A, Pisani E. Secretory immunoglobulin A and inhibitory activity of bacterial adherence to epithelial cells in urine from patients with urinary tract infections. Urol Res. 1990;18:305–8.
37. Hedges S, Stenqvist K, Lidin-Janson G, Martinell J, Sandberg T, Svanborg C. Comparison of urine and serum concentrations of interleukin-6 in women with acute pyelonephritis or asymptomatic bacteriuria. J Infect Dis. 1992;166:653–6.
38. Neutra M, Forstner J. Gastrointestinal mucus: synthesis secretion and function. In: Johnson L, editor. Physiology of the gastrointestinal tract. 2nd ed. New York: Raven Press; 1987. p. 975–1009.
39. Schlegel JU, Cuellar J, O'Dell RM. Bactericidal effect of urea. J Urol. 1961;86:819–22.
40. Hill MJ, Hudson MJ, Stewart M. The urinary bacterial flora in patients with three types of urinary tract diversion. J Med Microbiol. 1983;16:221–6.

41. Falagas ME, Vergidis PI. Urinary tract infections in patients with urinary diversion. Am J Kidney Dis. 2005;46(6):1030–7. https://doi.org/10.1053/j.ajkd.2005.09.008.
42. Keegan SJ, Graham C, Neal DE, Blum-Oehler G, N'Dow J, Pearson JP, Gally DL. Characterization of *Escherichia coli* strains causing urinary tract infections in patients with transposed intestinal segments. J Urol. 2003;169:2382–7.
43. Liu W, Shatagopam K, Monn F, et al. Risk for Clostridium difficile infection after radical cystectomy for bladder cancer: analysis of a contemporary series. Urol Oncol. 2015;33:503.e17–22.
44. Damle RN, Cherng NB, Flahive JM, et al. Clostridium difficile infection after colorectal surgery: a rare but costly complication. J Gastrointest Surg. 2014;18:1804.
45. Large MC, Kiriluk KJ, DeCastro GJ, et al. The impact of mechanical bowel preparation on postoperative complications for patients undergoing cystectomy and urinary diversion. J Urol. 2012;188:1801.
46. Mossanen M, Calvert JK, Holt SK, James AC, Wright JL, Harper JD, et al. Overuse of antimicrobial prophylaxis in community practice urology. J Urol. 2015;193(2):543–7.
47. Krasnow RE, Mossanen M, Koo S, Kubiak DW, et al. Prophylactic antibiotics and postoperative complications of radical cystectomy: a population based analysis in the United States. J Urol. 2017;198:297–304. https://doi.org/10.1016/j.juro.2017.02.3340.
48. Shah K, Pass LA, Cox M, et al. Evaluating contemporary antibiotics as a risk factor for Clostridium difficile infection in surgical trauma patients. J Trauma Acute Care Surg. 2012;72:691.
49. Keshavamurthy S, Koch CG, Fraser TG, et al. Clostridium difficile infection after cardiac surgery: prevalence, morbidity, mortality, and resource utilization. J Thorac Cardiovasc Surg. 2014;148:3157.
50. Hensgens MP, GoorhuisA DOM, et al. Time interval of increased risk for *Clostridium difficile* infection after exposure to antibiotics. J Antimicrob Chemother. 2012;67:742.
51. Valiquette L, Cossette B, Garant MP, et al. Impact of a reduction in the use of high-risk antibiotics on the course of an epidemic of *Clostridium difficile*–associated disease caused by the hypervirulent NAP1/027strain. Clin Infect Dis. 2007;45(Suppl 2):S112.
52. Muto CA, Blank MK, Marsh JW, et al. Control of an outbreak of infection with the hyper virulent Clostridium difficile BI strain in a university hospital using a comprehensive "bundle" approach. Clin Infect Dis. 2007;45:1266.
53. Cohen SH, Gerding DN, Johnson S, et al. Clinical practice guidelines for *Clostridium difficile* infection inadults: 2010 update by the Society For Healthcare Epidemiology of America (SHEA) and the Infectious Diseases Society of America (IDSA). Infect Control Hosp Epidemiol. 2010;31:431.
54. Dial S, Delaney JA, Barkun AN, et al. Use of gastric acid-suppressive agents and the risk of community-acquired *Clostridium difficile*-associated disease. JAMA J Am Med Assoc. 2005;294:2989.
55. Lowrance WT, Rumohr JA, Chang SS, et al. Contemporary open radical cystectomy: analysis of perioperative outcomes. J Urol. 2008;179:1313–8; discussion 1318.
56. Takeyama K. Incidence of and risk factors for surgical site infection in patients with radical cystectomy with urinary diversion. J Infect Chemother. 2005;11:177.
57. EAU Guidelines Urological Infections 2017 EAU; 2017.
58. Craig WA, Andes DR. Cephalosporins. In: Bennett JE, Dolin R, Blaser MJ, editors. Mandell, Douglas, and Bennett's principles and practice of infectious diseases. 8th ed. Philadelphia: Elsevier/Saunders; 2015.
59. Moellering RC Jr, Swartz MN. Drug therapy: the newer cephalosporins. N Engl J Med. 1976;294:24.
60. Mano R, Baniel J, Goldberg H, et al. Urinary tract infections in patients with orthotopic neobladder. Urol Oncol. 2014;32:50.e9.
61. Suriano F, Gallucci M, Flammia GP, et al. Bacteriuria in patients with an orthotopic ileal neobladder: urinary tract infection or asymptomatic bacteriuria? BJU Int. 2008;101:1576–9.
62. Paick SH, Park HK, Oh SJ, et al. Characteristics of bacterial colonization and urinary tract infection after indwelling of double-J ureteral stent. Urology. 2003;62:214–7.

63. Boni L, B. A. Infective complications in laparoscopic surgery. Surg Infect. 2006;7:s-109.
64. Mutoh M. Systemic inflammatory response syndrome in open versus laparoscopic adrenalectomy. Urology. 2004;64:422.
65. Studer UE, Zingg EJ. Ileal orthotopic bladder substitutes. What we have learned from 12 years' experience with 200 patients. Urol Clin North Am. 1997;24:781–93.
66. Steven K, Poulsen AL. The orthotopic Kock ileal neobladder: functional results, urodynamic features, complications and survival in 166 men. J Urol. 2000;164:288–95.
67. Wood DP Jr, Bianco FJ Jr, Pontes JE, Heath MA, DaJusta D. Incidence and significance of positive urine cultures in patients with an orthotopic neobladder. J Urol. 2003;169:2196–9.
68. Arai Y, Kawakita M, Terachi T, Oishi K, Okada Y, Takeuchi H, Yoshida O. Long-term follow-up of the Kock and Indiana pouch procedures. J Urol. 1993;150:51–5.
69. Bergman B. Studies on patients with ileal conduit diversion with special regard to renal infection. Scand J Urol Nephrol Suppl. 1978;(47):1–32.
70. Akerlund S, Campanello M, Kaijser B, Jonsson O. Bacteriuria in patients with a continent ileal reservoir for urinary diversion does not regularly require antibiotic treatment. Br J Urol. 1994;74:177–81.
71. Kim SP, Shah ND, Karnes RJ, et al. The implications of hospital acquired adverse events on mortality, length of stay and costs for patients undergoing radical cystectomy for bladder cancer. J Urol. 2012;187:2011–7.
72. Tal R, Sivan B, Kedar D, Baniel J. Management of benign ureteral strictures following radical cystectomy and urinary diversion for bladder cancer. J Urol. 2007;178:538–42.
73. Eisenberg MS, Thompson RH, Frank I, et al. Long-term renal function outcomes after radical cystectomy. J Urol. 2014;191:619–25.
74. Kumar A, Roberts D, Wood KE, et al. Duration of hypotension before initiation of effective antimicrobial therapy is the critical determinant of survival in human septic shock. Crit Care Med. 2006;34:1589–96.
75. Darouiche RO, et al. Bacterial interference for prevention of urinary tract infection: a prospective, randomized, placebo-controlled, double-blind pilot trial. Clin Infect Dis. 2005;41:1531. https://www.ncbi.nlm.nih.gov/pubmed/16231269
76. Sunden F, et al. *Escherichia coli* 83972 bacteriuria protects against recurrent lower urinary tract infections in patients with incomplete bladder emptying. J Urol. 2010;184:179. https://www.ncbi.nlm.nih.gov/pubmed/20473149

Prevention and Treatment of Infectious Complications After Urogenital Prosthesis Surgery

21

Michele Rizzo, Stefano Bucci, Nicola Pavan, Enrica Verzotti, Giacomo Di Cosmo, Paolo Umari, Carlo Trombetta, and Giovanni Liguori

21.1 Introduction

Prostheses are widely used in urogenital surgery for many decades and have gained a fundamental role in the management of multiple diseases with good results in terms of functionality, aesthetic outcomes, and patients' satisfaction.

It is remarkable that prosthetic device vary in terms of mechanical sophistication, costs, and surgical implantation techniques ranging from simple device widely used in urological practice like testicular prosthesis to highly sophisticated devices as inflatable penile prosthesis (IPP) and artificial urinary sphincter (AUS). Despite continuous implementations of devices and improvements of surgical implantation techniques, infective complications are still fearful and not uncommon events [1]. Incidence of infections reported by high-volume centers ranges from 1% to 2% for AUS [2, 3] and from 2% to 8% for IPP [4, 5] and growth further in the case of revision surgery [6]. Risk of infection depends on patients' individual features, perioperative strategies, implantation techniques, and prosthetic devices. Preventing these complications is imperative because the management of prosthesis infection requires removal of the device in most cases.

M. Rizzo (✉) · S. Bucci · N. Pavan · E. Verzotti · G. Di Cosmo · C. Trombetta · G. Liguori
Department of Urology, University of Trieste, Ospedale di Cattinara, Trieste, Italy
e-mail: michele.rizzo@asugi.sanita.fvg.it; stefano.bucci@asugi.sanita.fvg.it; Nicola.pavan@asugi.sanita.fvg.it; enrica.verzotti@asugi.sanita.fvg.it; giacomo.dicosmo@asugi.sanita.fvg.it; carlo.trombetta@asugi.sanita.fvg.it; giovanni.liguori@asugi.sanita.fvg.it

P. Umari
Division of Urology, Maggiore Della Carità Hospital, University of Eastern Piedmont, Novara, Italy
e-mail: paolo.umari@asugi.sanita.fvg.it

T. E. Bjerklund Johansen, T. Cai (eds.), *Guide to Antibiotics in Urology*,
https://doi.org/10.1007/978-3-319-92366-6_21

21.2 Patient Features

The importance of patients' features in the development of infective complication is often underestimated in clinical studies such as in clinical practices.

Before prosthetic implantation, patients should be categorized in relation to the presence of general and specific endogenous or exogenous risk factors for infective complications such as general health status according to American Society of Anesthesiology (ASA) score, diabetes mellitus, older age, impaired immune system, malnutrition, obesity, history of urogenital infection, indwelling catheters, bacterial burden, previous instrumentation, and genetic factors.

Some of these individual features are not modifiable, but some others are at least partially corrigible.

Habous et al. recently demonstrated a strong correlation between levels of glycated hemoglobin (HbA1c) and the risk of infective complications in a cohort of patients that underwent implantation of IPP for erectile dysfunction. Infection rates were as follows: 1.3% for patients with HbA1c <6.5%, 1.5% with HbA1c 6.5–7.5%, 6.5% with HbA1c 7.6–8.5%, 14.7% with HbA1c 8.6–9.5%, and 22.4% with HbA1c >9.5% ($p < 0.001$) [7]. PROPPR study collected 1019 patients from 11 medical centers in North America that underwent penile prosthesis implantation for erectile dysfunction; 20% of patients in this cohort were diabetic [8]. Lots of patients that require penile prosthesis for erectile restoration are diabetics. However, diabetes mellitus (DM) is a heterogeneous condition, and some patients present a well-controlled DM, while others present the most severe manifestations of the disease.

Nowadays, the blood level of glycated hemoglobin is still the best available marker for long-term DM control. Implant surgeons should know the importance of uncontrolled DM as a risk factor for infective complications of urogenital prosthesis surgery and should screen patients with an evaluation of HbA1c. Furthermore, surgeons should discuss with patients about the risks of infective complications connected with uncontrolled diabetes and should consider not proceeding with an implant procedure if glycosylated hemoglobin is more than 8.5%.

DM should be considered an individual modifiable risk factor of infective complications of surgery and, therefore, should be corrected before an elective surgical procedure.

21.3 Perioperative Strategies to Prevent Infective Complications of Prosthetic Urogenital Surgery

Many perioperative strategies have been proposed in order to reduce the risk of infective complication after urogenital implant surgery. These strategies include the skin preparation, the behavior protocols for all the surgical team components, and the antibiotic prophylaxis.

21.3.1 Skin Preparation

Most of infective complications after urogenital prosthesis implantation are surgical site infection due to skin-related staphylococci. For this reason, it is mandatory to reduce the microorganisms' presence on the skin at the time of surgery, therefore reducing the risk that the surgical wound will become contaminated and infected. Patients should shower or bathe (full body) with antimicrobial soap or an antiseptic agent on at least the night before the operative day [9]. Intraoperative, a penile, scrotal, and perineal scrub with an alcohol-based antiseptic agent should be performed. Yeung et al. demonstrated that chlorhexidine-alcohol was superior to the traditionally used povidone iodine in eradicating the skin flora at the surgical skin site before genitourinary prosthetic implantation [10]. Moreover, many experts sustain that the scrub procedure should last at least 10 min [10].

21.3.2 Antibiotic Prophylaxis

Antibiotic prophylaxis is only one of several measures to prevent infections and can never compensate for poor hygiene and operative technique. As known, antibiotics should never be used in fixed dosage, but every antibiotic regimen, both prophylactic and therapeutic, should be individualized and tailored on patients' features and surgical procedure. Given these previous considerations, good usage of antibiotic prophylaxes seems to reduce the incidence of infective complications after urogenital prosthesis implantation. Most of infective complications are caused by skin-related staphylococci; because of that, antibiotics used for prophylaxis must be chosen to target these bacteria as cephalosporin group 2 or 3 or penicillin (penicillinase stable). The use of gentamicin in association with the previously reported antibiotics seems to improve the prophylactic efficacy before inflatable penile prosthesis (IPP) implantation. According to the best evidence, gentamicin should be administered once a day at 5 mg/kg. Durations of perioperative antibiotic prophylaxis has not yet been adequately addressed; however, antibiotic regimens reported in high volume series last for about 1 week [11].

Gross et al. collected data from 25 centers of wound cultures retrieved at the time of explant/revision surgery for infected penile prosthesis. They identified a total of 204 organisms; 11% of these were *Candida* species [12]. According to these findings, implant surgeon should consider to enrich antibiotic prophylaxis with antifungals both locally and systemically.

21.3.3 Other Intraoperative Strategies

According to many experts, minimalizing foot traffic through the theatre can decrease the risk of infective complications. Furthermore, the vigorous washing of the cavity before device placement with antibiotic solutions is considered very important to both flush out and kill any present bacteria [13].

21.3.4 Surgical Procedure

Implantation techniques of urogenital prosthesis are still evolving, and, in order to reduce the risk of infection in implant surgery, some surgical strategies have been described. First of all, it is mandatory to decrease operative time as much as possible in order to reduce risks of device contamination and surgical site infection. As a matter of fact, skilled high-volume surgeons present a lower incidence of infective complications. Secondarily, it is imperative, during surgical implantation, to avoid any passage of microbes from the skin to the surgeons, the instruments, the devices, and the tissue where the prosthesis is going to be placed. Many strategies have been proposed, but the most effective seems the "no-touch technique" described by Eid [14]. Basically, the "no-touch technique" consists in covering the perineal and genital skin with a sterile drape before the skin incision and then applying a second sterile drape onto the surgical field once the book fascia has been exposed. This technique, combined with the substitution of all the gloves and the surgical instruments before the setting of the second sterile drape, minimizes the risk of contaminations. In a large series of patients who underwent IPP implantation using the "no-touch technique," the incidence of infective complications reported was less than 0.46% [14].

21.3.5 Device Features

Since their introduction, prosthetic devices have been evolving in order to achieve not only a better aesthetic and functional outcome but also to reduce the risks of contamination and infective complications. IIPs are probably the most sophisticated prosthetic devices used in urogenital surgery. The main manufacturers are AMS (American.

Medical Systems, Minneapolis, MN, USA) and Coloplast (Coloplast, Minneapolis, MN, USA). Both of these companies developed technologies to reduce the risk of prosthesis contamination during implant surgery. In 2001, AMS introduced a penile implant impregnated with rifampin and minocycline (InhibiZone®). This technology permits a continuous antibiotic release from the surface of the device with bactericidal effects toward the majority of contaminating bacteria on the implant surface and the surrounding tissue. In 2002, Mentor (now Coloplast) introduced a penile prosthesis precoated with hydrophilic polyvinyl pyrrolidone (Titan®). This hydrophilic coating is designed to inhibit bacterial adherence on the surface of the penile implant. Both these technologies have resulted in the decrease of infective complications. Titan® systems could be coated with different antibiotic solutions; however, the most effective in reducing infectious complication is the associations of rifampin and gentamicin [15]. The superiority of one system over the other has not yet been demonstrated.

21.4 Treatment of Infective Complications After Urogenital Prosthesis Surgery

Conservative management of infective complications is almost never possible. Bacteria that contaminated the device produce a slime-like material called biofilm. Biofilm is an exopolysaccharide and plays an important role in the pathogenesis of infection. It provides nutrition to the bacteria, interferes with phagocytosis, blocks response to antibiotics, and facilitates adhesion, aggregation, and polymicrobial interaction. When the biofilm deposition begins, the colonization of the device is not reversible. Because of the treatment of infections, complications require an early diagnosis, the prompt start of antibiotic therapy, and the removal of the prosthesis.

21.5 Conclusion

Prosthetic surgery represents an important treatment option of multiple urologic conditions. The risk of infective complication after urogenital prosthetic surgery depends on patients' individual features, perioperative strategies, implantation techniques, and prosthetic devices. Many strategies have been developed to prevent colonization of the device and reduce the risk of infections. Centers that plan prosthetic implantations should be based on these strategies and protocols in order to prevent, as far as possible, infective complications.

References

1. Henry GD, Wilson SK. Updates in inflatable penile prostheses. Urol Clin North Am. 2007;34(4):535–47. https://doi.org/10.1016/j.ucl.2007.08.015.
2. Nam RK, Herschorn S, Loblaw DA, et al. Population based study of long-term rates of surgery for urinary incontinence after radical prostatectomy for prostate cancer. J Urol. 2012;188(2):502–6. https://doi.org/10.1016/j.juro.2012.04.005.
3. Lee R, Te AE, Kaplan SA, Sandhu JS. Temporal trends in adoption of and indications for the artificial urinary sphincter. J Urol. 2009;181(6):2622–7. https://doi.org/10.1016/j.juro.2009.01.113.
4. Carson CC. Penile prosthesis implantation and infection for Sexual Medicine Society of North America. Int J Impot Res. 2001;13(Suppl 5):S35–8. https://doi.org/10.1038/sj.ijir.3900775.
5. Petero VG, Diokno AC. Comparison of the long-term outcomes between incontinent men and women treated with artificial urinary sphincter. J Urol. 2006;175(2):605–9. https://doi.org/10.1016/S0022-5347(05)00243-0.
6. Jarow JP. Risk factors for penile prosthetic infection. Int Urol Nephrol. 2003;35(2):209–13. https://doi.org/10.1023/B:UROL.0000020300.23522.49.
7. Habous M, Tal R, Tealab A, Soliman T, Nassar M, Mekawi ZMS, Abdelwahab O, Elkhouly M, Kamr H, Remeah A, Binsaleh S, Ralph DMJ. Defining a glycated haemoglobin (HbA1c) level that predicts increased risk of penile implant infection. BJU Int. 2017;121:10. https://doi.org/10.1111/bju.14076.

8. Henry GD, Karpman E, Brant W, et al. The who, how and what of real-world penile implantation in 2015: the PROPPR Registry Baseline Data. J Urol. 2016;195(2):427–33. https://doi.org/10.1016/j.juro.2015.07.109.
9. Berríos-Torres SI, Umscheid CA, Bratzler DW, et al. Centers for Disease Control and Prevention guideline for the prevention of surgical site infection, 2017. JAMA Surg. 2017;152(8):784. https://doi.org/10.1001/jamasurg.2017.0904.
10. Yeung LL, Grewal S, Bullock A, Lai HH, Brandes SB. A comparison of chlorhexidine-alcohol versus povidone-iodine for eliminating skin flora before genitourinary prosthetic surgery: a randomized controlled trial. J Urol. 2013;189(1):136–40. https://doi.org/10.1016/j.juro.2012.08.086.
11. Xie D, Gheiler V, Lopez I, Nehrenz GM Sr, Klopukh B, Bianco FPP, E. G. Experience with prophylactic gentamicin during penile prosthesis surgery: a retrospective comparison of two different doses. J Sex Med. 2017;14(9):1160–4. https://doi.org/10.1016/j.jsxm.2017.06.014.
12. Gross MS, Phillips EA, Carrasquillo RJ, et al. Multicenter investigation of the micro-organisms involved in penile prosthesis infection: an analysis of the efficacy of the AUA and EAU guidelines for penile prosthesis prophylaxis. J Sex Med. 2017;14(3):455–63. https://doi.org/10.1016/j.jsxm.2017.01.007.
13. Abouassaly R, Angermeier KW, Montague DK. Risk of infection with an antibiotic coated penile prosthesis at device replacement for mechanical failure. J Urol. 2006;176(6):2471–3. https://doi.org/10.1016/j.juro.2006.08.010.
14. Eid JF. Penile implant: review of a "no-touch" technique. Sex Med Rev. 2016;4(3):294–300. https://doi.org/10.1016/j.sxmr.2016.01.002.
15. Dhabuwala C, Sheth S, Zamzow B. Infection rates of rifampin/gentamicin-coated titan Coloplast penile implants. Comparison with inhibizone-impregnated AMS penile implants. J Sex Med. 2011;8(1):315–20. https://doi.org/10.1111/j.1743-6109.2010.02068.x.

Part VI

Practical Guidelines on Antibiotic Treatment of Urinary Tract Infections

Practical Guidelines on Antibiotic Treatment of Urinary Tract Infections

22

Truls E. Bjerklund Johansen, Tommaso Cai, Kurt G. Naber, José Medina-Polo, Laila Schneidewind, Gernot Bonkat, Bela Koves, Ana-María Tapia-Herrero, Florian M. E. Wagenlehner, and George G. Zhanel

T. E. Bjerklund Johansen (✉)
Department of Urology, Oslo University Hospital, Oslo, Norway

Institute of Clinical Medicine, University of Oslo, Oslo, Norway

Institute of Clinical Medicine, University of Aarhus, Aarhus, Denmark
e-mail: tebj@uio.no

T. Cai
Department of Urology, Santa Chiara Regional Hospital, Trento, Italy

K. G. Naber
Department of Urology, Technical University of Munich, Munich, Germany
e-mail: kurt.naber@nabers.de

J. Medina-Polo
Department of Urology, Health Research Institute, Hospital Universitario 12 de Octubre, Madrid, Spain
e-mail: jose.medina@salud.madrid.org

L. Schneidewind
Department of Urology, University Medical Center Rostock, Rostock, Germany
e-mail: Laila.Schneidewind@med.uni-rostock.de

G. Bonkat
alta uro AG, Merian Iselin Klinik, Center of Biomechanics & Calorimetry, University of Basel, Basel, Switzerland
e-mail: Bonkat@alta-uro.com

B. Koves
Department of Urology, University of Szeged, Szeged, Hungary

A.-M. Tapia-Herrero
Department of Urology, Complejo Asistencial de Zamora, Zamora, Spain

F. M. E. Wagenlehner
Clinic for Urology, Pediatric Urology and Andrology, Justus Liebig University, Giessen, Germany
e-mail: florian.wagenlehner@chiru.med.uni-giessen.de

G. G. Zhanel
Department of Medical Microbiology and Infectious Diseases, Max Rady College of Medicine, Rady Faculty of Health Sciences, University of Manitoba, Winnipeg, Canada
e-mail: ggzhanel@pcsinternet.ca

T. E. Bjerklund Johansen, T. Cai (eds.), *Guide to Antibiotics in Urology*,
https://doi.org/10.1007/978-3-319-92366-6_22

22.1 Introduction

Previous chapters in this book have introduced the reader to epidemiological and microbiological aspects, clinical presentation forms, and diagnostic workup of urinary tract infections (UTI). The editors' ambition is to provide relevant information to anyone with an interest in the field of UTI. In particular, we want to provide guidance to clinicians on how to treat patients presenting with a suspected UTI. The core questions in treatment are which antibiotic, which dose, and which duration.

The first step in the clinical decision-making is to assess the severity of the situation and decide if the patient needs treatment at all. This implies taking a careful medical history and doing basic exams. The second step is to decide if the patient can be treated in an outpatient setting, usually with oral or intramuscular antibiotics or if hospitalization is needed for further diagnostic workup and intravenous administration of antibiotics. The third step is to decide which antibiotics to administer. Reasoning follows a complex algorithm also involving antibiotic stewardship principles and ends up with a few prioritized treatment alternatives.

International and national guidelines provide guidance on diagnostic workup and treatment.

However, every patient is unique and therefore the clinician must take the ultimate responsibility for what are often difficult treatment decisions. The aim of this chapter is to introduce the reader to the principles and limitations of guidelines and to give practical recommendations on antibiotic type, route of administration, dosing, and duration in the treatment of different severity types of urinary tract infections.

22.2 Clinical Decision-Making in Antibiotic Treatment of UTI

The reason for the elaborate decision process is that initial antibiotic treatment is always empiric versus directed therapy once a causative pathogen is identified and the susceptibility pattern is known. The algorithm of clinical decision-making starts with an identification of the antibiotics that are available for clinical use at a given site and time. Unfortunately, there are countries with limited access to antibiotics, and there are countries that do not allow the use of certain antibiotics. The rest of the algorithm is in principle an elimination process (Fig. 22.1.).

Pathogen characteristics. The clinician must consider which is (are) the most likely pathogen(s) and their likely resistance to the available antibiotics [1, 2]. The spectrum of causative microorganisms and their resistance depend on the geographical region and the clinical setting [3]. For example, the rate of *E. coli* infections is about half as frequent in a healthcare setting as in a community setting. This means that non-*E. coli* urinary tract pathogens are relatively more frequent in a healthcare setting. Likewise, the resistance rates of pathogens are much higher in healthcare-acquired infections than in community-acquired infections [4]. In addition, the resistance rates to the most commonly used antibiotics are much higher in the south of Europe and in the southern states of the USA than in the northern parts [5].

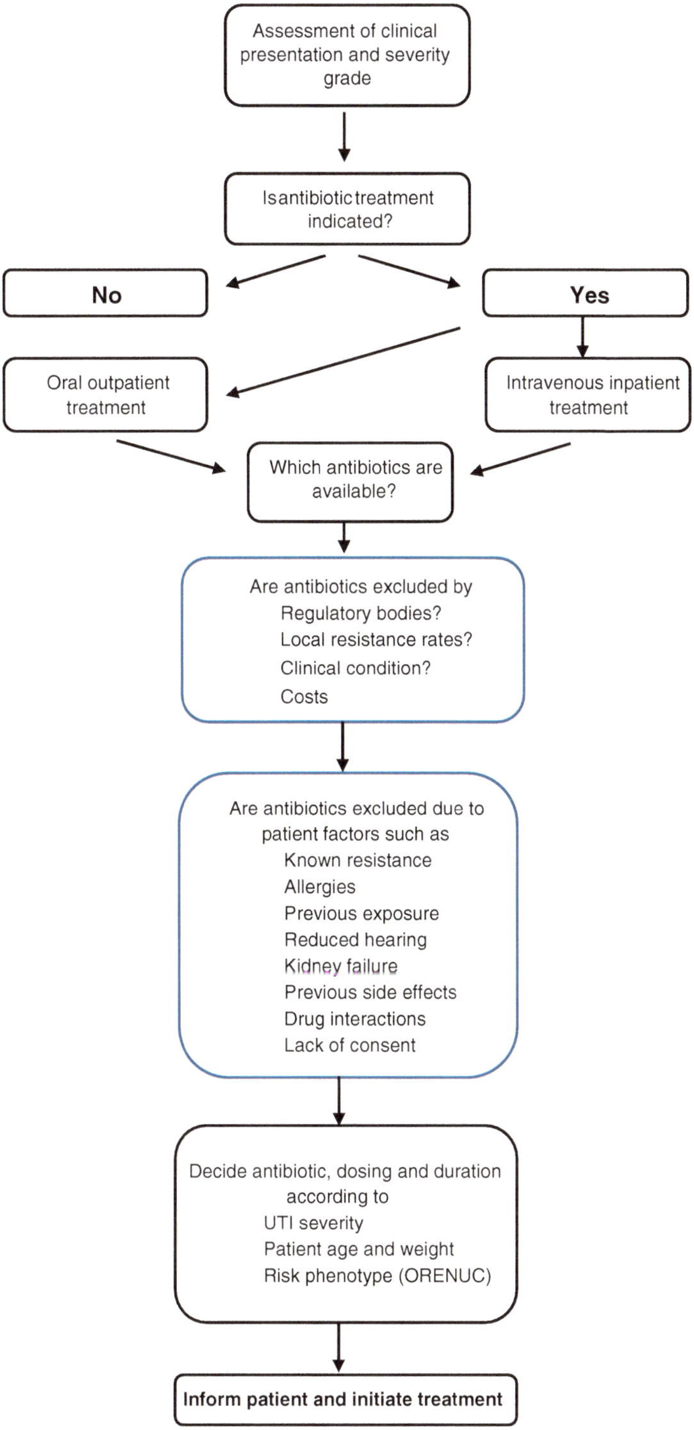

Fig. 22.1 Algorithm for clinical decision in selecting empiric antibiotic treatment for UTIs

Clinicians should be aware that in 2019 and 2020, the European Committee on Antibiotic Susceptibility Testing (EUCAST) changed the definitions of susceptibility categories S, I, and R [6]. Each susceptibility category is now defined by "breakpoints" specific for each bacterial species and antibiotic agent. The breakpoint is defined by the minimum inhibitory concentration (MIC) and describes the amount of antibiotic needed to inhibit the growth of the specific bacterial pathogen. Therefore, the interpretation of old data on rates of S, I, and R might need to be changed. While we used to interpret "I" as resistant the new definition replaces "I" with "susceptible, increased exposure." This means that there is a high likelihood of therapeutic success if exposure to the agent is increased by adjusting the dosing regimen or by its concentration at the site of infection. The change means that microbiologists extend their evaluation from a mere laboratory finding to an evaluation of the likelihood of bacteriological and clinical efficacy by also considering pharmacokinetic and pharmacodynamic data [7].

Patient characteristics. As the number of alternative antibiotics is reduced, the clinician must also consider toxicity data and the evidence for efficacy of antibiotics in the relevant severity type of UTI [1]. The clinical implication of the new EUCAST definition depends on the severity grade of the UTI, and in case of severe pyelonephritis or urosepsis, the new "I" does not necessarily mean a high likelihood of success. In severe UTI, we would not recommend treatment with an antibiotic classified as susceptible at increased exposure. Finally, yet importantly, the clinician must consider the history of the patient with regard to previous courses of antibiotics and culture results as well as side effects, allergies, and drug interactions. Risk factors, such as recurrent UTI, urinary stones, and catheters, also influence the evaluation of the most likely pathogen and its potential resistance [8]. Whoever pays for the antibiotic treatment, costs are an issue. The costs of last-line intravenous antibiotics are high and vary significantly.

Antibiotic stewardship. The O'Neil report from 2016 increased awareness of antibiotic resistance and the need for antibiotic stewardship [9]. Antibiotic resistance depends on the total consumption of antibiotics through a mechanism called the collateral effect. In acute care hospitals, 20–50% of prescribed antibiotics are either unnecessary or inappropriate [10]. This means that the clinician must consider the risk of adverse ecological effects each time she or he prescribes an antibiotic. Unintended societal consequences of antibiotic use are selection of virulent organisms, emergence of resistant bacterial strains, altered gut microbiome, healthcare-associated infections including *Clostridium difficile,* and adverse effects [11, 12].

Antibiotic therapy of severe UTI might be lifesaving and is clearly indicated. Antibiotic therapy is also recommended in low-severity UTI such as cystitis in women, because clinical success is significantly more likely in women treated with antibiotics compared with placebo [13].

22.3 Development of UTI Guidelines

In 1972, Archie Cochrane published his book *Effectiveness and Efficiency*, which described the lack of controlled trials supporting many practices that had previously been assumed to be effective [14]. In 1990, David Eddy first introduced the term "evidence-based" in an article in JAMA (Journal of the American Medical Association) that laid out the principles of evidence-based guidelines and population-level policies [15].

Early guidelines. The European Association of Urology (EAU) developed its first international guidelines on UTI in 2000. Six urologists with a documented interest and publication experience in the field of UTI met in person on several occasions and wrote UTI guidelines. The members were familiar with recent scientific literature from either authoring, reviewing, or reading the most important and impactful publications. The group organized regular scientific symposia with international opinion leaders to discuss recent papers. Privately, members subscribed to the most influential journals and built their own libraries with several hundred printed copies of the most important papers. Everyone had their own archive system. Some stored papers in alphabetical order according to the family name of the first author. Others numbered papers with corresponding punch cards with up to 200 holes to indicate categories and search terms. By inserting knitting needles through the holes, relevant papers could be retrieved within seconds. Group members had a good overview of relevant papers. For a well-defined topic such as antibiotic treatment of pyelonephritis, this usually meant about 10 papers. Early guidelines development was a very low-cost project.

Archiving of papers. The National Library of Medicine (NLM) made Medline freely available in 1997, and PubMed became a free archive in 2000 [16]. Today, PubMed stores more than 35 million citations and abstracts dating back to 1966. Each year, 1 million new papers are added to the PubMed database corresponding to 3–5000 new publications each day [16]. Librarians at the National Library of Medicine tag every biomedical article to be indexed by their PubMed information system with terms from the MeSH terminology or thesaurus, a biomedical conceptual hierarchy with over 27,000 terms. MeSH is an acronym for *Me*dical *S*ubject *H*eadings, which are organized in a "tree" with 16 main branches, i.e., anatomy, diseases, and drugs [17].

Retrieving relevant papers. Retrieval of papers from the vast NLM database follows the archiving process in the opposite direction. To facilitate the literature search and help find relevant evidence, guideline developers use a specialized framework, called PICO, to formulate the research question. PICO stands for *P*atient, *I*ntervention, *C*omparison, and *O*utcome [18]. The PICO framework can be expanded to PICOTT by adding information about the *T*ype of question being asked (therapy, diagnosis, prognosis, harm, etc.) and the best *T*ype of study design for that particular question. The initial search outcome usually contains several thousand abstracts, which undergo structured and systematic review by two or more guideline associates. They score papers according to study criteria, check for bias, and ascribe levels of evidence. Evaluation of inconsistencies, heterogeneity, and bias require special statistical methods (I^2-test) [19]. In the end, there might be only a handful of papers left for scrutiny. If more than two randomized controlled studies are available, they may undergo meta-analysis and be presented in a forest plot [20]. Retrieval of papers that are relevant for guidelines development is a very resource-demanding and high-cost process.

Relevant papers in urology. UTIs are diagnosed by clinical symptoms and evidence for presence of a pathogen [21]. In order to be relevant, papers must have included patients with a well-defined clinical condition (i.e., pyelonephritis, cystitis, and urethritis), setting (community- or hospital-acquired infection), and gender (male/female). Patient groups must be similar in terms of risk factors or phenotypes that will influence treatment outcomes (recent antibiotic treatment, hospitalization, diabetes mellitus, immunodeficiency, urinary tract obstruction, and presence of catheters and stents). Main outcomes of clinical studies are rates of symptom relief and eradication of causative microorganisms. Unless the type of pathogen and it's resistance profile are among inclusion criteria, both variables will be major confounders. Because antibiotic resistance has increased over time, 20–30-year-old studies may have limited relevance today. Thirty years ago, we did not know about resistance or long-term side effects of fluoroquinolones. Today, resistance rates are as high as 50% in certain regions, and groups such as the EMA (European Medical Agency) have banned the use of fluoroquinolones in infections with low severity grade because of side effects [22]. Likewise, the resistance rate of *E. coli* to co-trimoxazole is now more than 20% in certain regions, which is above the threshold for giving this antibiotic on empirical basis. The meaning of these confounders is that it can be difficult to design and interpret the outcome of studies on antibiotic treatment of UTI. Studies from one region at a given time might not be relevant in other regions and times.

22.4 Antibiotic Treatment of UTI

Guidance on antibiotic treatment is a core element of all guidelines on UTI. In the present section, we present a narrative review of guidelines recommendations developed by different international societies and institutions. The European Association of Urology (EAU) guidelines are regarded the most influential UTI guidelines in the world. More than 60 countries have adopted these guidelines. Below, we compare EAU recommendations with recommendations in other international and selected national guidelines. Recommendations are presented according to clinical severity grade and risk factors. The evidence base is discussed briefly.

22.4.1 Cystitis

EAU recommendations on antibiotic treatment of cystitis in women are presented as first-line treatment and alternative treatment (Table 22.1).

Table 22.1 EAU guidelines recommendations on antibiotic treatment of cystitis in women [23]. Severity grades refer to the ORENUC grading which is presented in Chap. 5

Cystitis (severity grade 1)		
First-line treatment		
Antibiotic	Daily dose	Number of days
Fosfomycin trometamol	3 g SD	1
Nitrofurantoin macrocrystal	50–100 mg qid	5
Nitrofurantoin monohydrate/macrocrystals	100 mg bid	5
Nitrofurantoin microcrystal prolonged release	100 mg bid	5
Pivmecillinam	200 mg tid	3–5
Alternative treatment		
Antibiotic	**Daily dose**	**Number of days**
Cephalosporins (e.g., cefadroxil) or comparable	500 mg bid	3
Trimethoprim[a]	200 mg bid	5
TMP/SMX[a]	160/800 mg bid	3

Bid Twice a day, *tid* Three times a day, *qid* Four times a day, *SD* Single dose, *TMP/SMX* Trimethoprim/sulfamethoxazole

[a]Only if the local resistance rate for *E. coli* is <20%

Evidence base. The EAU guidelines strongly recommend prescribing fosfomycin trometamol, pivmecillinam, or nitrofurantoin as first-line treatment of uncomplicated cystitis in women [23]. Four papers published in 1996, 2000, 2007, and 2015, respectively, support this recommendation [24–27]. The paper from 2000 is a review paper discussing two Scandinavian comparative studies on pivmecillinam [26]. The paper from 2007 compares the cure rates of nitrofurantoin and co-trimoxazole [24]. The paper from 2015 is a review of the effects of nitrofurantoin based on trials performed during the period of 1970–1990 [27]. Hence, the evidence base for the first-line recommendations are either very old or the comparator is less relevant.

The evidence base for recommendations on alternative antibiotics consists of two papers, a US-based guideline from 1999, meant to be updated after 2 years, and a review paper published in 2002 [28, 29]. The EAU guidelines recommend against using aminopenicillin/clavulanic acid and against using oral cephalosporins. One of the two papers supporting this recommendation is from 2005 [30]. The other is from 2012 [31]. In the first study, amoxiclavulanate was inferior to ciprofloxacin, and in the second paper, cefpodoxime did not meet inferiority criteria against ciprofloxacin. Hence, in both studies, the comparator is no longer relevant as oral treatment of cystitis.

Modifications by risk factors. Presence of risk factors indicates a more thorough diagnostic workup and longer treatment duration. For details, we refer the reader to the full text version of EAU guidelines [23].

Recommendations in other guidelines. To obtain an international overview, we reviewed guidelines presented in the WHO EML-handbook (Essential Medicines

List Antibiotic Book) [32], American guidelines (IDSA, Infectious Disease Society of America) [33], Asian guidelines [34], selected national European guidelines from the UK (NICE, National Institute of Clinical Excellence) [35], and German guidelines [36] (Table 22.2).

While German guidelines are largely consistent with EAU guidelines, the other guidelines differ with regard to the use of fosfomycin, co-trimoxazole, fluoroquinolones, and β-lactams in the treatment of cystitis in adult women without risk factors. German guidelines also recommend nitroxoline among antibiotics to be used in the treatment of uncomplicated cystitis and also hint that nonantibiotic, symptomatic treatment may be considered in cases with mild or moderate symptoms [36]. Interestingly, there are significant differences between national European guidelines in terms of recommended antibiotics, routes of administration, and duration of treatment [37]. This reflects the complexity of guideline development and differences in weighting of factors that influence clinical decision-making.

22.4.2 Mild Pyelonephritis

Mild pyelonephritis may be treated with oral antibiotics in an outpatient setting or with parenteral treatment in an inpatient setting. In Table 22.3, we present EAU recommendations on oral antibiotic treatment of mild pyelonephritis. In Table 22.4, we present recommendations on oral treatment in other guidelines.

Evidence base. EAU recommendations on oral treatment of pyelonephritis are based on three papers, one published in 2010 and two published in 2018 [33, 38, 39]. The paper from 2010 is an update of the IDSA guideline from 1999 [33]. The first paper from 2018 is a systematic review with rather weak conclusions that are not consistent with a strong recommendation on the use of fluoroquinolones and cephalosporins as oral treatment [38]. The second paper from 2018 has studied short- and long-term treatment with four different antibiotics and emphasizes that the risk of reinfection is much higher after short-treatment courses [39].

Modifications by risk factors. Patients with significant risk factors should be regarded as having severe pyelonephritis and should be treated as inpatients with intravenous antibiotics.

Recommendations in other guidelines. We reviewed recommendations in the WHO handbook, the IDSA American guidelines, as well as UK and German guidelines [32, 33, 36, 40]. The recommendations on oral, outpatient treatment of mild pyelonephritis are presented in Table 22.4.

EAU recommendations on intravenous antibiotic treatment of both mild and severe pyelonephritis are presented as first-line, second-line, and last-line alternatives. Second- and last-line treatments are meant for severe pyelonephritis (Table 22.5).

Evidence base. EAU guideline recommendations on first- and second-line intravenous treatment of pyelonephritis are based on one review paper by a single author from 2012 [41]. Recommendations on last-line alternatives are based on 12 papers published in the period 1999–2018 [42–53]. Ten papers report on nine studies, all of

Table 22.2 Recommendations on antibiotic treatment of cystitis in international and selected national guidelines

Guideline	Antibiotics								Ref
	Nitrofurantoin	Nitroxoline	Co-trim[a]	Fosftrom[b]	Pivm[c]	Fluoroquinolones[d]	β-lactams	Trim[e]	
WHO EML	X		X				X[f]		32
US (IDSA)	X mono hydrate		X	X	X	X	X[g]		33
Asian First choice	X macro crystal		X	X + fosf calcium			X[h]		34
Asian alternative						Cipro-, levofloxacin	X[i]		34
UK (NICE) First choice	X				X			X	35
UK (NICE) Sec choice	X			X	X				35
German First choice	X + RT = slow release	X		X					36
German alternative			X			X + norfloxacin	Cefpodoxime-proxetil		33

[a]Co-trimoxazole
[b]Fosfomycin trometamol
[c]Pivmecillinam
[d]Ofloxacin, ciprofloxacin, levofloxacin
[e]Trimethoprim
[f]Amoxicillin/clavulanate (=co-amoxiclav)
[g]Amoxicillin/clavulanate, cefdinir, cefaclor and cefpodoxime-proxetil
[h]Amoxicillin/clavulanate, cefaclor, cephalexin
[i]Cefdinir, cefpodoxime-proxetil, cefcapene pivoxil

Table 22.3 EAU recommendations on oral antibiotic treatment of mild pyelonephritis [23]

Mild pyelonephritis (severity grade 2)			
Empirical oral treatment			
Antibiotic	Daily dose	Number of days	Comments
Ciprofloxacin	500–750 mg, bid	7	Fluoroquinolone resistance should be less than 10%
Levofloxacin	750 mg, qd	5	
Trimethoprim sulfamethoxazole	160/800 mg, bid	14	If such agents are used empirically, an initial intravenous dose of a long-acting parenteral antibiotic (e.g., ceftriaxone) should be administered
Cefpodoxime	200 mg, bid	10	
Ceftibuten	400 mg, qd	10	

Bid Twice a day, *tid* Three times a day, *qid* Four times a day

which are organized and sponsored by pharmaceutical companies [42–51]. All studies are phase II or III RCTs (randomized controlled trials) on patients with complicated UTIs and multiresistant pathogens, with many centers from Eastern European countries. One paper reports an investigator-initiated study on transition from parenteral to oral antibiotics [52]. This study had no sponsors. The last paper is a review paper by a single author from 2010 [53]. All papers were published in high-impact journals.

Modifications by risk factors. Risk factors influence antibiotic selection toward broad-spectrum antibiotics and longer-treatment courses.

Recommendations in other guidelines. The recommendations on intravenous inpatient treatment of both mild and severe pyelonephritis are presented in Table 22.6. We reviewed recommendations in the WHO handbook, the IDSA American guidelines, as well as UK and German guidelines [33, 35, 36, 40].

22.4.3 Urosepsis

The definition of urosepsis is "a dysregulated host immune response to an infection in the urogenital tract" [54]. The diagnosis is based on evidence for failure of one or more organs by means of SOFA score [55]. Effective antibiotics must be administered as soon as possible after samples of urine and blood have been taken for culture, preferably within 1 h of diagnosis. Early antibiotic treatment is always empirical and must provide a broad coverage. The intravenous alternatives are the same as for severe pyelonephritis, but adding an aminoglycoside is more common, and ertapenem 1 g, qd, should also be considered [23]. The Surviving Sepsis Campaign has provided recommendations on resuscitation and adjunctive measures [54]. For a broader coverage of the antibiotic treatment of urosepsis, the reader is referred to Chap. 12.

Table 22.4 Recommendations on oral antibiotic treatment of mild pyelonephritis in international and selected national guidelines

Guideline	Antibiotic					Ref
	Fluoroquino-lones[a]	Co-trimoxazole	Cephalosporin	β-lactams	Trimethoprim	
WHO EML	Ciprofloxacin					32
US (IDSA)	X	X				33
UK (NICE)	X		Cefalexin	Co-amoxiclav	X	40
German	X		Cefpodoxime-proxetil, ceftibuten			36

[a]Ciprofloxacin, levofloxacin

Table 22.5 EAU recommendations on intravenous antibiotic treatment of mild and severe pyelonephritis [23]

Mild pyelonephritis (severity grade 2)		
Empirical intravenous treatment		
First-line treatment		
Antibiotic	Daily dose	Comments
Ciprofloxacin,	500–750 mg, bid	
Levofloxacin	750 mg, qd	
Cefotaxime	2 g, tid	Not studied as monotherapy in acute uncomplicated pyelonephritis
Ceftriaxone	1-2 g, qd	Lower dose studied, but higher dose recommended
Severe pyelonephritis (severity grade 3)		
Second-line parenteral treatment of mild pyelonephritis and empirical treatment of severe pyelonephritis		
Antibiotic	**Daily dose**	**Comments**
Cefepime	1–2 g, bid	Lower dose studied, but higher dose recommended
Piperacillin/tazobactam	2.5–4.5 g, tid	
Gentamicin	5 mg/kg, qd	Not studied as monotherapy in acute uncomplicated pyelonephritis
Amikacin	15 mg/kg qd	
Last-line alternative treatment		
Antibiotic	**Daily dose**	**Comments**
Imipenem/cilastatin	0.5 g, qid	These agents should only be used as directed therapy once culture results demonstrate a resistant pathogens
Meropenem	1 g, tid	
Ceftolozane/tazobactam	1.5 g, tid	
Ceftazidime/avibactam	2.5 g, tid	
Cefiderocol	2 g, tid	
Meropenem-vaborbactam	2 g, tid	
Plazomicin	15 mg/kg, qd	

Bid Twice a day, *qd* Once daily, *tid* Three times a day, *qid* Four times a day, *MDR* Multidrug-resistant

22.5 Comments and Conclusions

Guidelines are written to be read by specialists as well as general practitioners (GPs). Recently, however, primary care physicians in the USA and Europe estimated that if they were to read and implement guidelines from all specialties, there would be no time left for patients within regular working hours. Specialists are also in a time crunch. GPs urged guideline developers to find other ways of communicating guidance and introduced the new concept "time needed to treat" [56]. It is being

Table 22.6 Recommendations on treatment of both mild and severe pyelonephritis in international and selected national guidelines

Guideline	Empirical IV antibiotics						Ref
	Fluoro[a]	Aminogly[b]	Penicillin broad[c]	Cephalo[d]	Cefotaxime	Carbapenem	
WHO EML	Cipro + iv/im 5 = ceftriaxone				X and/or 2 = gentamicin iv/im and/or 2 = amikacin iv/im		32
US (IDSA)	X	X		Ceftriaxone			33
UK (NICE)	Cipro	Amikacin co-amoxiclav, gentamicin		Ceftriaxone	X		40
German First choice	X			Ceftriaxone	X		36
German Sec choice		Amikacin, gentamicin	X[e]	X[f]		Erta-, mero-, and imipenem/cilastatin	36

[a]Fluoroquinolones (ciprofloxacin or levofloxacin)
[b]aminoglycoside
[c]broad-spectrum penicillins
[d]cephalosporin
[e]Piperacillin/tazobactam, amoxicillin/clavulanate
[f]Cefepime, ceftazidime, ceftazidime/avibactam, ceftolozane/tazobactam

said that the annual versions of EAU guidelines have become too heavy to carry and too expensive to send. The increase in the total volume of guidelines happens in parallel with a volume increase in patient documents. The medical community needs to find cost-effective ways to define, store, retrieve, read, and implement key information.

Cost-effective guidelines development. Decision-making in antibiotic treatment of UTI follows a complex algorithm. The structure of the algorithm and the evaluation steps are defined by general medical principles that don't change very often. Principles must be learned, but detailed practical recommendations can be easily looked up at points of care by means of modern search technologies. Principles do not need to be updated every year and guideline panels must differentiate between lasting principles and new findings that influence practical recommendations (e.g., game changers).

Retrieval of papers that are relevant for guideline development is resource-demanding, and guideline panels spend huge amounts of time on scoring medical articles. Systematic reviews are the most expensive tasks. We have argued that panel members already know recent publications currently used as references for guideline recommendations, as these are published in high-impact journals read by panel members. Guideline panels must therefore consider carefully when to undertake systematic reviews.

Weaknesses of the evidence base. Guideline recommendations are not applicable to every patient in every situation. To make good decisions, the clinician also needs sound clinical judgment and knowledge about risk factors. We believe differences between national and international guideline recommendations reflect differences in weighting of study results according to regional or local conditions, such as resistance and availability of antibiotics. Unclear inclusion criteria in studies may give different grading of evidence. For example, "complicated UTI" is a very heterogeneous group as compared to studies of patients with the same risk factor, such as male sex, diabetes mellitus, immunosuppression, catheter, etc. Unclear classification and inclusion criteria cause bias in treatment groups, and antibiotic resistance is a major confounder in studies on antibiotic treatment of UTI.

Identification of knowledge gaps. Our analysis of the evidence base shows that most articles behind recommendations on first-line treatments are very old. This is a strong signal that we need new studies. Almost all evidence on new treatments are from phase II or phase III studies (c–d). This is a sign that we also need more phase III and phase IV studies. Recent experience with ciprofloxacin underlines the importance of phase IV studies [21].

Ten out of twelve RCTs on second- or last-line treatment of severe UTIs in EAU guidelines predominantly included sites and patients from Eastern Europe [42–51]. We need to discuss if the way investigators are reimbursed in these studies might lead to selection bias. If inclusion criteria are unclear, such as "pyelonephritis and complicated UTI," and investigators have a financial interest in recruiting, then there is a risk of including patients with less severe infections, which might skew study results. Therefore, stratification algorithms such as the ORENUC classification could introduce more transparent and comparable measures. The pharmaceutical industry initiated, sponsored, and published all the above studies [42–51]. Having said this, studies are extremely difficult and expensive to perform nowadays and would not have been possible without the support of the pharmaceutical industry. All data in the above studies are accurate, and they do describe the percentage of bacteremia.

Expensive RCTs are not necessarily the best studies to provide all the information we currently need. Once the pathogen is identified and directed therapy is initiated, results from mere observational studies can provide valuable information on clinical cure and pathogen eradication rates. Guideline panels are in a unique situation to identify knowledge gaps in the field of UTI. The situation demonstrates the close interdependence between the medical community and the pharmaceutical industry.

The way forward. It is time for clinicians and pharma companies to meet and discuss alternative ways to spend time and money to the best of all stakeholders. An interesting alternative is to run prospective registries, where clinical severity and risk factors could be better defined and inform prospective registry embedded RCTs, also outside former Eastern Europe and at lower costs. In the era of antibiotic stewardship, we need to act faster and smarter [9].

References

1. Bartoletti R, Cai T, Wagenlehner FM, Naber K, Johansen TEB. Treatment of urinary tract infections and antibiotic stewardship. Eur Urol Suppl. 2016;15:81. https://doi.org/10.1016/j.eursup.2016.04.003.
2. Tandogdu Z, Kakariadis ETA, Naber K, Wagenlehner F, Johansen TEB. Appropriate empiric antibiotic choices in health care associated urinary tract infections in urology departments in Europe from 2006 to 2015: a Bayesian analytical approach applied in a surveillance study. PLoS One. 2019;14(4):e0214710.
3. Tandogdu Z, Cek M, Wagenlehner F, Naber K, Tenke P, Ostrum E, Bjerklund Johansen TE. Resistance patterns of nosocomial urinary tract infections in urology departments: 8-year results of the Global Prevalence of Infections in Urology study. World J Urol. 2014;32(3):791–801. https://doi.org/10.1007/s00345-013-1154-8.
4. Wagenlehner F, Tandogdu Z, Bartoletti R, Cai T, Cek M, Kulchavenya E, Koves B, Naber K, Perepanova T, Tenke P, Wult B, Bogenhard F, Bjerklund Johansen TE. The global prevalence of infections in urology study: a long-term, worldwide surveillance study on urological infections. Pathogens. 2016;5(1):10.
5. https://arpsp.cdc.gov/profile/antibiotic-resistance/fluoroquinolone-resistant-ecoli
6. https://www.eucast.org/newsiandr
7. https://www.eucast.org/fileadmin/src/media/PDFs/EUCAST_files/Guidance_documents/To_clinical_colleagues_on_recent_changes_in_clinical_microbiology_susceptibility_reports_9_July2021.pdf
8. Bjerklund Johansen TE, Botto H, Cek M, Grabe M, Tenke P, Wagenlehner FME, Naber KG. Critical review of current definitions of urinary tract infections and proposal of an EAU/ESIU classification system, Chapter 16: Classification of urinary tract infections. In: Naber KG, Scaeffer AJ, Heyns CF, Matsumoto T, Shoskes DA, Bjerklund Johansen TE, editors. Urogenital infections (textbook 1182pp). International Consultation on Urological Diseases (ICUD) and European Association of Urology; 2010. p. 979–93. ISBN: 978-90-79754-41-0, Arnheim.

9. Antimicrobial Resistance: Tackling a Crisis for the Health and Wealth of Nations. 2014. The Review on Antimicrobial Resistance Chaired by Jim O'Neill December 2014. 1.pdf (amr-review.org)
10. Hulscher ME, et al. Antibiotic prescribing in hospitals: a social and behavioural scientific approach. Lancet Infect Dis. 2010;10:167.
11. Dellit TH, et al. Infectious Diseases Society of America and the Society for Healthcare Epidemiology of America guidelines for developing an institutional program to enhance antimicrobial stewardship. Clin Infect Dis. 2007;44:159.
12. Edlund C, Ternhag A, Ståhlgren GS, Edquist P, Balkhed ÅÖ, Athlin S, Månsson E, Tempé M, Bergström J, Giske CG, Hanberger H, on behalf of the Temocillin Study Group. The clinical and microbiological efficacy of temocillin versus cefotaxime in adults with febrile urinary tract infection, and its effects on the intestinal microbiota: a randomised multicentre clinical trial in Sweden. Lancet Infect Dis. 2021. Published online October 28, 2021.; https://doi.org/10.1016/S1473-3099(21)00407-2.
13. Falagas ME, et al. Antibiotics versus placebo in the treatment of women with uncomplicated cystitis: a meta-analysis of randomized controlled trials. J Infect. 2009;58:91.
14. effectiveness-and-efficiency-web-final.pdf (nuffieldtrust.org.uk)
15. Eddy DM. What do we do about costs? JAMA. 1990;264(9):1161–5. https://doi.org/10.1001/jama.1990.03450090099038.
16. https://www.nlm.nih.gov/medline/medline_history.htmom
17. https://www.nlm.nih.gov/bsd/disted/meshtutorial/introduction/index.html
18. Richardson WS, Wilson MC, Nishikawa J, Hayward RS. The well-built clinical question: a key to evidence-based decisions. ACP J Club. 1995;123:A12–3.
19. Fletcher J. What is heterogeneity and is it important? BMJ. 2007;334:94.
20. Deeks JJ, Higgins JPT, Altman DG. Chapter 9: Analysing data and undertaking meta-analyses. In: Higgins JPT, Green S, editors. Cochrane handbook for systematic reviews of interventions version 5.1.0 [updated March 2011]. The Cochrane Collaboration; 2011. www.cochrane--handbook.org.
21. Horan TC, Andrus M, Dudeck MA. CDC/NHSN surveillance definition of health care-associated infection and criteria for specific types of infections in the acute care setting. Am J Infect Control. 2008;36(5):309–32.
22. https://www.ema.europa.eu/en/documents/referral/quinolone-fluoroquinolone-article-31-referral-disabling-potentially-permanent-side-effects-lead_en.pdf.
23. Bonkat G, Bartoletti R, Bruyere F et al. EAU guidelines on urological infections. EAU Guidelines Office, Arnhem, The Netherlands. http://uroweb.org/guidelines/compilations-of-all-guidelines/
24. Gupta K, et al. Short-course nitrofurantoin for the treatment of acute uncomplicated cystitis in women. Arch Intern Med. 2007;167:2207.
25. Lecomte F, et al. Single-dose treatment of cystitis with fosfomycin trometamol (Monuril): analysis of 15 comparative trials on 2,048 patients. Giorn It Ost Gin. 1997;19:399.
26. Nicolle LE. Pivmecillinam in the treatment of urinary tract infections. J Antimicrob Chemother. 2000;46(Suppl 1):35.
27. Huttner A, et al. Nitrofurantoin revisited: a systematic review and meta-analysis of controlled trials. J Antimicrob Chemother. 2015;70:2456.
28. Gupta K, et al. Outcomes associated with trimethoprim/sulphamethoxazole (TMP/SMX) therapy in TMP/SMX resistant community-acquired UTI. Int J Antimicrob Agents. 2002;19:554.
29. Warren JW, et al. Guidelines for antimicrobial treatment of uncomplicated acute bacterial cystitis and acute pyelonephritis in women. Infectious Diseases Society of America (IDSA). Clin Infect Dis. 1999;29:745.
30. Hooton TM, et al. Amoxicillin-clavulanate vs ciprofloxacin for the treatment of uncomplicated cystitis in women: a randomized trial. JAMA. 2005;293:949.
31. Hooton TM, et al. Cefpodoxime vs ciprofloxacin for short-course treatment of acute uncomplicated cystitis: a randomized trial. JAMA. 2012;307:583.

32. World Health Organization (WHO). The WHO essential medicines list antibiotic book: improving antibiotic AWaReness. November 2021, pp. 1–424. DRAFT.
33. Gupta K, et al. International clinical practice guidelines for the treatment of acute uncomplicated cystitis and pyelonephritis in women: a 2010 update by the Infectious Diseases Society of America and the European Society for Microbiology and Infectious Diseases. Clin Infect Dis. 2011;52:e103.
34. Choe HS, Lee SJ, Yang SS, et al. Summary of the UAA-AAUS guidelines for urinary tract infections. Int J Urol. 2018;25:175–85.
35. National Institute for Health and Care Excellence (NICE). Urinary tract infection (lower): antimicrobial prescribing. England: Public Health England; 2018. p. 1–39.
36. Kranz J, Schmidt S, Lebert C, et al. The 2017 update of the German clinical guideline on epidemiology, diagnostics, therapy, prevention, and management of uncomplicated urinary tract infections in adult patients. Part II: therapy and prevention. Urol Int. 2018;100:271–8.
37. Malmros K, Huttner BD, McNulty C, et al. Comparison of antibiotic treatment guidelines for urinary tract infections in 15 European countries: results of an online survey. Int J Antimicrob Agents. 2019;54:478–86.
38. Cattrall JWS, et al. A systematic review of randomised clinical trials for oral antibiotic treatment of acute pyelonephritis. Eur J Clin Microbiol Infect Dis. 2018;37:2285.
39. Berti F, et al. Short versus long course antibiotic therapy for acute pyelonephritis in adults: a systematic review and meta-analysis. Italian J Med. 2018;12:39.
40. National Institute for Health and Care Excellence (NICE). Pyelonephritis (acute): antimicrobial prescribing. England: Public Health England; 2018. p. 1–30.
41. Hooton TM. Clinical practice. Uncomplicated urinary tract infection. N Engl J Med. 2012;366:1028.
42. Arakawa S, et al. The efficacy and safety of tazobactam/ceftolozane in Japanese patients with uncomplicated pyelonephritis and complicated urinary tract infection. J Infect Chemother. 2019;25:104.
43. Armstrong ES, et al. Outcomes of high-dose levofloxacin therapy remain bound to the levofloxacin minimum inhibitory concentration in complicated urinary tract infections. BMC Infect Dis. 2016;16:710.
44. Huntington JA, et al. Efficacy of ceftolozane/tazobactam versus levofloxacin in the treatment of complicated urinary tract infections (cUTIs) caused by levofloxacin resistant pathogens: results from the ASPECT-cUTI trial. J Antimicrob Chemother. 2016;71:2014.
45. Carmeli Y, et al. Ceftazidime-avibactam or best available therapy in patients with ceftazidime-resistant Enterobacteriaceae and Pseudomonas aeruginosa complicated urinary tract infections or complicated intra-abdominal infections (REPRISE): a randomised, pathogen-directed, phase 3 study. Lancet Infect Dis. 2016;16:661.
46. Sims M, et al. Prospective, randomized, double-blind, phase 2 dose-ranging study comparing efficacy and safety of imipenem/cilastatin plus relebactam with imipenem/cilastatin alone in patients with complicated urinary tract infections. J Antimicrob Chemother. 2017;72:2616.
47. Wagenlehner FM, et al. Ceftazidime-avibactam versus Doripenem for the treatment of complicated urinary tract infections, including acute pyelonephritis: RECAPTURE, a phase 3 randomized trial program. Clin Infect Dis. 2016;63:754.
48. Kaye KS, et al. Effect of meropenem-vaborbactam vs piperacillin-Tazobactam on clinical cure or improvement and microbial eradication in complicated urinary tract infection the TANGO I randomized clinical trial. JAMA. 2018;319:788.
49. Wunderink RG, et al. Effect and safety of meropenem-vaborbactam versus best-available therapy in patients with carbapenem-resistant Enterobacteriaceae infections: the TANGO II randomized clinical trial. Infect Dis Ther. 2018;7:439.
50. Wagenlehner FME, et al. Once-daily plazomicin for complicated urinary tract infections. N Engl J Med. 2019;380:729.
51. Portsmouth S, et al. Cefiderocol versus imipenem-cilastatin for the treatment of complicated urinary tract infections caused by Gram-negative uropathogens: a phase 2, randomised, double-blind, non-inferiority trial. Lancet Infect Dis. 2018;18:1319.

52. Mombelli G, et al. Oral vs intravenous ciprofloxacin in the initial empirical management of severe pyelonephritis or complicated urinary tract infections: a prospective randomized clinical trial. Arch Intern Med. 1999;159:53.
53. Pitout JD. Infections with extended-spectrum beta-lactamase-producing Enterobacteriaceae: changing epidemiology and drug treatment choices. Drugs. 2010;70:313.
54. Singer M, Deutschman CS, Seymour CW, et al. The third international consensus. Definitions for sepsis and septic shock (Sepsis-3). JAMA. 2016;315:801–10.
55. Vincent JL, Moreno R, Takal J, et al. Working group on sepsis-related problems of the European society of intensive care medicine: the SOFA (Sepsis-related Organ Failure Assessment) score to describe organ dysfunction/failure. Intensive Care Med. 1996;22(7):707–10.
56. Johansson M, Guyatt G, Montori V. Guidelines should consider clinicians' time needed to treat. BMJ. 2023;380:e072953. https://doi.org/10.1136/bmj-2022-072953. Published: 03 January 2023.

GPSR Compliance

The European Union's (EU) General Product Safety Regulation (GPSR) is a set of rules that requires consumer products to be safe and our obligations to ensure this.

If you have any concerns about our products, you can contact us on ProductSafety@springernature.com

In case Publisher is established outside the EU, the EU authorized representative is:

Springer Nature Customer Service Center GmbH
Europaplatz 3
69115 Heidelberg, Germany

Batch number: 10726060

Printed by Printforce, the Netherlands